Instant Clinical Diagnosis in Ophthalmology

Glaucoma

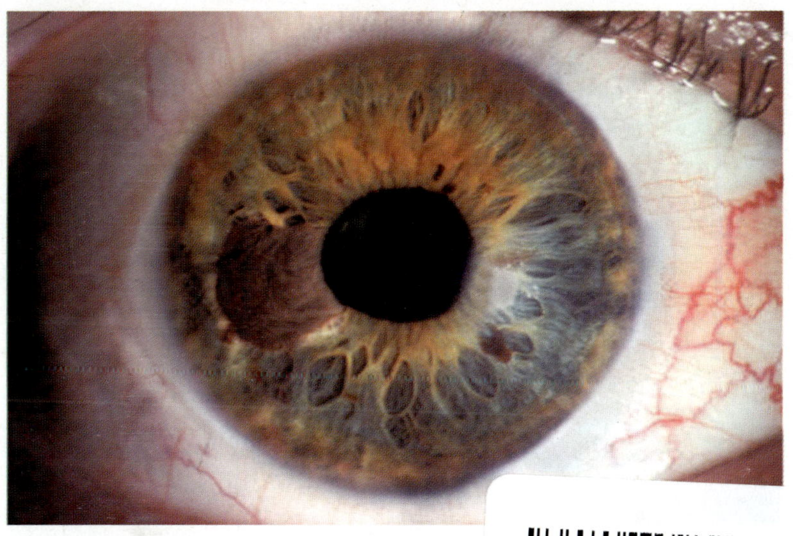

Instant Clinical Diagnosis in Ophthalmology
Glaucoma

Series Editors

Ashok Garg
MS PhD FIAO(Bel) FRSM FAIMS ADM FICA
International and National Gold Medalist
Chairman and Medical Director
Garg Eye Institute and Research Centre
235-Model Town, Dabra Chowk
Hisar-125005, Haryana, India

Emanuel Rosen
MD
Medical Director
Rosen Eye Associates
Harbour City, Salford Quays
M50 3 BH
UK

Editors

Shlomo Melamed
MD PhD
Professor of Ophthalmology
Sackler Medical School
Tel-Aviv University
Head and Chairman
Sam Rothberg Glaucoma Centre
Tel HaShomer, Israel

Tanuj Dada
MD
Associate Professor of Clinical
Ophthalmology, Dr RP Centre
for Ophthalmic Sciences
AIIMS, Ansari Nagar
New Delhi-110029
India

Ahmad K Khalil
MD PhD
Professor of Ophthalmology, Medical Director
Saridar Clinic Tower, Apt 67-C, 92, Tahrir St.
Dokki Square, Cairo, Egypt-12411

Foreword

Robert N Weinreb

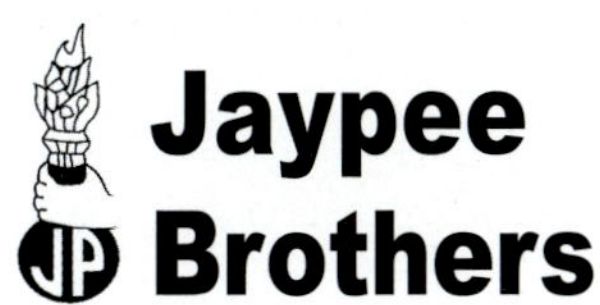

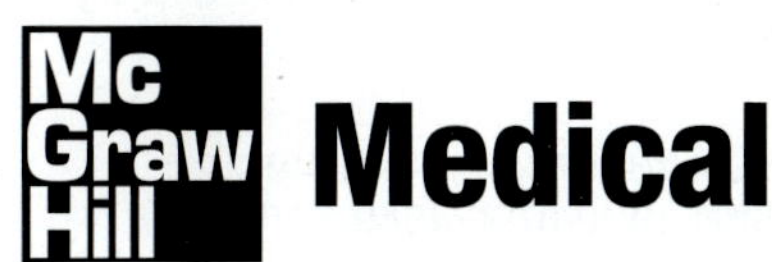

First published in India in 2009 by

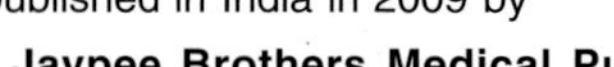

Jaypee Brothers Medical Publishers (P) Ltd.

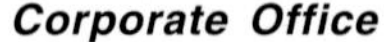

Corporate Office

4838/24 Ansari Road, Daryaganj, **New Delhi** - 110002, India, +91-11-43574357

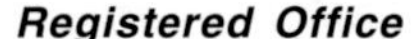

Registered Office

B-3 EMCA House, 23/23B Ansari Road, Daryaganj, **New Delhi** 110 002, India
Phones: +91-11-23272143, +91-11-23272703, +91-11-23282021,
+91-11-23245672, Rel: +91-11-32558559 Fax: +91-11-23276490, +91-11-23245683
e-mail: jaypee@jaypeebrothers.com, Website: www.jaypeebrothers.com

First published in USA by The McGraw-Hill Companies, 2 Penn Plaza, New York, NY 10121. Exclusively worldwide distributor except South Asia (India, Nepal, Sri Lanka, Bhutan, Pakistan, Bangladesh, Malaysia).

ISBN-13: 978-0-07-174949-7
ISBN-10: 0-07-174949-7

Dedicated to

- My Respected Param Pujya Guru Sant Gurmeet Ram Rahim Singh Ji for his blessings and motivation.
- My Respected Parents, teachers, my wife Dr Aruna Garg, son Abhishek and daughter Anshul for their constant support and patience during all these days of hard work.
- My dear friend Dr. Amar Agarwal, a renowned International Ophthalmologist for his constant support, guidance and expertise.

— Ashok Garg

- The memory of my step daughter Nicola Ross whose enjoyed benefits from refractive surgery were cut short by a tragic fatal illness.

— Emanuel Rosen

- To my loving wife Shuvit.

— Shlomo Melamed

- The Revered Sufi Saint Hazoor Maharaj Gurmeet Ram Rahim Singh Ji, Dera Sacha Sauda Ashram, Sirsa, Haryana, India.

— Tanuj Dada

- To the memory of great father, whose open mindedness and guidance will always be there.
- To my mother, my first teacher and supporter, to my wife for her encouragement and patience, to my sons, Hassan and Omar with love.

— Ahmad K Khalil

Contributors

Ahmed Mostafa Abdelrahman MD FRCS
Assistant Professor Ophthalmology
Cairo University
8-Morad Street (Morad Tower)
Apart 409, Giza, Egypt

Ahmed Galal MD PhD
Vissum/Instituto Oftalmologico
De Alicante, Alicante, Spain

Ahmad K Khalil MD PhD
Associate Professor of Ophthalmology
Saridar Clinic Tower
92, Tahrir St, Dokki, Cairo, Egypt

Andre Mermoud MD
Prof of Ophthalmology
Jules Gonin Eye Hospital
CH-1004, Lausanne, Switzerland

Ashok Garg MS PhD FRSM
Medical Director
Garg Eye Institute and Research Centre, 235-Model Town
Dabra Chowk, Hisar-125005
India

Bojan Pajic MD
Chief, Cornea and Refractive Surgery
Deptt, Vision Care, Klinik Pallas
Louis Giroud Str. 20, 4600 Olten
Switzerland

Boris Malyugin MD PhD
Chief of Department of Contract and Implant Surgery, Dy. Director General
S. Fyodorov Eye Microsurgery
Complex State Institution
127486 Moscow
Beskudnikovsky blvd 59A
Russia

Cyres K Mehta MS FSVH FAGE
Director and Consultant
Mehta International Eye Institute
Seaside, 147, Colaba Road
Mumbai-400005
India

Daljit Singh MS DSc
Director
Dr Daljit Singh Eye Hospital
57, Joshi Colony, Amritsar-143001
India

Ehud I Assia MD
Deptt of Ophthalmology
Meir Hospital, Sapir Medical Centre
Tsharnihovski St., 44281, Kafar, Saba
Israel

Emanuel Rosen MD FRCS
Rosen Eye Associates
Harbour City, Salford Quays
M50 3 BH
UK

G Marchini MD
Head of Eye Clinic
Deptt of Neurological and Visual Sciences
University of Verona
Borgo Trento Hospital
P.Ie. A. Stefani, 1, 37126 Verona
Italy

Guillermo Avalos Urzua MD
Terranova No. 676-101
Col. Providencia
Guadalajara, Jal,
Mexico CP-44630

Jens Funk MD
Prof of Ophthalmology
Augenklinik-Universitatsklinikum
Killianstr. 5, 79106 Freiburg
Germany

Jerome Bovet MD
Consultant Ophthalmic Surgeon
FMH Clinique de I'oeil
15, Avenue du Bois-de-la-Chapelle
CH-1213 Onex
Switzerland

Jes Mortensen MD
Consultant, The Eye Deptt.
Orebro University Hospital
SE-70185, Orebro
Sweden

Jorge L Alio MD PhD
Director
Instituto Oftalmologico De Alicante
Avda. Denia 111, 03015
Alicante
Spain

Jose L Rodriguez Prats MD
Instituto Oftalmologico De Alicante
Avda. Denia 111, 03015
Alicante
Spain

JT Lin PhD
Professor Institute of Electro Optics
National Taiwan University
268-1 (11F)
Han Sheng E Rd
Banciao
Taiwan-22066

Kaweh Mansouri MD
Jules Gonin Eye Hospital
Lausanne
Switzerland

Keiki R Mehta MS DO FIOS
Chairman and Medical Director
Mehta International Eye Institute
147, Shahid Bhagat Singh Road
Colaba Road
Mumbai-400005
India

KP Takhchidi MD
Director General
S. Fyodorov Eye Microsurgery
Complex State Institution
127486 Moscow
Beskudnikovsky blvd 59A
Russia

Kiranjit Singh MS
Dr Daljit Singh Eye Hospital
57, Joshi Colony, Amritsar-143001
India

Madhu Nagar MS FRCOph
Consultant Ophthalmologist
Clayton Eye Hospital
Wakefield, West Yorkshire
UK

Maria da Leiz Freitas MD
R Crasto, 708-4050-243, Porto
Portugal

Mordechai Goldenfeld MD
The Sam Rothberg Glaucoma Centre
Goldschleger Eye Institute
Sheba Medical Centre
Tel-Hashomer
Israel

M Marraffa MD
Deptt of Neurological and Visual Sciences
University of Verona
Borgo Trento Hospital
P.Ie. A. Stefani, 1, 37126 Verona
Italy

Mona Pache MD
Augenklinik-Universitatsklinikum
Killianstr. 5, 79106 Freiburg
Germany

Nicola Freeman MD
Sr. Consultant Ophthalmic Surgeon
Deptt of Ophthalmology
Faculty of Health Sciences
University of Stellenbosch
Tygerberg Academic Hospital
Cape Town
South Africa

Nikolay N Ereskin MD
Consultant
SN Fyodorov Eye Microsurgery Complex, Moscow
Russia

Pascal Rozot MD
Consultant Ophthalmic Surgeon
Clinique Moniticelli, Marsilles,
France

P Ceruti MD
Deptt of Neurological and
Visual Sciences
University of Verona,
Borgo Trento Hospital,
P.Ie. A. Stefani, 1, 37126 Verona
Italy

Peter WT de Waard MD
The Rotterdam Eye Hospital
Schiedamse Vest 180
3011-BH-Rotterdam
Netherlands

Ranjit S Dhaliwal MS
Director, Eye Infirmary, Hira Mahal
Radha Soami Marg, Nabha-147201
India

Ranjit H Maniar MS
17, Vithal Court, 6th Floor, 151, August Kranti Marg, Mumbai-400036
India

RC Nagpal MS
Professor of Ophthalmology
Himalayan Institute of Medical Sciences, Swami Ram Nagar
Jolly Grant, Dehradun -248140
Uttaranchal, India

R Morbio MD
Deptt of Neurological and Visual Sciences
University of Verona
Borgo Trento Hospital, P.Ie. A. Stefani 1, 37126 Verona, Italy

Roberto G Carassa MD
Director Glaucoma Service
Deptt of Ophthalmology and
Visual Sciences, University Hospital
S. Raffaele via Olgettina 60
20132 Milano, Italy

Shalini Mohan MD
Senior Registrar
Dr RP Centre for Ophthalmic Sciences
AIIMS, Ansari Nagar,
New Delhi-110029
India

Shibal Bhartiya MD
Senior Research Associate,
Dr RP Centre for Ophthalmic Sciences
AIIMS, Ansari Nagar, New Delhi
India

Shlomo Melamed MD
Prof of Ophthalmology
Sackler Medical School
Tel Aviv University
Head and Chairman
Sam Rothberg Glaucoma Centre
Goldschleger Eye Institute,
Sheba Medical Centre, Tel-Hashomer
Israel

Shweta Jindal MD
Resident
Dr RP Centre for Ophthalmic Sciences
AIIMS, Ansari Nagar
New Delhi-110029
India

Tanuj Dada MD
Associate Professor
Clinical Ophthalmology
Dr RP Centre for Ophthalmic Sciences
AIIMS, Ansari Nagar
New Delhi-110029
India

Vivek Kadambi MD DOMS
Director
Laser Vision Netralaya
Chinmaya Hospital
CMH Road
Bangalore-560038
India

V Velayutham MS
Regional Institute of Ophthalmology
Government Ophthalmic Hospital
Egmore
Chennai
India

Foreword

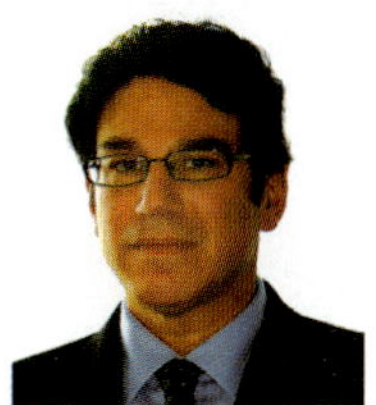

It seems like yesterday that I began a career in glaucoma and first contemplated what might transpire during the ensuing decades. At times, it has seemed that what has been learned through basic research has been inadequate to justify it's time and effort. Also the pace of translational clinical research often has appeared to be so slow, and certainly not fast enough to have a major impact on glaucoma blindness. There still are fundamental issues relating to glaucoma that have to be addressed, including some very basic ones. The absence of a clear definition of glaucoma is the one that most consistently irks me. It is, perhaps, the most basic of issues in glaucoma and is at the core of what we do in the laboratory. More significantly, it is central to how we daily diagnose and manage our glaucoma patients. *Plus ca change, plus la meme chose*? Or are we on the precipice of paradigm changes for both diagnosis and treatment that will impact significantly the prognosis for retaining vision and quality of life with glaucoma. From my vantage point, I suspect that it is the latter.

Never before have we had better tools to elucidate glaucoma pathophysiology, as well as to better diagnose, better monitor progression, and better treat glaucoma. And never before have we had the desire and commitment to do so. New instruments for imaging the optic disk, retinal nerve fiber layer and anterior segment have emerged that provide objective analyses that clearly are superior to subjective examinations of the past. There also has been the introduction into clinical practice of new medical and surgical therapies, albeit they all still have limitations.

Many of these advances are described in this text, particularly the innovative surgical approaches that promise to revolutionize our care.

Despite having all this new information so nicely packaged and available in this book, it still will be a daunting task for an interested reader to be constantly updating their knowledge and clinical skills. In addition to being grounded in the fundamentals of glaucoma, high quality glaucoma care requires access to timely and informed information. One needs then to critically evaluate the provided information, place it in the context of one's own clinical experience and translate it into clinical practice. Evidence-based medicine, consensus and clinical experience are all complementary for the most thoughtful clinicians.

I congratulate Dr. Ashok Garg, editors and authors who have contributed to this timely book.

Dr Robert N Weinreb MD
Distinguished Professor of Ophthalmology
Director
Hamilton Glaucoma Center
University of California, San Diego
La Jolla, California 92093
United States
Ph.: 001 858 534-8824.
e-mail : weinreb@eyecenter.ucsd.edu

Preface

In modern day busy and fast life ophthalmologists are glued to their clinical and surgical practice and have little time to read large volume books. The need of hour is to have pocket size ready recokner enriched with complete and up-to-date information of the diseases in a most comprehensive manner. At present very few quality ready reference books are available at an International level.

After detailed research regarding the needs of ophthalmologists we have developed a series of 10 volume ready reference books termed as Instant Clinical Diagnosis in Ophthalmology. This series covers Oculoplastic and Reconstructive Surgery, Retina, Lens, Glaucoma, Refractive Surgery, Pediatric Ophthalmology, Strabismus, Anterior Segment Diseases, Cornea and Neuro-ophthalmology. Present series has been designed to provide up-to-date information of concerned disease in a comprehensive and a lucid manner along with high quality clinical photographs in an easy to read format. International masters of concerned subjects have contributed chapters in this series covering pathophysiology, clinical signs and symptoms, investigations, differential diagnosis, treatment and prognosis in a simplified manner.

This volume deals with important clinical entity, glaucoma, which is one of the major causes of blindness worldwide. This volume consists of latest information on various clinical glaucoma conditions, their diagnosis and management in an easy to ready format for the benefit of readers. A number of leading international glaucoma experts have shared their experiences in form of chapters covering all aspects of glaucoma. We are glad to provide complete and latest information of glaucoma in a comprehensive manner in this book for quick look and as a ready reckoner.

We are highly thankful to our publisher M/s Jaypee Brothers Medical Publishers Pvt. Ltd. especially Shri Jitendar P Vij (CEO), Mr. Tarun Duneja (Director, Publishing) and all staff members for their dedication and hard efforts put in the preparation of high quality series of Instant Clinical books.

We hope this 10 volume set of ready reference pocket size books shall provide complete and useful clinical information to ophthalmologists all around the world and shall help them to accurately and precisely diagnose, treat and manage their clinical cases confidently to the satisfaction and expectations of their valued patients. We also hope this ready reckoner shall serve as useful companion on every clinician desk.

Editors

Contents

SECTION 1: CLINICAL GLAUCOMA

SECTION 2: SPECIAL GLAUCOMA SURGICAL TECHNIQUES

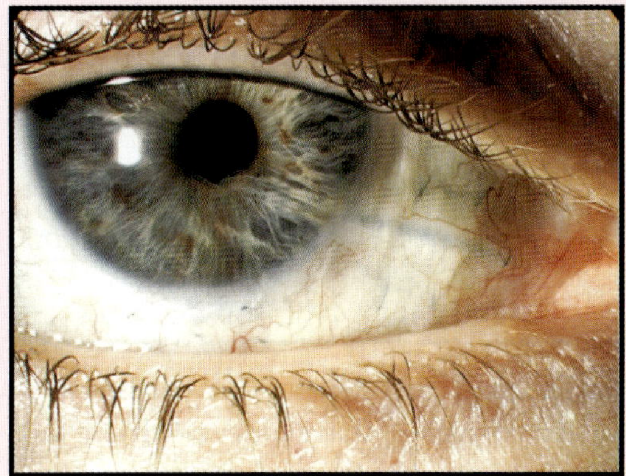

SECTION 1

CLINICAL GLAUCOMA

1

Early Onset Developmental Glaucoma (Primary Congenital Glaucoma)

Ahmad K Khalil (Egypt)

INTRODUCTION

Developmental glaucoma is a glaucoma caused by maldevelopment of the eye's aqueous outflow system. Depending on the severity of this maldevelopment the resultant elevated intraocular pressure may occur at birth or anytime thereafter. Most cases present at birth (congenital) or within the first year of life (infantile), and on these entities, we refer as early onset developmental glaucoma (EODG). Due to the elastic nature of the embryonic tissues, the eye ball stretches and enlarges in congenital cases, with subsequent Descemet's membrane ruptures, corneal edema and cloudiness. Pressure on the elastic optic nerve head and lamina cribrosa leads to early (distension) cupping, but eventually functional loss and glaucomatous optic atrophy ensue .

The disease is bilateral in 75% of the cases, males more commonly affected (65%). There is sporadic occurrence in 90% of the cases, the remainder; autosomal recessive with variable penetrance. Its incidence is 1:10,000 births in the West and 1:2500 births in the Middle East. More than 80% present before 1 year.

Genetically, EODG appears to be a genetically heterogeneous disorder in that there is an unequal sex distribution and fewer numbers of affected siblings. To date, 2 loci have been found for EODG: GLC3A (chromosome 2p21) and GLC3B (chromosome 1p36).

CLINICAL SIGNS AND SYMPTOMS

Epiphora, photophobia and blepharospasm are often the first symptoms to alarm the parents. Any of these symptoms warrants careful examination with glaucoma in mind. I have seen infants with a moderate degree of glaucoma who were referred because of persistent epiphora after nasolacrimal probing.

Grayish discoloration (cloudiness of the cornea) is usually the presenting symptom of more advanced cases.

Corneal enlargement without cloudiness is a less often presenting symptom, as it is often thought by parents as a beauty sign, rather than an abnormal alerting sign.

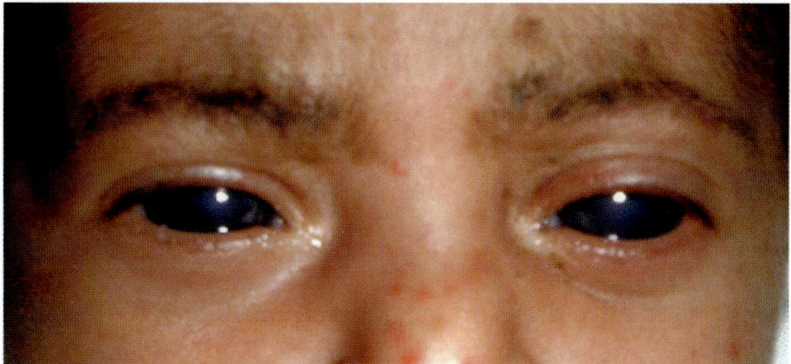

Fig. 1: Classically described EODG with photophobia, epiphora, corneal enlargement and cloudiness

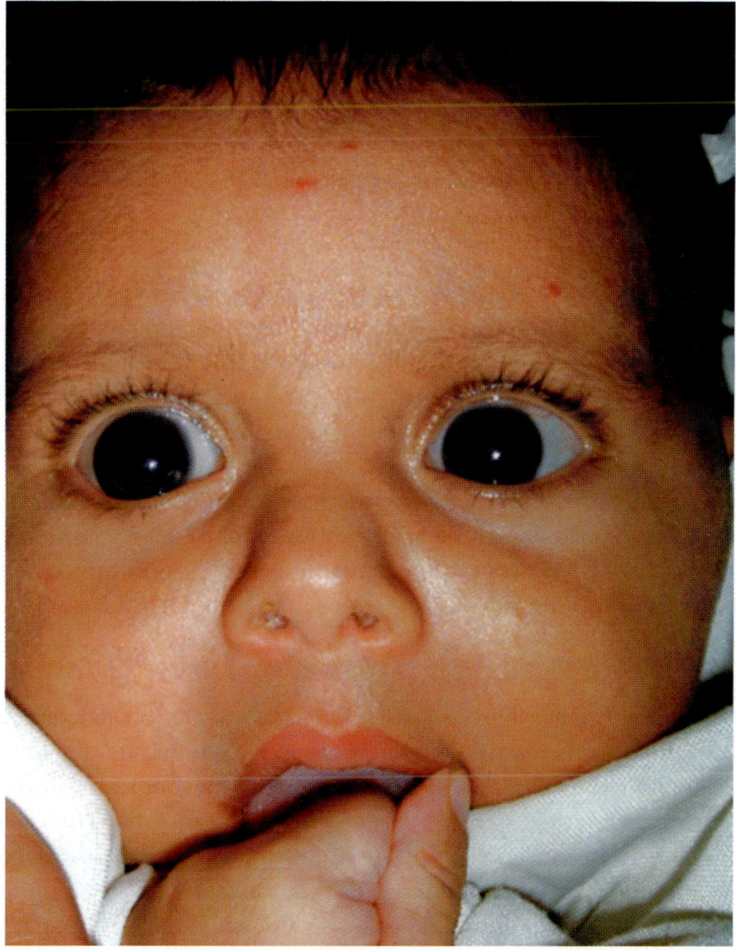

Fig. 2: Parents are often peaceful with larger corneas of their infants seeing it as a sign of beauty, and often overlooking the mild corneal cloudiness seen in the right eye of this infant

EXAMINATION

The normal IOP in the newborn well falls in the 1 digit mmHg readings. The disc has almost no cup. The cornea is clear, its horizontal diameter in a full-term newborn is 10 to 10.5 mm and increases to the adult diameter of approximately 11.5 to 12 mm by 2 years of age.

IOP

Examination is ideally done under general anesthesia, where it would be possible to make a full examination at no haste. This is at least necessary for a first full examination for decision making and a couple of follow up examinations as thought necessary. Follow up examinations can then adequately be made with sedation (chloral hydrate), and with proper training afterwards, without sedation as early as the second year of life.

Most general anesthetics tend to lower IOP readings, and a knowledge of the anesthetic used and its behavior is needed. A hand-held applanation tonometer, is a good device in this regard. Lid and canthal pressure can lead to false high IOP readings with forceful opening of the eye lids.

Cornea

Using the surgical microscope or a portable slit lamp, early corneal edema or more pronounced clouding and breaks in Descemet's membrane should be looked for. A diameter greater than 12 mm in an infant is highly suggestive of EODG. Developmental anomalies of the cornea and iris must be noted because they may alter diagnosis and treatment. Corneal clouding is usually reversible after IOP control.

Rupture lines of Descemet's membrane (Haab's striae) with associated localized areas of edema can be seen in moderate to severe untreated cases. Glassy lines can be seen long after glaucoma control, and might be the only indication of self limited IOP rise episodes in infancy.

The Optic Nerve Head

A cup/disc ratios greater than 0.3 in an infant is suggestive of glaucoma. Changes in the optic disc occur readily with changes in IOP in infants due to increased tissue elasticity which translates IOP increase into mechanical distortion in the disc supporting elements. Globe enlargement further magnifies this mechanical cupping. This cupping is easily reversible typically within 4-6 weeks after normalization of IOP. The younger the child, the faster the reversibility. If left untreated, neuronal loss eventually ensues, with irreversible damage. Together with regression of photophobia, reversibility of optic disc cupping is one of the best criteria for surgical success in most cases.

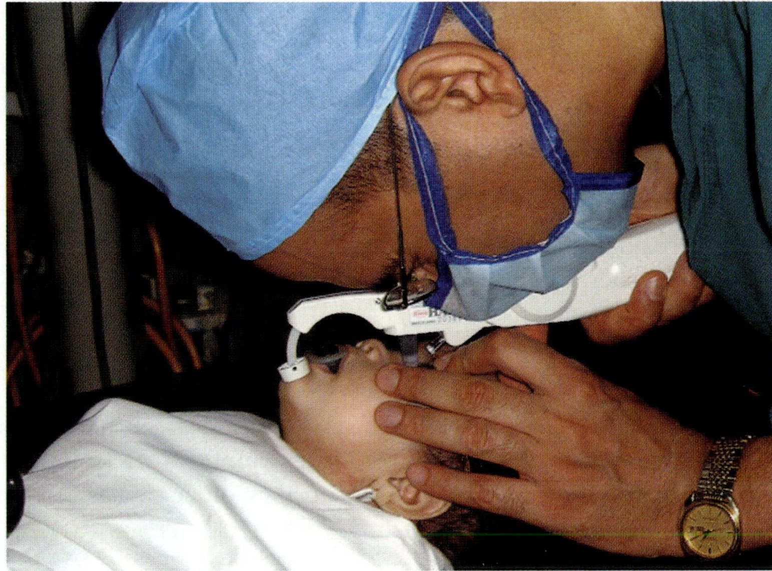

Fig. 3: Measuring the IOP under general anesthesia using the Perkins tonometer in the operation theater. For follow up examinations, a mask anesthesia with an oral airway is usually adequate

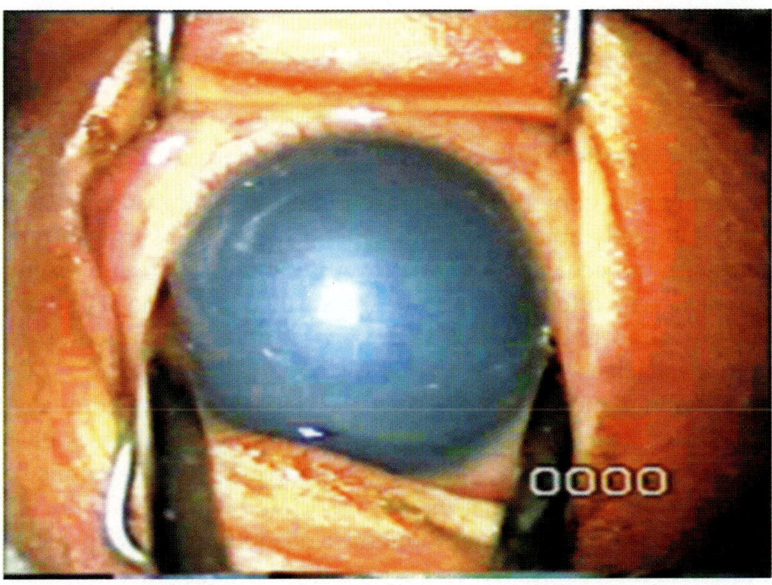

Fig. 4: Measuring of the white to white corneal diameter

Gonioscopy

Gonioscopy is performed by use of a gonioprism, a Koeppe or a barkan operating lens (a truncated koeppe lens) and binocular microscope for the evaluation of goniodysgenesis.

Axial Length Measurements

Measuring the axial length was proposed as a diagnostic and follow-up procedure. It is generally thought, however that corneal diameter is a more sensitive tool in this context.

Differential Diagnosis

Mild to moderate cases can easily be confused by entities which increase corneal diameter (megalocornea), cases with corneal cloudiness (sclerocornea, dystrophies like Meesman's and Reis-Buckler), or other causes of epiphora (NLD obstruction).

MANAGEMENT

Surgery is the first line of therapy for EODG for the following reasons: 1) Since this type of glaucoma results from abnormal anatomical development of the anterior chamber angle, anatomical or surgical correction is recommended. 2) Accumulated experience shows the effectiveness of surgery. 3) It is difficult to determine the effectiveness of medical therapy in infants and children because the procedure is complicated and may require anesthesia. The long-term effectiveness and complications of different anti-glaucoma drugs have not been well studied.

Surgical Management

Trabeculotomy and goniotomy remain the first line surgical procedures for EODG. They directly attack the faulty site with minimal surgical trauma, as compared with trabeculectomy, hence inviting much less tissue reaction and fibrosis which very often compromise the surgical outcome. The absence of external aqueous filtration precludes delayed filtering bleb-related complications, such as infection, hypotony, and leaks.

Trabeculotomy and goniotomy seem to be in some ways equivalent, and both are particularly successful in previously unoperated cases of EODG. Goniotomy, however, does not have a good success rate when done below 1 month or over 2 years of age. It is usually associated with a relatively high rate of recurrence, and multiple goniotomies are needed to achieve a success rate similar to that of trabeculotomy. Trabeculotomy is probably a more demanding technique with which it may be more difficult to achieve a technically perfect procedure than it is with goniotomy, but it is the preferred choice of the author of this chapter, with a 5-year cumulative success rate of 92%.

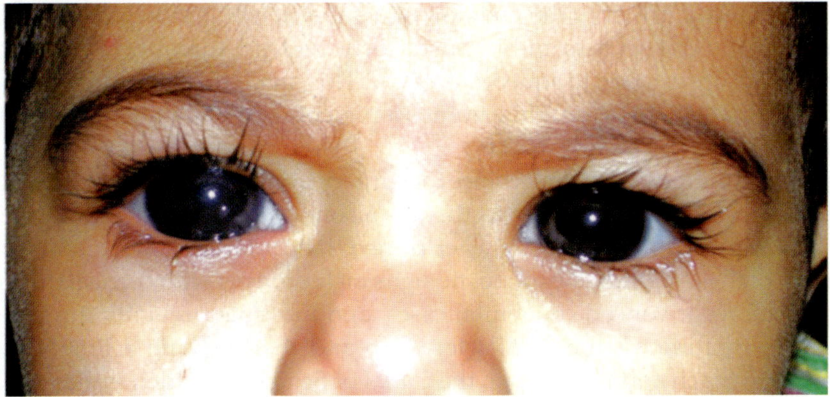

Fig. 5: Corneal cloudiness clearing in the left eye 5 days after surgery as compared to the right still cloudy non-operated eye (watering is caused by child crying rather than epiphora)

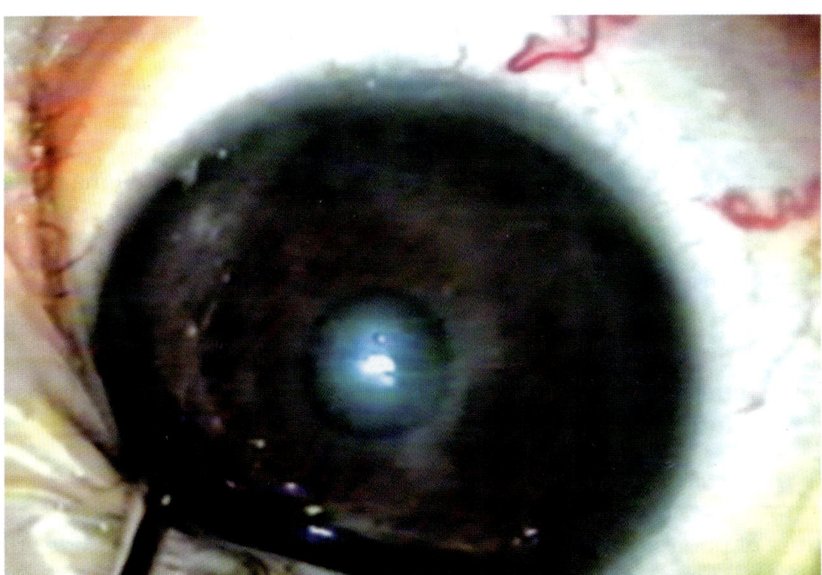

Fig. 6: Rupture lines of Descemet's membrane (Haab's striae) with associated localized areas of edema

Goniotomy involves the creation of a superficial incision into uveal TM, allowing the iris root to move posteriorly and presumably relieving the mechanical obstruction to aqueous outflow. This procedure is performed under direct visualization through a gonioscopic contact lens and the operating microscope.

Trabeculotomy is my first choice for surgery in all cases of EODG, regardless any previous surgery, as long as there is a sound non-scarred 120 degrees of limbic circumference. A properly performed trabeculotomy gives good results in most of these eyes. Bad prognostic signs include; eyes with corneal diameter 14.5 or more, advanced congenital cases, and multiple previous surgeries. It involves creating a superficial sclera flap and then making a limbal radial incision to reach and incise open the Canal of Schlemm, which is then probed on either side by specially designed probes. When these are rotated into the AC, they sever the malformed trabecular/angle tissue.

Trabeculectomy: The decision to perform this procedure must be made carefully because in infants and children, filtering bleb formation may be difficult despite intraoperative use of antimetabolites. Even after filtering blebs are successfully formed, the patients may be exposed to the risk of postsurgical infections for the rest of their life.

Deep Sclerectomy

No much role as it leaves the trabecular beams, which are the main site for resistance to outflow in EODG, untouched.

Aqueous Shunt Implantation

The enhanced success with aqueous shunt devices is associated with a higher likelihood of postoperative complications. They can probably used as a last resort in refractory cases with multiple previous surgeries and compromised angle structures.

MEDICAL TREATMENT

Because of poor efficacy, a greater potential for adverse systemic side effects, medical treatment is used as an auxiliary means to temporarily control IOP till surgery is performed or in the rare instance when repeated surgeries fail to control IOP. **Brimonidine** should be used with caution in young children because of the potential for CNS depression.

Prognosis

Even after successful surgery with IOP control and regression/stabilization of optic disc cupping, regular follow-up and rehabilitation measures will be necessary to achieve a favorable outcome and prognosis. It is near meaningless to save an eye from sight threatening glaucoma, and lose it.

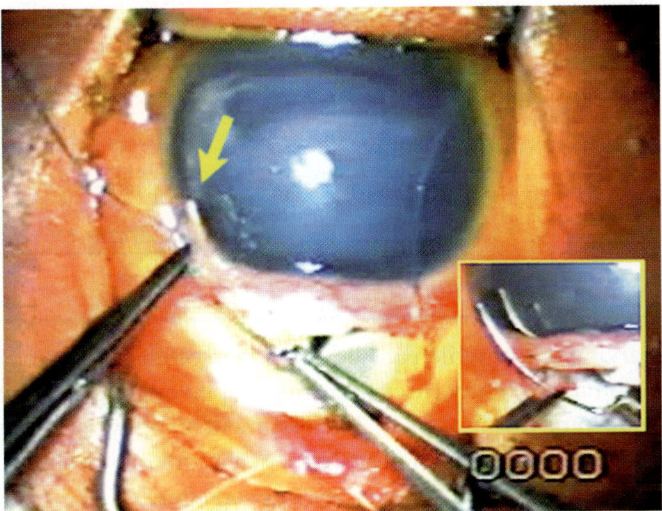

Fig. 7: The second trabeculotomy probe is being rotated into the AC

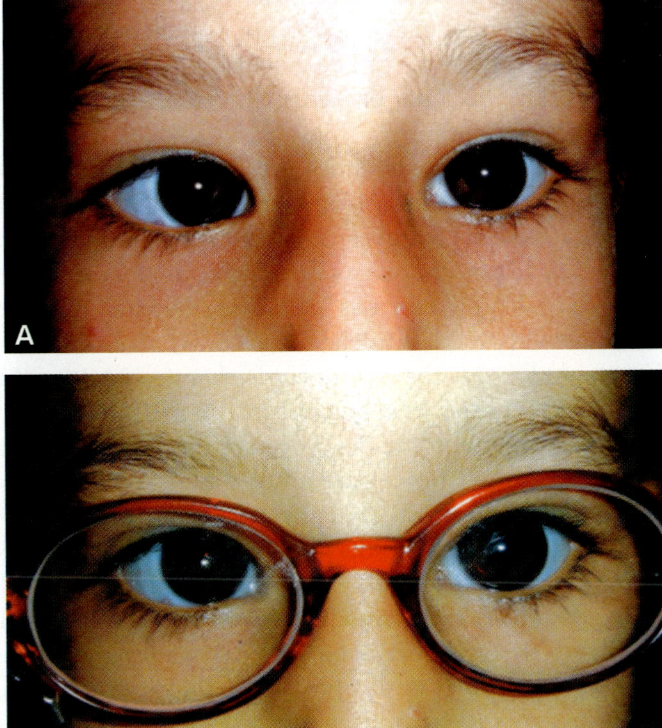

Figs 8A and B: 3 years after bilateral successful trabeculotomy for EODG, this case presented with anisometropia (one eye myopic, the other low hyperopic) and strabismus. Glasses correction and amblyopia management could achieve a bilateral 0.8 visual acuity

2

Late (Adult) Onset Developmental Glaucoma

Ahmad K Khalil (Egypt)

INTRODUCTION

This is an evolving entity which would include in older literature entities like juvenile glaucoma and many cases of primary open angle glaucoma (POAG). This type of glaucoma results from maldevelopment of the eye's aqueous outflow system, but as the extent of such morphological anomalies is slight; the age of onset is delayed until late teens, twenties, or even later.

CLINICAL SIGNS AND SYMPTOMS

Accidental discovery of a moderately high IOP or optic disc cupping in a late teen who is known not to be glaucomatous in previous examinations is not uncommon. Onset and diagnosis can be even delayed to the age of forties or fifties. Less frequently, patients presents by visual complaint caused by advanced visual loss and cupping.

IOP rise ranges between low twenties to mid forties. Sudden IOP rise can occur which brings the patient complaining of headache. Cupping can be seen in these subacute cases, and I have seen a patient in his mid-forties presenting with high IOP, and optic disc cupping of 0.6 which was reversed on IOP control to 0.3. This denotes the rapid onset as well as the residual elasticity of optic nerve head structures up to this adult age.

The hallmark of LODG is the typical angle changes. **Maldevelopment of the angle (gonio-dysgenesis)** with anterior insertion of the iris root into the trabecular area and/or embryonic iris processes reaching to Schwalbe's line and the corneal periphery. **Corneal diameter** is typically within the normal adult size. Finding of a larger corneal diameter or endothelial (Haab's) striae/lines denote an infantile onset of a milder glaucoma. LODG should be considered when evaluating cases with presenile cataracts, as it can be the inciting factor.

Regular glaucoma tests including diurnal variations, visual field testing, and nerve fiber layer analysis, should be pursued in all cases. Most structural tests do not still have a normative database for younger individuals, but even though; such tests can still be done for future comparison and potential progression evaluation with evolving newer technology.

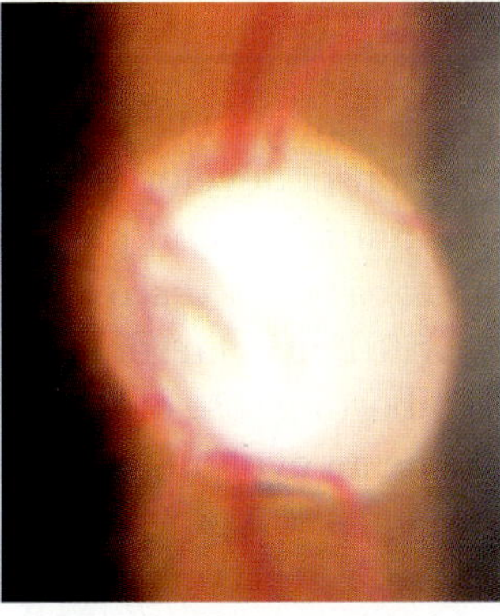

Fig. 1: Advance cupping in a recently diagnosed case of LODG, female age 19 years

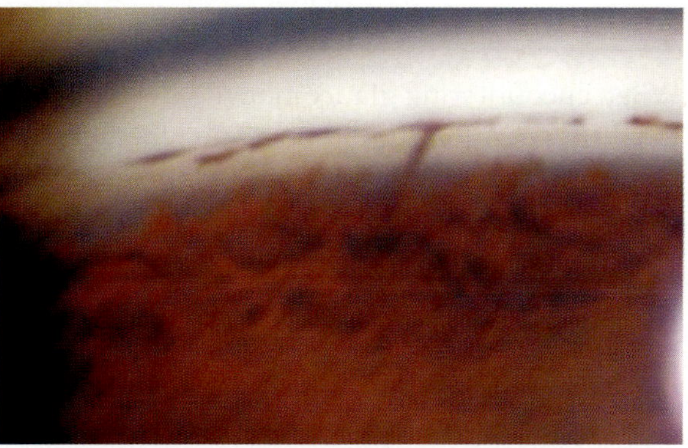

Fig. 2: Gonio-dysgenesis; anterior insertion of iris root into anterior trabecular area

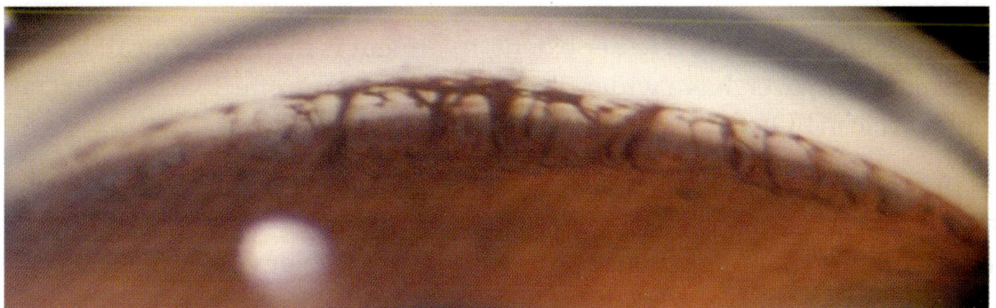

Fig. 3: Gonio-dysgenesis; embryonic iris processes bridging and covering most of the angle structures and reaching to the corneal periphery

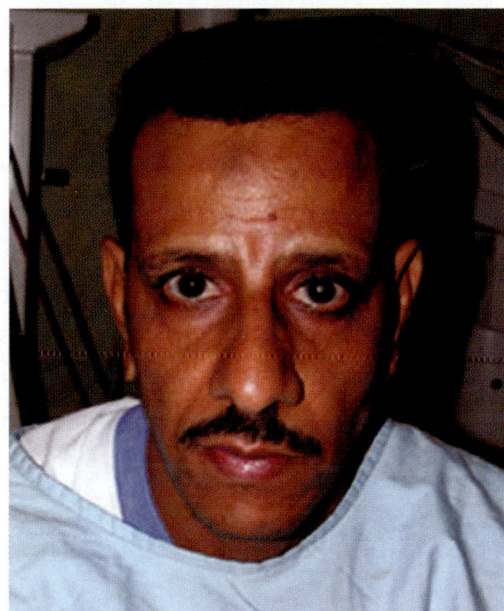

Fig. 4: A case presenting with left pre-senile cataract, gonio-dysgenesis and a pressure in the mid 40s were found

DIFFERENTIAL DIAGNOSIS

When encountering glaucoma with developmental angle changes in an adult, the differentiation should be made whether this is a late onset developmental glaucoma or a self limited mild glaucoma developed in infancy and passed unnoticed, whether this is a newly developed glaucoma or a newly discovered glaucoma! This becomes particularly important in cases with borderline findings like a 20 mmHg IOP, a 0.6 C/D ratio. This can be a self aborting case of EODG which does not require more than follow-up, and can be an evolving case of LODG which requires immediate attention and management. As mentioned above, the presence of corneal enlargement and/or Haab's striae denotes an earlier onset. When uncertain, closer follow-up is advised for IOP fluctuations and visual field changes.

TREATMENT

Similar to EODG but to a lesser extent, treatment is mainly surgical. Medical treatment, however, has a wider place here and is more effective than that very limited role in EODG.

SURGICAL OPTIONS

Trabeculotomy: Similar to EODG as the main pathology is in the trabecular area, trabeculotomy remains the preferred surgical option regardless the age of the patient. Different from trabeculotomy in the newborn, Schlemm's Canal should be sought more anteriorly in the limbus area, as there is less ocular stretch. For the same reason, the canal is also deeper and narrower. After probing both cut ends of the canal simultaneously with trabeculotomy probes, they are rotated into the AC severing the faulty trabecular tissue.

PROGNOSIS

When detected at an early stage, the prognosis is favorable, as it usually responds well to medical and surgical management. The major negative prognostic factor in cases with LODG, however, is that it inflicts an age range, for which, more often than not, IOP measurement is skipped even during professional ophthalmological examination, and cases can be diagnosed when one eye has an almost total visual field loss, and the other has an advanced loss.

Trabeculectomy: Can have a role in this population when trabeculotomy can not be performed. The addition of antimetabolites is more warranted in younger age populations.

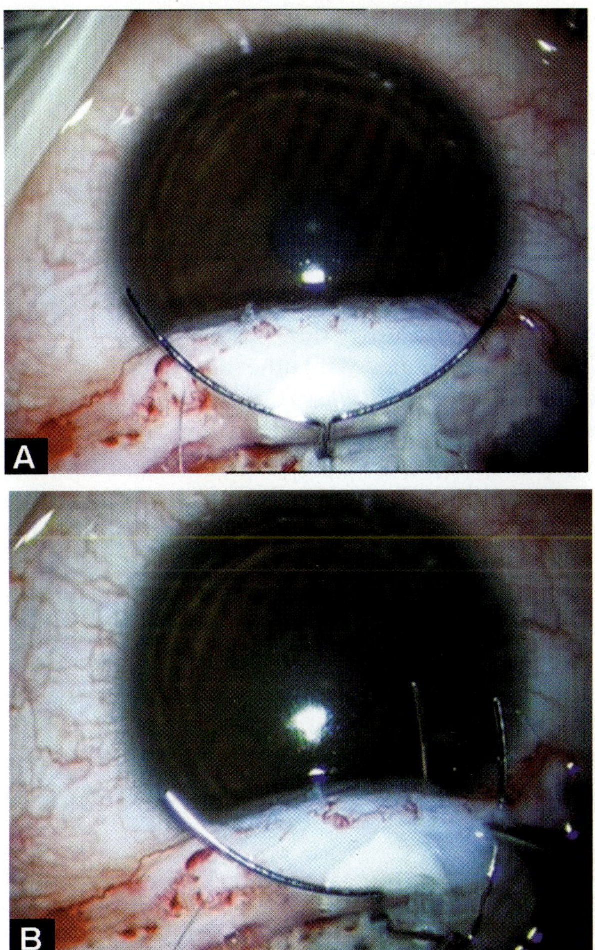

Figs 5A and B: Trabeculotomy in an adult eye: (A) Both trabeculotomes in place, a limb inside Schlemm's Canal and the outer guiding limb conforming with the limbal circumference. (B) The first trabeculotome is rotated into the AC

3

Primary Infantile Glaucoma

Maria Da Luz Freitas (Portugal)

INTRODUCTION

The term *Developmental Glaucoma* includes primary congenital glaucoma and glaucoma associated with other developmental anomalies, either ocular or systemic. Glaucoma associated with other anomalies, either ocular or systemic may be inherited or acquired. *Primary Congenital or Infantile Glaucoma* is evident either at birth or within the first few years of life. This condition is believed to be caused by dysplasia of the anterior chamber angle without other ocular or systemic abnormalities. *Secondary infantile glaucoma* is associated with inflammatory, neoplastic, hamartomatous, metabolic, or other congenital abnormalities of the eye.

Developmental glaucoma occurs in about 1 in 10.000 live births and *Primary Congenital or Infantile Glaucoma* is believe to occur 1 in 30.000 births; 60% are diagnosed by the age of 6 months and 80% within the first year of the life. Approximately 65% of patients are male, and the involvement is bilateral in 70% of cases. Most cases occur sporadically.

Various classifications of the *Development Glaucoma* have been used. Hoskins *et al* have suggested an anatomic classification. Clinically identifiable anatomic

Table 1: Hoskins's anatomic classification of developmental glaucomas

I. Isolated trabeculodysgenesis (malformation of trabecular meshwork in the absence of iris or corneal anomalies)
   A. Flat iris insertion
      1. Anterior insertion
      2. Posterior insertion
      3. Mixed insertion.

II. Iridotrabeculodysgenesis (trabeculodysgenesis with iris anomalies)
   A. Anterior stromal defects
      1. Hypoplasia
      2. Hyperplasia
   B. Anomalous iris vessels
      1. Persistence of tunica vasculosa lentis
      2. Anomalous superficial vesssels
   C. Structural anomalies
      1. Holes
      2. Colobomata
      3. Aniridia

III. Corneotrabeculodysgenesis (usually has associated iris anomalies)
   A. Peripheral
   B. Midperipheral
   C. Central
   D. Cornea size

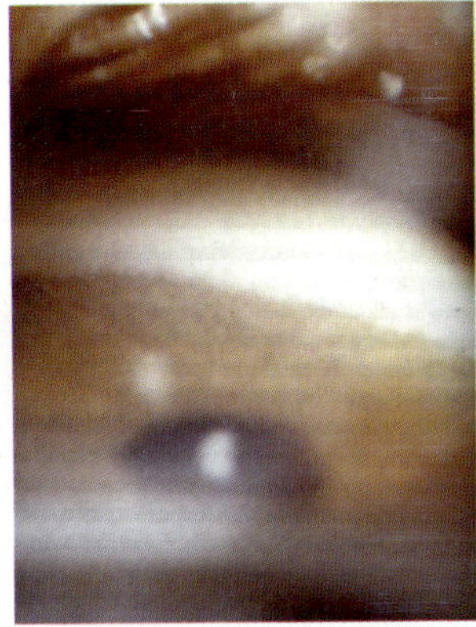

Fig. 1: Anterior insertion

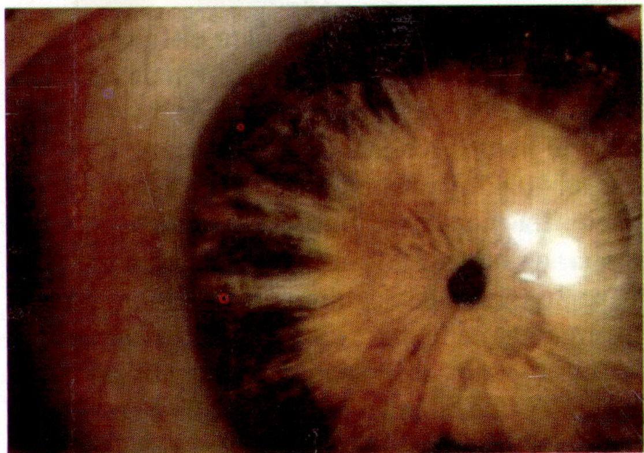

Fig. 2: Hypoplasia iris

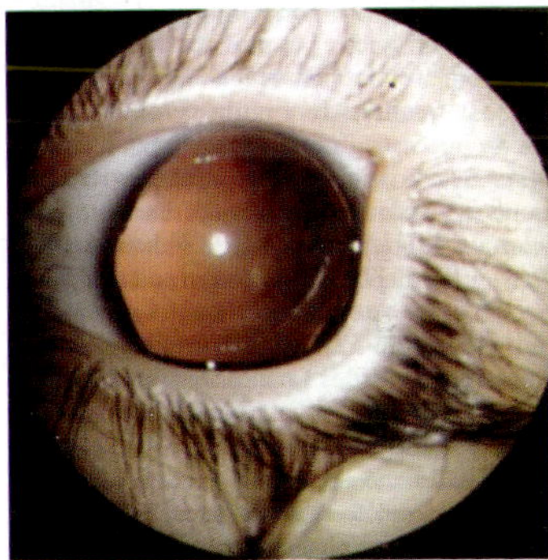

Fig. 3: Aniridia congenita

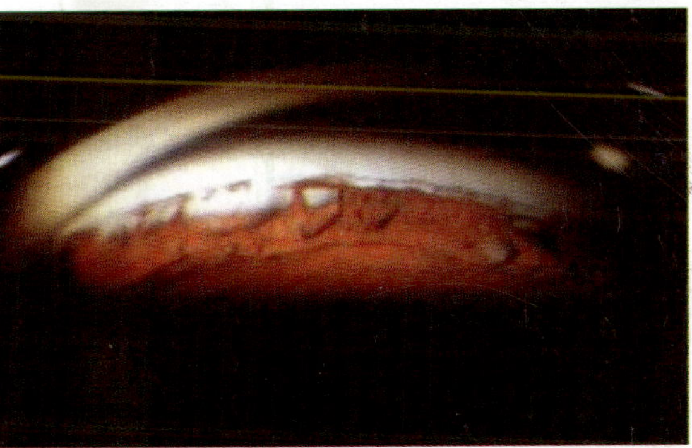

Fig. 4: Axenfeld syndrome

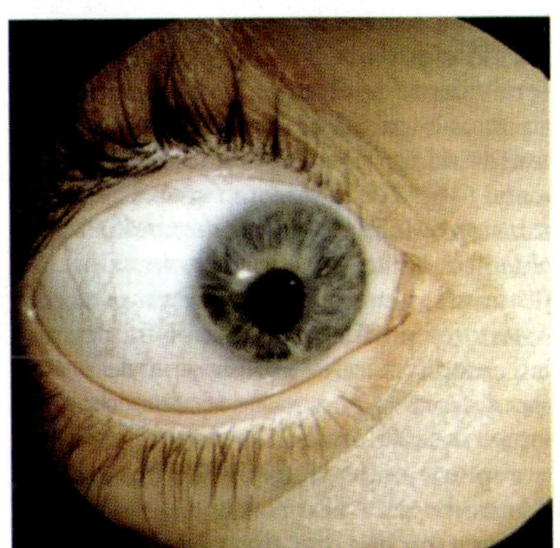

Fig. 5: Axenfeld-Rieger syndrome

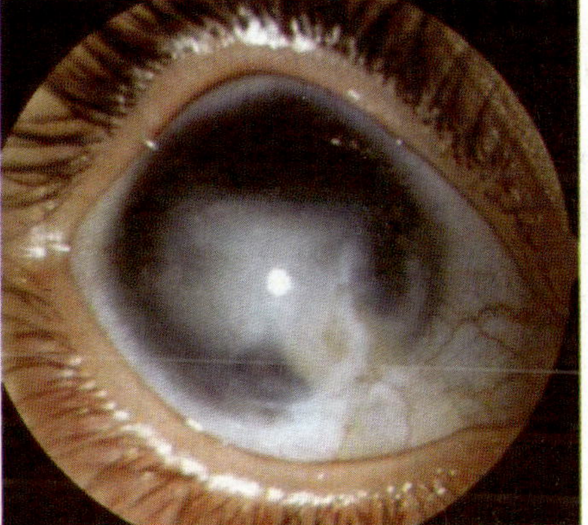

Fig. 6: Peters anomaly

defects of the eye were chosen as the basis for this system because they are readily apparent on examination and do not require supplemental information. The goniodysgenesis that leads to glaucoma occurs in a variety of ways and may involve one or more of the three angle structures: the trabecular meshwork, the iris and the cornea, so the extent of maldevelopment is indicated by the presence or absence and degree of trabeculodysgenesis, iridodysgenesis and corneodysgenesis. These defects occur in a variety of combinations with attributes that have therapeutic and prognostic significance.

PATHOPHYSIOLOGY

Although the exact mechanism of *Primary Infantile Glaucoma* remains unproven, it is generally related to an iridocorneal angle malformation, with an obstacle to aqueous humor outflow. Some investigators have suggested that a cellular or membranous abnormality in the trabecular meshwork is the primary pathologic mechanism. This abnormality is described as either an anomalous impermeable trabecular meshwork or a Barkan membrane covering the trabecular meshwork. Other investigators have emphasized a more widespread anterior segment anomaly, including abnormal insertion of the ciliary muscle. Many of these features suggest a development arrest in the late embryonic period.

CLINICAL FEATURES

Diagnosis of *Infantile Glaucoma* depends on careful clinical evaluation, including IOP measurement, measurement of corneal diameter, gonioscopy, measurement of axial length by ultrasonography and retinoscopy, and ophthalmoscopy.

Characteristic findings of *Infantile Glaucoma* include the classic triad of presenting symptoms in the newborn: *epiphora, photophobia and blepharospasm*. External eye examination may reveal *buphthalmos* with corneal enlargement greater than 12 mm in diameter during the first year of life (the normal horizontal corneal diameter is 9.5-10.5 mm in the full-term newborns and smaller in premature newborns). Corneal edema may range from mild haze to dense opacification of the corneal stroma because of elevated IOP (corneal edema is present in 25% of affected infants at birth and in more than 60% by the sixth month). Tears in Descemet's membrane called *Haab's striae* may occur acutely as a result of corneal stretching.

Critical evaluation of infants requires an examination under anesthesia. Most general anesthetic agents and sedatives lower IOP, so the normal IOP in an infant under anesthesia may range form 10 to 15 mmHg, depending on the tonometer. Measurement of corneal diameter with a caliper, gonioscopy, measurement of axial length by ultrasonography and ophthalmoscopy under anesthesia is recommended.

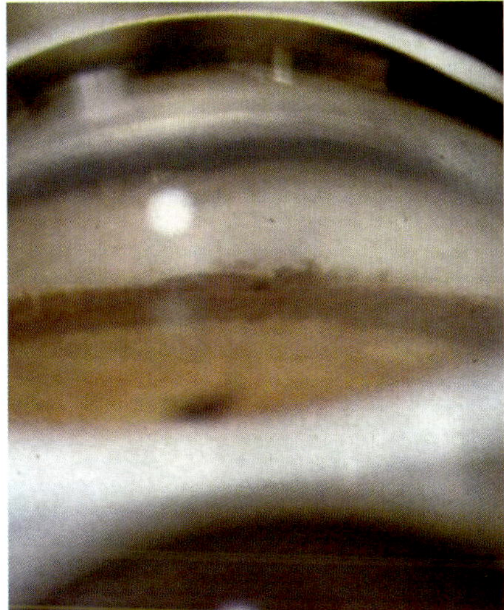

Fig. 7: Abnormal angle

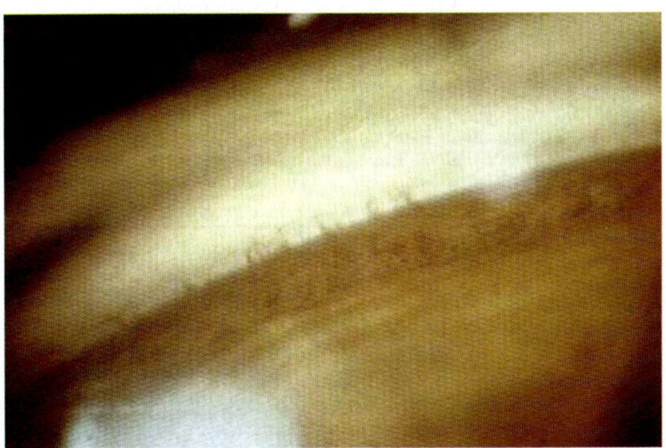

Fig. 8: Iris process

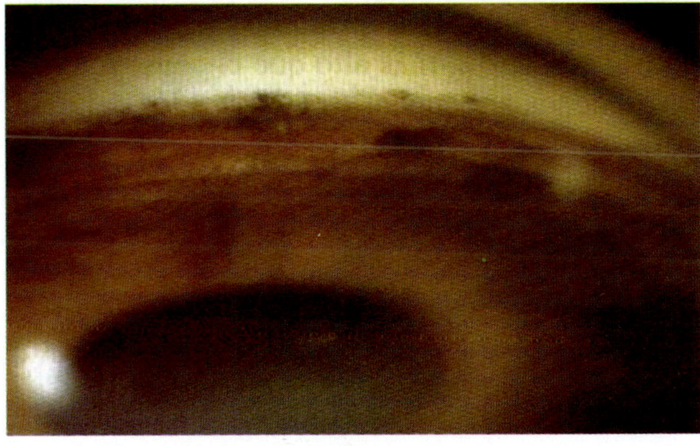

Fig. 9: Pigmented angle

Table 2: Clinical evaluation chart

	Right Eye	Left Eye
Name:		
Birthday:		
Corneal		
Edema		
Horizontal diameter		
Vertical diameter		
Gonioscopy		
Iris		
Lens		
IOP (type of tonometer)		
Ultrasonography		
AC		
Axial length		
Paquimetry		
Ophthalmoscopy		

In *Primary Infantile Glaucoma*, the anterior chamber is characteristically deep with normal iris structure. Findings include a high and flat iris insertion, absence of angle recess, peripheral iris hypoplasia, tenting of the peripheral iris pigment epithelium and thickened uveal trabecular meshwork. The angle is typically open, with a high insertion of the iris root that forms a scalloped line as a result of abnormal tissue with a shagreened, glistening appearance. This tissue holds the peripheral iris anteriorly. The angle is usually avascular, but loops of vessels from the major arterial circle may be seen above the iris root. The normal anterior chamber angle in childhood is different from the adult angle. Many of the findings just listed are nonspecific, and it may by difficult to distinguish the gonioscopic findings in infantile glaucoma from a normal infant angle.

Visualization of the optic disc may be facilitated by using a direct ophthalmoscope and a direct gonioscopic or fundus lens on the cornea. The optic nerve head of a normal infant is pink with a small physiologic cup. Glaucomatous cupping in childhood resembles the cupping in adulthood, with preferential loss of neural tissue in the superior and inferior poles. In childhood, the scleral canal enlarges in response to the elevated IOP, causing enlargement of the cup. Cupping may be reversible if IOP is lowered, and progressive cupping indicates poor control of IOP.

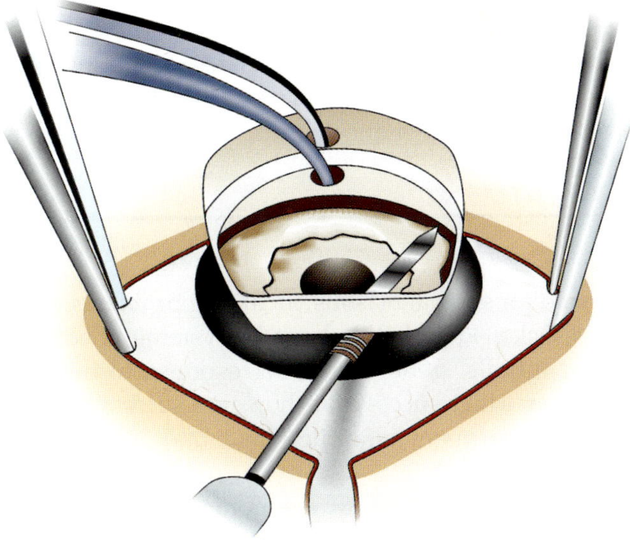

Fig. 10: Goniotomy using a Barkan lens and Swan goniotomy knife

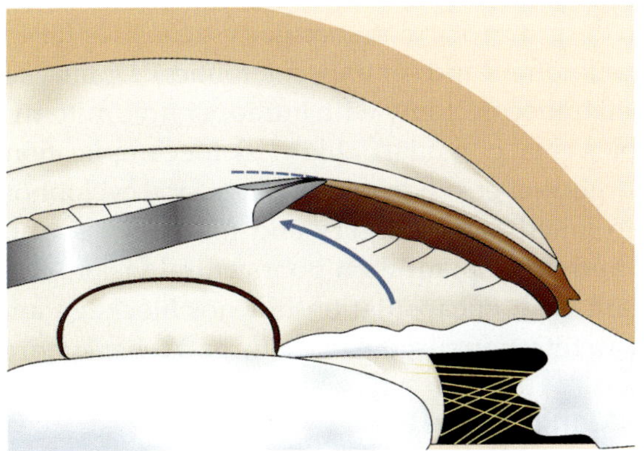

Fig. 11: Correct location and depth of the goniotomy incision

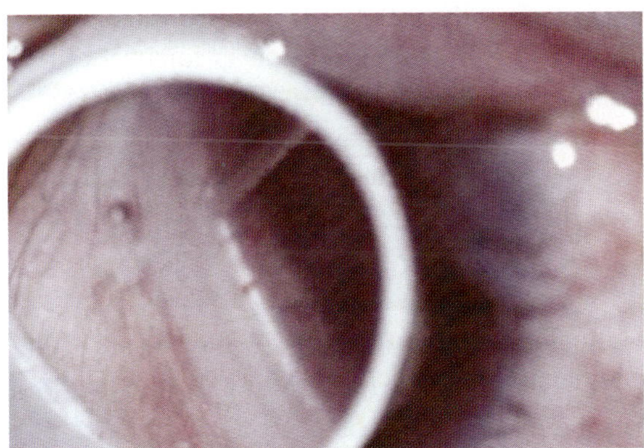

Fig. 12: Goniotomy using a Swan-Jacob lens

Medications have limited long-term value for *Infantile Glaucoma* in most cases, and the preferred therapy is surgical. If there are high suspect of glaucoma, the parents must be inform and the surgical procedure must be done immediately after the first examination under anesthesia.

SURGICAL TREATMENT

Introduction

Surgery is preferred for several reasons, including problems with compliance with medications, lack of knowledge about the systemic effects of medications in the infant and infants' generally poor response to medications. Most important, surgery has a high success rate (however, success rates vary markedly among the anatomic forms of infantile glaucoma) and a low incidence of complications.

In children under 2 to 3 years of age goniotomy or trabeculotomy are recommended. Trabeculotomy is recommended for children over 2 to 3 years of age and for all children in whom corneal clouding prevents adequate visualization of the angle. Combined trabeculotomy-trabeculectomy is recommended in the group of iridotrabeculodysgenesis or failed previous angle surgery (2 or < goniotomies and/or trabeculotomies). Drainage implant surgery is done after failed trabeculectomy with intraoperative mitomycin C and when there is reasonable visual potential or high risk for complications with filtration surgery (e.g., Sturge-Weber syndrome). Transscleral cyclophotocoagulation is recommended in failed angle surgery and minimal visual potential, failed trabeculectomy and/or implant with poor central vision, IOP too high after glaucoma implant with encapsulation but not blockage and high risk for complications with filtration surgery (e.g. Sturge-Weber syndrome).

Preoperative Management

Some time medications play an auxiliary role before the surgery. Oral carbonic anhydrase inhibitors, primary acetazolamide, have effectively reduced elevated IOP. When administered orally with food or milk three or four times dairy (total dose 10 to 20 mg/kg/day), acetazolamide is fairly well tolerated. Topical dorzolamide together with apraclonidine 0,5% could be used in select cases. In goniotomy and trabeculotomy, to obtain miosis, pilocarpine 1% should be placed onto the eye to be operated upon just before surgery to protect the crystalline lens from injury during surgery.

Angle Surgery

The introduction of angle surgery made a revolution in infantile glaucoma procedures. In fact, the poor prognosis of infantile glaucoma changed dramatically with the introduction of goniotomy by Otta Bakan in 1938 (Gk. *gonio*, "angle", and *tomein*, "to cut"). Although the instrumentation has since

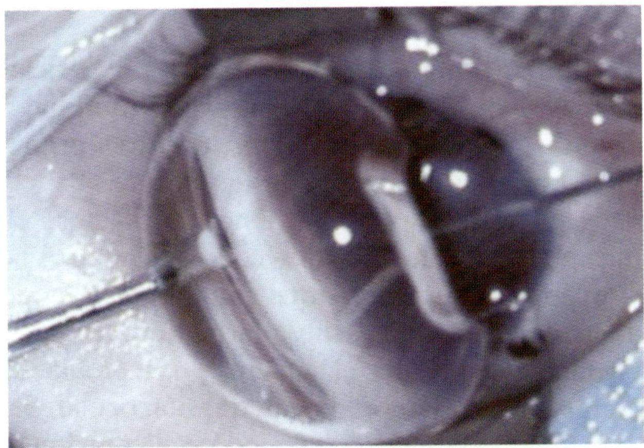

Fig. 13: Goniotomy using a Worst lens

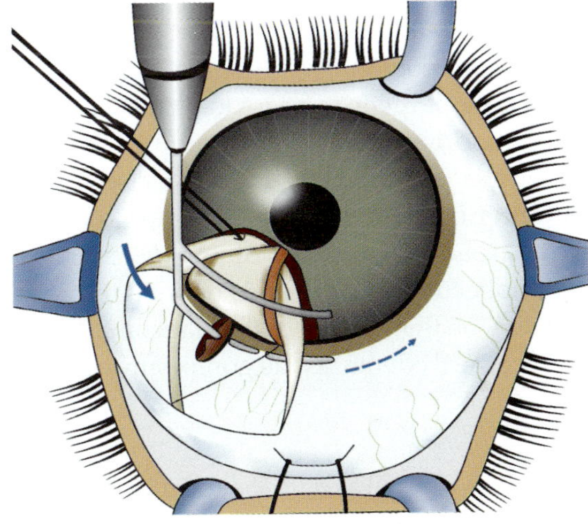

Fig. 14: Trabeculotomy under a limbus-based conjunctival and partial-thickness scleral flap

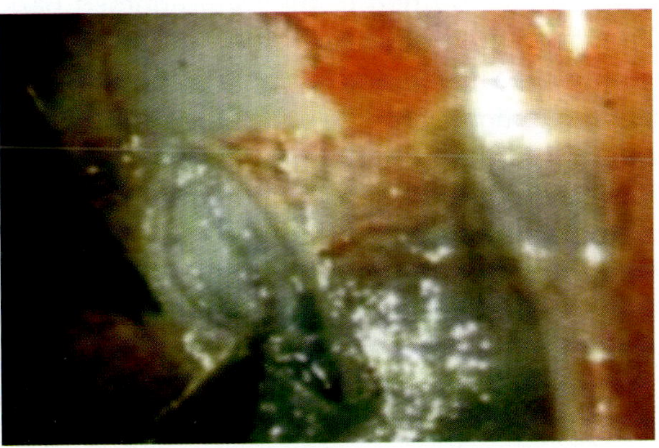

Fig. 15: Radial incision of the Schlemm's canal

been refined and the operating microscope now permits more precise visualization of the angle structures, the operation has remained essentially unchanged.

A further advance in management came in the 1960s with the introduction of trabeculotomy by Allen and Burian and Smith, which was popularized by Harms and Dannheim.

Both goniotomy and trabeculotomy have their staunch advocates. Trabeculotomy is our preferred operation for the following reasons:

- Trabeculotomy has a documented higher success than goniotomy. The latter controls intraocular pressure is about 74% of the eyes having glaucoma of all degrees of severity, although control may be as high as 85% if eyes with corneal clouding are excluded.
- Trabeculotomy is technically easier for a well-trained microsurgeon because it does not require the introduction of sharp instruments across the anterior chamber, which increases the risk of damage to other ocular tissues. It can be performed with the same accuracy in advanced cases in which the cornea is edematous or scarred and there is poor visibility in the anterior chamber
- There no need for the surgeon to adapt to the visual distortion produced by the operating gonioprism
- A trabeculotomy is anatomically more precise in creating an opening between the anterior chamber and Schlemm's canal, and there is the advantage to associate a viscocanulostomy
- The success of trabeculotomy depends only on the type of angle anomaly and not dependent on the severity of the glaucoma, the size of the cornea, or the presence of corneal edema, as the goniotomy does.

Goniotomy

The aim of goniotomy is to open a route for aqueous humor to exist the anterior chamber into Schlemm's canal by removing obstructing tissue and it is performed using a surgical goniolens and a goniotomy knife. There are several available goniolenses, in addition to the round-domed Barkan goniolens, including the Lister modification, which includes irrigation, or the Swan-Jacobs lens, which incorporates a handle and facilitates use of a microscope, or Worst lens. Numerous modifications of Barkan's goniotomy knife have been described, including attached fiber optics for intraocular illumination. A non-tapered Swan knife enters the anterior chamber easily and cuts in either direction. Alternatively, a disposable 23- or 25-gauge needle attached to a syringe containing viscoelastic may used in place of a knife, allowing the anterior chamber to be deepened before incision and to be maintained upon instrument removal. The perform goniotomy safely and effectively, corneal clarity must be sufficient to allow an adequate view of the angle structures. The surgeon usually sits opposite the portion of the angle to be operated, with the patient's head slightly rotated away from the surgeon. Viscoelastic may placed onto the central cornea just

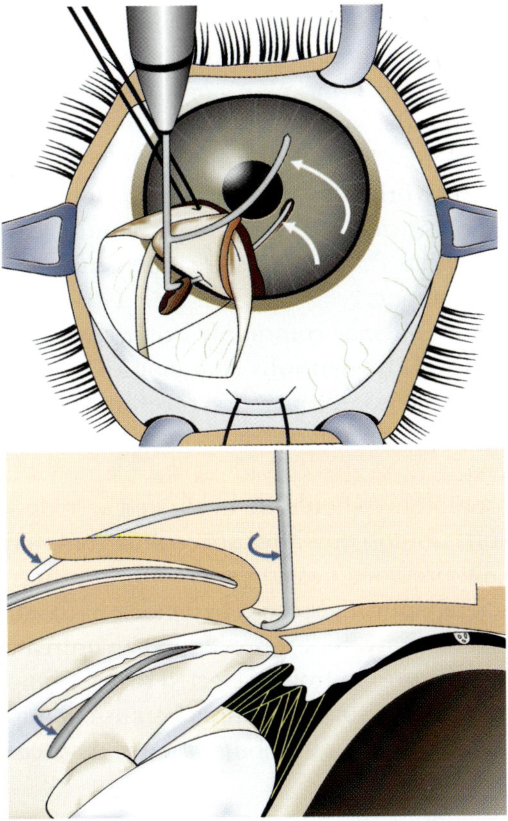

Fig. 16: Rotation of the trabeculotome into the anterior chamber

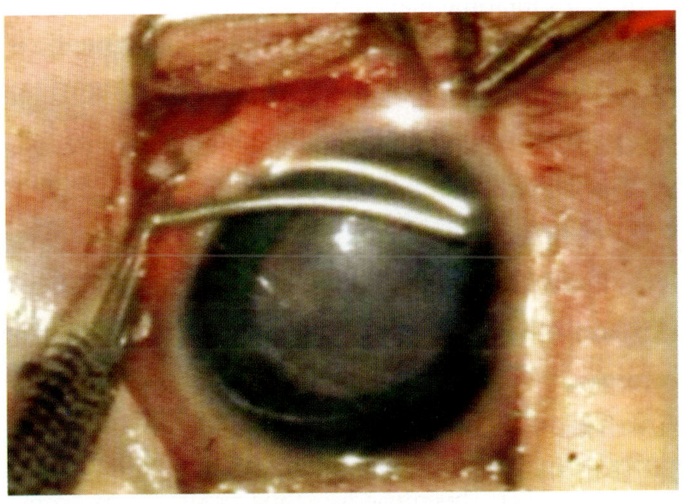

Fig. 17: Trabeculotomy

before placing the operating goniolens. The goniolens may be stabilized with a nontoothed fine forceps in the positioning holes of the lens, or it may be modified to include a handle. The goniotomy knife or needle is placed through peripheral clear cornea 1 mm from the limbus, opposite the midpoint of the intended goniotomy, in a plane parallel to the iris. It is guided over the iris tissue to engage trabecular meshwork in its anterior third, just posterior to Schwalbe's line. A circumferential incision is then made for about 4 to 5 clock hours. The incision must be superficial. Postoperative treatment includes the use of topical antibiotic, steroid, and miotic.

Mild to moderate hyphemas commonly occur after goniotomy, but they almost always clear rapidly without sequelae over several days. Other complications following goniotomy are rare and include iridodialysis, cyclodialysis, small peripheral anterior synechiae in the incised angle, damage to the crystalline lens.

The results of goniotomy should be evaluated weekly in the immediate postoperative period. Gonioscopy after successful goniotomy often reveal a widened angle in the previous incision site, with improved visibility of the ciliary band and scleral spur. Because 4 to 5 clock hours of angle tissue are incised with single goniotomy, repeat procedures in untreated portions of the angle may enhance pressure control in selected cases. Goniotomy may fail to control infantile glaucoma in some instances because of improper placement and depth of the angle incision, or the obliteration of the incision by peripheral synechiae.

The success of goniotomy in controlling glaucoma varies with the etiology of the glaucoma. The best results – 80% to more than 90% success after one or two procedures—are achived in infants with primary infantile glaucoma presenting between 3 months and 1 year of age. Success rates are much lower for cases of primary infantile glaucoma presenting either at birth or after 12 months of age (about 30 to 50%). The success of goniotomy depends also on the size of the cornea, or the presence of corneal edema.

The need to use a multiple lens system (operating microscope, goniotomy lens, lens-cornea-fluid meniscus and cornea) to visualize the angle, as well as the above changes in the cornea that reduce visualization, combine to make goniotomy a difficult and hazardous procedure. To improve visualization the corneal epithelium may be removed. Use of prismatic lenses to view the angle also usually requires tilting of the operating microscope, further reducing its resolution power.

Trabeculotomy

The surgical techinique of trabeculotomy is performed by cannulating Schemm's canal from external approach and then tearing through the trabecular meshwork into the anterior chamber. This procedure thus creates a direct communication between the anterior chamber and Schlemm's canal.

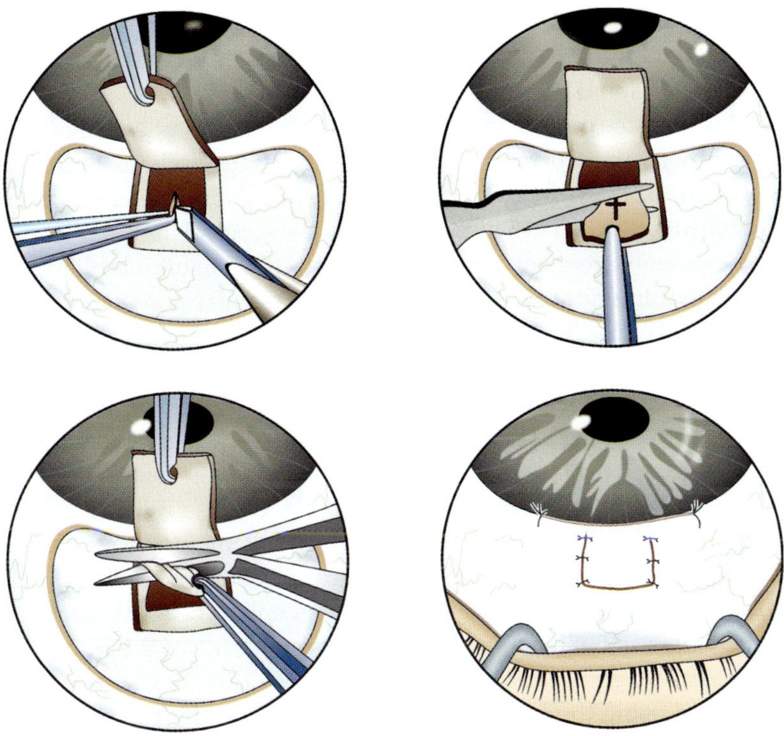

Fig. 18: Technique for combined trabeculotomy-trabeculectomy

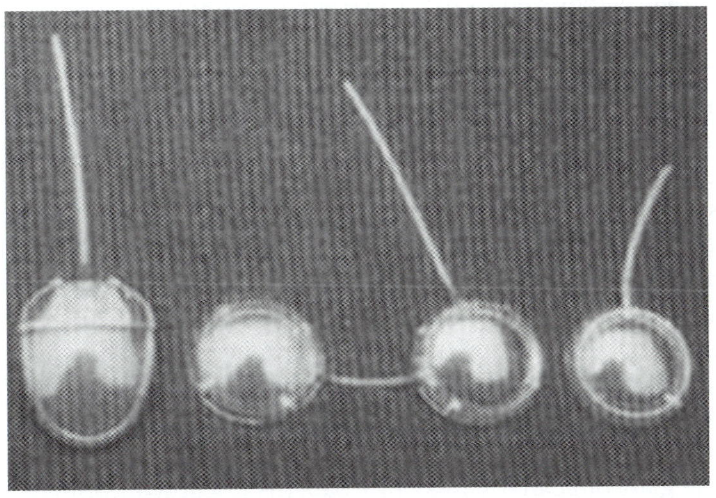

Fig. 19: Ahmed valve Implant, double-plate and single-plate Molteno Implant

In the surgical technique described by McPherson, a limbal based conjunctival flap and a partial-thickness triangular or rectangular scleral flap are created as for standard trabeculectomy.

Alternatively, the procedure may be easier to perform under a small fornix-based conjunctival peritomy. After partial-thickness scleral flap has been created, a radial scratch incision is made in the bed of the scleral flap across the sclerolimbal junction (2.5 to 3 mm posteriorly the surgical limbus). This scratch incision is gradually deepened under high magnification until Schlemm's canal is identified just anterior to the circumferential fibers of the sceral spur (near the posterior aspect of the limbal "gray zone").

Often a small amount of blood or aqueous humor refluxes through the cut ends of Schlemm's canal, and the internal wall of the canal appear slightly pigmented. To confirm the identity of the canal, a Grieshaber cannula should threat easily to both the left and right sides of the radial incision. If resistence is met, the radial incision must be deepened, or a second parallel radial incision must be done. Once the canal has been located, I like to do viscocanalostomy with Grieshaber cannula with and sodium hyaluronate at 1.4%. This procedure turns the introduction of the trabeculotome easier,enlarging the Schlemm's canal and destroying any bands. After this, the internal arms of the trabeculotome should be passed gently into the canal as far as possible without meeting resistence, and using the parallel external arm as a guide. The internal arm is then gently rotated into the anterior chamber, with care to avoid entry into the peripheral cornea or beneath the iris plate. Rotation of the trabeculotome into the anterior chamber tears through the intervening trabecular meshwork and requires very little force. Rotation should be halted once about 75 to 80% of the internal arm of the trabeculotome is visible in the anterior chamber. The trabeculotome is removed from the eye along its path. In similar fashion, the trabeculotome should be placed into the other side of the radial incision and the procedure repeated. The scleral flap and the conjunctive are then sutured with 8-00 polyglactin. Subconjunctival antibiotic and steroid may be given at the end of surgery.

Postoperatively, patients are treated with topical antibiotics and steroids. While small hyphema occurs commonly after trabeculotomy, rarer complications include inadvertent filtering blebs, choroidal detachement, iridotomy, damage of the lens, false passages into the anterior chamber or suprachoroidal space, and infection.

The effects of trabeculotomy should be determined 3 to 4 weeks after surgery. This procedure may be repeated in the different portion of the angle if the effect is inadequate following the first procedure.

Success rates varying from 73 to 100% have been reported for trabeculotomy in infantile glaucoma. In a series of 71 patients (most with primary infantile glaucoma), Akimoto and colleagues reported total success probabilities of one or more trabeculotomies of 92.5% and 76.5% at 5 and 10 years, respectively.

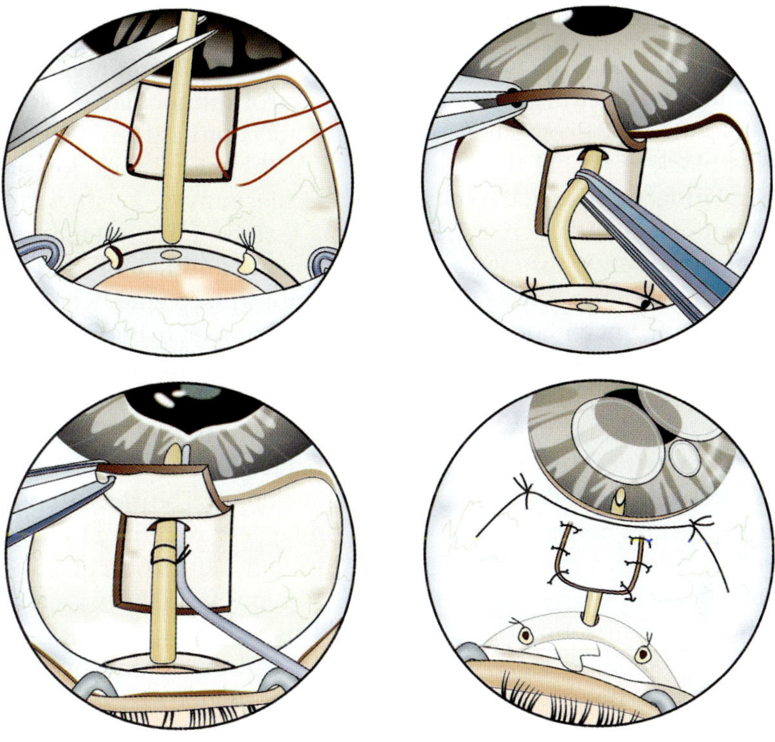

Fig. 20: Surgical steps for synthetic drainage implants

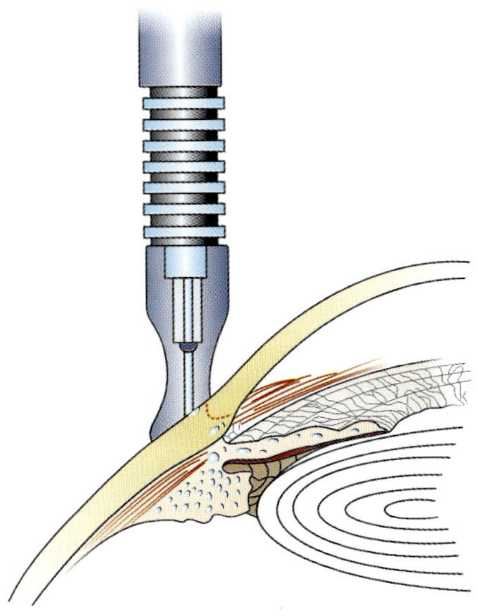

Fig. 21: G-Probe

Combined Trabeculotomy-Trabeculectomy

If Schlemm's canal has not been successfully cannulated or if previous similar trabeculotomy procedures have failed to control intraocular pressure, the trabeculotomy can be combined with a trabeculectomy by removal of a full-thickness block of limbal tissue in the bed of the scleral flap, followed by peripheral iridectomy as in the standard trabeculectomy.

Penetration into the anterior chamber is made slowed. The anterior chamber is entered at one corner through a small opening by careful dissection through Descemet's membrane, allowing aqueous humor to seep slowly out until the eye becomes soft, but without losing the anterior chamber. In buphthalmic eyes, the zonules may be stretched and, with penetration into the anterior chamber, vitreous can prolapse through the chamber. The risk of this complication can be reduced by slowly reducing intraocular pressure before completing the trabeculectomy. After the eye has softened, air or balanced salt solution is injected into the anterior chamber to maintain a moderate depth. The iridecotmy should be made carefully because vitreous may prolapse through a stretched and ruptured zonule and erupt through the iridectomy. If this occurs, a limited vitrectomy must be performed, removing all vitreous from the iridectomy and the immediately surrounding iris surface. This is best accomplished using sponges and Vannas scissors. The scleral flap and the conjunctiva are then sutured with 8-00 polyglactin. Subconjunctival antibiotic and steroid may be given at the end of surgery. If antimetabolites are used, I prefer limbus-based conjunctiva-Tenon's capsula flap, and is closed with continuous suture.

The postoperative management for the trabeculotomy, combined trabeculotomy-trabeculectomy or isolated trabeculectomy is the same. Intraocular pressure is checked in the office or by examination under anesthesia within 6 weeks of the surgical procedure. A cycloplegic is used in combined trabeculotomy-trabeculectomy or isolated trabeculectomy if there is a significant postoperative inflammation.

Some surgeons advocate combined trabeculotomy-trabeculectomy as the first surgery for infantile glaucoma.

Trabeculectomy

Filtering surgery is usually done when goniotomy and trabeculotomy either failed or are unlike to succeed. Poor outcome from trabeculectomy is most likely multifactorial, but several authors have reported much higher rates of success using primary trabeculectomy in children with glaucoma, mostly in infantile cases. Although subconjunctival 5-fluoruracil has been administered postoperatively in children after trabeculectomy, resulting in successful filtration, its administration usually requires multiple sequential anesthesias and is limited by corneal epithelial toxicity, as in the adults. The intraoperative use of mitomycin C has greatly enhanced the success of trabeculectomy in controlling glaucoma, presumable by limiting postoperative scaring by Tenon's capsula and scleral fibroblasts. The success of mitomycin C augmented trabeculectomy in chidren is much higher in those who are older and phakic. Hence several authors independently found young age and aphakia to be negative predictors of success. I do not use mitomycin C in a very young children, because the response is extremely variable, with some patients scarring rapidly despite antifibrotic therapy and others developing hypotony with large avascular filtration blebs.

Synthetic Drainage Implants

Drainage implant surgery is done when it is a children whom failed trabeculectomy with intraoperative mitomycin C and reasonable visual potential or high risk for complications with filtration surgery (e.g. Sturge-Weber syndrome). All modern drainage implant devices have the same basic design, which typically consist of a silicone tube that extends from the anterior chamber to a plate, disc, or encircling element beneath conjunctiva and Tenon's capsule. The edge of the external plate has a ridge, through which the distal end of the tube inserts onto the upper surface of the plate. The ridge decreases the risk of obstruction of the posterior opening of the tube with the surrounding tissue and fibrous capsule. The plates of the glaucoma drainage devices have large surface areas and promote the formation of the filtering bleb posteriorly, near the equator.

Performance of similar drainage devices can vary significantly, depending on the size, shape, and materials from which the external component and tube are constructed. One of the most fundamental design differences is the way the device has an open, unobstructed drainage tube or one that contains a pressure-regulating valve. Baerveldt, Molteno, and Schocket implants are the examples of open tube implants. Ahmed and Krupin implants are designed to have a flow-restricting valve mechanism.

Molteno Implant is the prototype drainage implant device and has had the longest and most extensive clinical experience since it was introduced by Molteno in 1969.

Ahmed glaucoma valve implant has a mechanism to decrease early postoperative hypotony by providing resistance to the flow and therefore regulating the pressure within a desired range. In this valved drainage implant design, a silicone tube is connected to a silicone sheet valve, which is held in a polypropylene body. The valve mechanism consist of two thin silicone elastomer membranes, which allows one-way regulation of the flow with a goal of keeping the IOP between 8 and 10 mmHg in the early postoperative period. The inlet cross section of the chamber is wider than the outlet, which offers a theoretical small pressure differential between the anterior chamber and subconjunctival space, which is claimed to enable the valve to remain open even when only a small difference in pressure exist.

Only Molteno and Ahmed glaucoma valve implants are usually used in children eyes. Although certain variations of surgical techniques are required for implantation of the different implants, the basic surgical principles apply in general to all drainage implant devices.

Adequate surgical expose is dependent on proper placement of a traction suture. A 6-0 polyglactin or silk traction suture on a spatulated needle is placed through superficial cornea near the superior limbus and attached to the drape beneath the eye. A fornix-based conjunctive-Tenon's capsule flap is created, usually in the superotemporal quadrant, to expose the scleral bed. The initial conjunctival incision may be made approximately 2-3 mm from the limbus, to create a limbal based flap and to permit easier closed suture. The flap is slightly elevated to allow for blunt dissection between Tenon's and episclera with blunt Westcott scissors. Because it is necessary to have surgical exposure to or beyond the equator of the globe, radial relaxing incisions should be placed on one or both sides of the conjunctival flap. A muscle hook is then used to isolate the two rectus muscles on either side of the surgical site. With Ahmed valve implant it is necessary to irrigate balanced salt solution though the tube using 27-gauge cannula, before the insertion into the anterior chamber, to ensure that the valve opens properly. The external plate is then tucked posteriorly into sub-Tenon's space one sutured to sclera with 8-00 nylon sutures through the anterior positional holes of the plate. The anterior, border depending on the size of the globe, must be 6 to 8 mm posterior the limbus. After the plate been sutured a lamellar scleral flap must been dissected with 6x4 mm. Preplaced sutures at the corners of the flap will be looped out of the way. The tube of the flap is trimmed to size at its anterior end (2 to 3 mm into the anterior chamber). The anterior end of the tube is inserted into the anterior chamber via the needle track using a nontoothed forceps and is secured to the sclera with a loose nylon suture. The scleral falp is sutured back in place. The conjunctiva is then sutured back its original position using polyglactin sutures. Subconjunctival steroids and antibiotic are injected.

With Molteno implant, restriction of aqueous flow to avoid severe early postopearative hypotony can be achieved by using a two-stage implantation technique, in which the external plate is placed in the subconjunctival space without inserting the tube into the anterior chamber. The tube is inserted 6 to 8 weeks later, after the fibrous capsule has formed around the external plate. A more popular technique is to occlude the tube, this provides the advantage over the two-stage technique of avoiding a second operation. The tube can be occluded in different ways: a ligature of 6-0, 7-0, or 8-0 polyglactin before inserting it into the anterior chamber; an adjustable suture could be done.

Complications of drainage implantion in children include tube malposition, flat anterior chamber, tube obstruction by iris or vitreous, cataract, cornea-tube touch, choroidal detachment, corneal edema and corneal abrasion.

Cyclodestructive Procedures

The surgical procedures previously described all share the goal of increasing aqueous outflow from the eye. Cyclodestructive procedures reduce the rate of aqueous production by injuring the ciliary processes.

Indications for cyclodestructive procedures is usually reserved for situations in which repeated filtration surgery are failure and when there is severely buphthalmic eye with extensive optic nerve pathology and a poor visual prognosis.

The success of the cyclodestructive procedures is also modest (about 50%), results are often unpredictable, but with lower reported incidence of phthisis bulbi and hypotony. The cyclodestructive procedures used are cyclocryotherapy and transscleral cyclophotocoagulation.

Cyclocryotherapy presumably destroys the ability of ciliary processes to produce aqueous humor by the biphasic mechanism of intracellular ice crystal formation and ischemic necrosis.

The mechanism by which transscleral cyclophotocoagulation lowers IOP is not fully understood. The prevailing theory is that it reduces aqueous production by damaging the pars plicata, although it is not clear whether this due to direct destruction of the ciliary epithelium or reduced vascular perfusion. In ours days it is available the *neodymium:YAG* and the *semiconductor diode* lasers. Advantages of these laser techniques over cyclocryotherapy include less transient IOP rise, a less exuberant uveitic response, and less pain postoperative.

Cyclocryotherapy

Cyclocryotherapy has been used as therapy for infantile glaucomas for many years, and is applied with a similar technique to that used in adults. In children, cryotherapy should be applied to a maximum of 180 degrees of the circumference of the eye at one session, using six or seven freezes (60 seconds each at -80° C) with the anterior edge of a 2.5 mm diameter cryoprobe placed 1 to 1.5 mm from the limbus, in a nonbuphthalmic eye, and placed 1.5 to 2 mm from the limbus in a buphthalmic eye. Placement of the probe directly over the 3- and 9-o' clock positions should be avoided to prevent damage to the long posterior ciliary vessels. In addition to limited success rates, the risk includes not only hypotony or phthisis, but also uveitis, cataract formation, and attendant visual loss. Al Faran et al reported 30% success after one or more treatments in a large series of children with advanced infantile glaucoma.

Transscleral Cyclophotocoagulation

Neodymium:YAG Lasers

Neodymium:yttrium aluminum garnet (Nd:YAG) lasers, with a wavelength of 1,064 nm, are useful for transscleral cyclophotocoagulation because they transverse the sclera with relatively low absorption and scatter. They may be operated in a continuous-wave mode, and be delivered by a contact probe, fiberoptic system.

Continuous-wave mode. The SLT CL60 (Surgical Laser Technologies) provides contact probe delivery in a continuous-wave of 0.1 to 10 seconds. A 2.2 mm sappire-tipped, handheld probe, which is focused at 1.5 to 2 mm in air, is coupled to a fiberoptic delivery system. The unit can provide powers in excess of 10 W. the SLT is the unit on which most of the early experience with contact, continuous-wave Nd:YAG transscleral cyclophotocoagulation is based. A subsequent instrument, the Microruptor 3 (MR3) also provides continuous-wave Nd:YAG laser energy, which can be delivered by either a 600 mm, flat tip, quartz fiber probe or a slit-lamp.

This technique has been performed primary with the SLT, using exposure times of 0.5 to 0.7 seconds. The laser focus is fixed by the design of the probe tip, which is held perpendicular to the surface of the conjunctiva with the anterior edge of the probe 0.5 to 1.5 mm behind the limbus; 32 to 40 applications of 7 to 9 W for 0.5 to 0.7 seconds are applied for 360 degrees, often sparing the 3 and 9 o' clock positions. Limited experience with Nd:YAG contact transscleral cyclophotocoagulation in young children with advanced, uncontrolled glaucoma suggest effective pressure reduction in approximately 40% after a single 360 degrees treatment.

Semiconductor Diode Lasers

Although semiconductor diode lasers, with a range of wavelengths between 750 and 850 nm, do not transverse the sclera as efficiently as Nd:YAG lasers, they have the advantage of greater absorption by uveal melanin. In addition, they have the advantage of solid-state construction with compact size, lower maintenance requirements, and no special requirement for electric outlet or water cooling. The Oculight SLx (Iris Medical Instruments) is a continuous-wave, contact delivery diode laser with a wavelength of 810 nm, a maximum power output of 2.5 to 3.0 W, and a maximum duration of 9.9 seconds. The probe (G-Probe) consists of a 600 mm quartz fiberoptic, protruding 0.7 mm from a handpiece, which is fabricated to center the fiberoptic 1.2 mm behind the surgical limbus and parallel to the visual axis. The back of the G-Probe pushes the limbus away from the surgical site, and the sides can be used to aide in spacing the laser applications. Initial settings are 1,750 mW and 2 seconds. If a popping sound is heard with the initial application, the power is reduced by increments of 250 mW until no pop is heard. If no pop is heard with the initial application, the power is increased by the increments until the sound is heard and then reduced by one increment. The laser applications are spaced circumferentially by placing the side of the G-probe footplate adjacent to the indentation mark of the previous fiberoptic placement. The original protocol involved 18 applications for 270 degrees, avoiding the 3- and 9-o'clock positions because this reduce the chances of occluding the long posterior ciliary vessels and thus reduce the chance of anterior segment ischemia. The rate success of this technique is of 30 to 75% after one or more treatments.

Postoperative inflammation can be a significant problem, requiring special prophylactic measures. One approach is to give a subconjunctival injection of a short acting steroid at the end of the procedure and to prescribe topical atropine and steroid for approximately 10 days. Postoperative pain also tends to be mild, with many patients requiring no analgesic. The most significant complication associated with transscleral cyclophotocoagulation is loss of visual acuity. The precise mechanisms are not fully understood, but likely causes include macular edema associated with the inflammatory. Maximum pressure reduction is typically achieved in 1 month, and it is usually desirable to wit at least this long before retreating.

LONG-TERM FOLLOW-UP

Patients with infantile glaucoma require follow-up examinations for life.

Long-term medical therapy in children can be difficult because of side effects and compliance problems. Medical therapy is used primary in difficult cases that have not responded well to surgical intervention.

PROGNOSTIC FACTORS

It appears that the surgical prognosis for patients with infantile glaucoma is best when the onset of the disease occurs between the first and the twenty-four month of life. The reasons for this are unclear. Earlier cases with onset at birth may represent a more severe developmental disorder. Later, possibly changes of trabecular tissues or apposition and compression of the wall of Schlemm's canal or impermeability of the canal's inner wall play a role.

Various factors, such as the age of onset, may affect the prognosis. On the other hand, surgery is generally more successful when performed as early as possible. It is generally accepted that the success of goniotomy is not as good in eyes with significant buphthalmos.

The appearance of the anterior chamber angle is of great prognostic significance. In the group of isolated trabeculodysgenesis, the angle anomaly may be result of incomplete development of tissue derived from neural crest cells. These patients have the best prognosis for either goniotomy or trabeculotomy, over 90% achieving intraocular pressure control. In the group of iridotrabeculodysgenesis, the anomaly involves the peripheral iris and the trabecular meshwork and is the result of a cicatricial process in the periphery of the anterior chamber angle. These patients have a far poorer prognosis with surgery, particularly goniotomy or trabeculotomy, which have success rates approximately 30%. Patients undergoing trabeculectomy, combined trabeculotomy-trabeculectomy have success rate of approximately 50%. When filtration surgery fails, a glaucoma drainage implant or cyclodestructive procedure would be indicated. Some surgeons consider drainage implants as the primary procedure in these patients. In the group of corneotrabeculodysgenesis (Axenfeld-Rieger syndrome and Peters' anomaly, for example) the prognosis is also poor with trabeculotomy or goniotomy and better with trabeculectomy, but many of these patients also finally require a drainage implant or cyclodestructive procedure. However, even with the use of a drainage implant, the prognosis for successful surgery in groups 2 and 3 probably not exceed 60%.

4

Open Angle Glaucoma

Mordechai Goldenfeld, Shlomo Melamed (Israel)

INTRODUCTION

Open Angle Glaucoma (OAG)—Definition

A chronic optic neuropathy caused by a group of diseases and characterized by:

Damage to the optic nerve that is usually, but not always, caused by high intraocular pressure (IOP) which causes characteristic morphological changes to the optic nerve. These changes may lead to typical visual field defects over time, and if not treated can eventually lead to blindness. The disease process may be arrested or slowed by lowering of intraocular pressure (IOP). Damage caused by glaucoma cannot be reversed and is permanent, and is caused by a progressive retinal ganglion cell loss.

There are different types of open angle glaucomas and all share the common feature of having an open anterior chamber angle. In order to differentiate between these subtypes a morphological description of the glaucoma is used. When evidence of a morphological change is lacked, the glaucoma is defined as primary open angle glaucoma (POAG).

Open Angle Glaucoma Subtypes

- Low tension glaucoma.
- Pigmentary glaucoma.
- Exfoliation glaucoma (PXFG)
- Inflammatory glaucoma
- Fuchs's Heterochomic cyclitis
- Glaucomatocyclitic crisis—Posner-Schlossman syndrome
- Steroid induced Glaucoma
- Intraocular bleeding and hyphema
- Ghost-cell glaucoma
- Uveitis glaucoma hyphema syndrome (UGH)
- Steroid induced glaucoma
- Phacolytic glaucoma
- Tumor related glaucoma
- Sturge Weber syndrome.

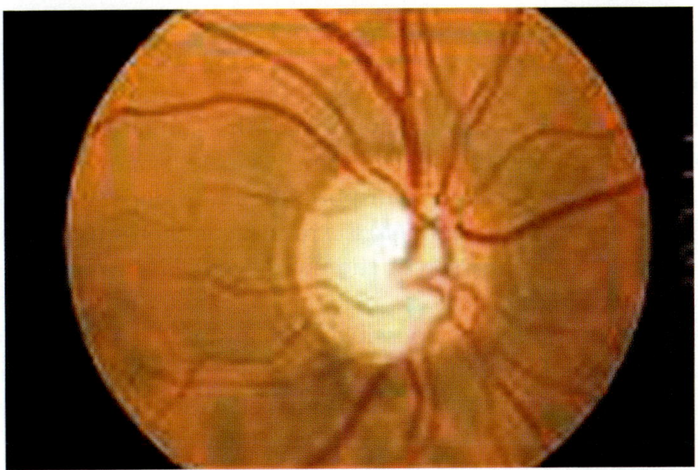

Fig. 1: Glaucomatous disc with inferior notching

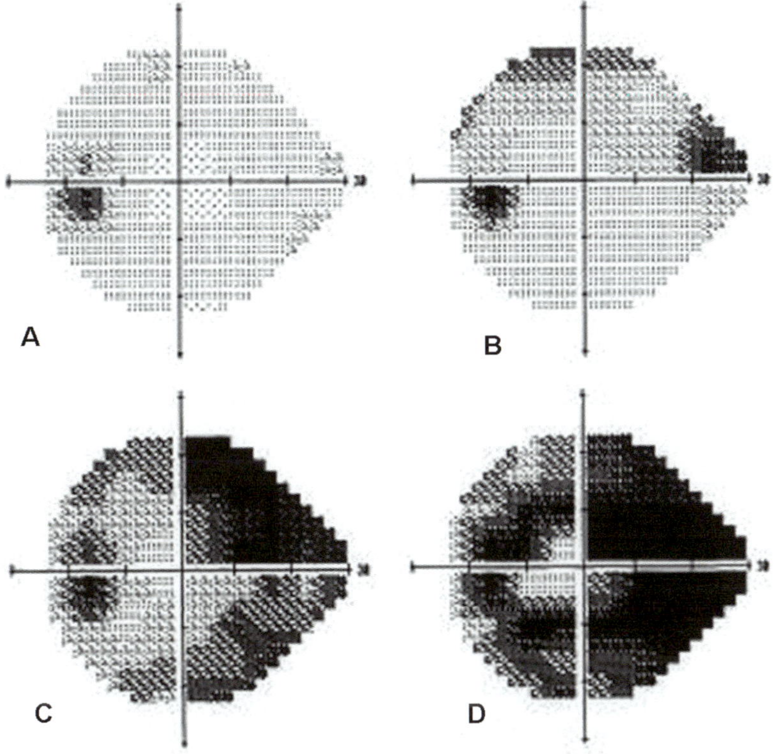

Figs 2A to D: Typical visual field progression from Normal (A) Superior nasal step (B) Superior and inferior arcuate scotoma to a tubular visual field defect (C and D)

PRIMARY OPEN ANGLE GLAUCOMA

Pathophysiology

- The mechanical theory—elevated IOP distorts the lamina cribrosa, crushing the axons of the optic nerve and disturbing the axoplasmic flow through the lamina. The axoplasmic flow transports the brain derived neurotrophic factor (BDNF) which is essential to the retinal ganglion survival, from the lateral geniculate nucleus. A reduction of the axoplasmic flow eventually kills the retinal ganglion cells.
- The vascular theory offers two possible mechanisms, the first is supplanting the mechanical theory, assuming that the elevated IOP exerts pressure of the small caliber vessels of the eye; the second explanation is that a reduction in the diastolic perfusion pressure reduces the blood flow to the optic nerve thus depriving the ganglion cells of oxygen and nutrients.

Demographics

More than 3 million people are bilaterally blind from POAG worldwide, and more than 2 million people will develop POAG each year. Estimates from the World Health Organization suggest that if 100 million people are glaucoma suspects, over 20 million suffer from glaucoma, and over five million people are blind as a result of glaucoma. Approximately 70% of glaucoma is found in developing countries. It is estimated that two thirds of those blind are cases of POAG, but the majority of the remainder being cases of angle closure glaucoma (particularly common in China and the Far East). The prevalence of OAG is about 2%. Glaucoma is the most common cause of blindness among people of African descent. Prevalence of POAG is 3-4 times higher in blacks than in Caucasians, and blacks are up to 6 times more susceptible to optic disc nerve damage than Caucasians. They are more likely to develop glaucoma early in life, and they tend to have a more aggressive form of the disease.

CLINICAL SIGNS AND SYMPTOMS

There are no symptoms in OAG or POAG, and POAG patients are virtually asymptomatic. Patients my become aware to the presence of the disease either due to a severe visual field loss or vision loss late in course of the disease when the loss is felt, or during a routine eye examination like during a renewal of a driving permit. Others may experience the first sign of a visual impairment with sudden loss of vision due to a central retinal vein occlusion (CRVO). Elevated IOP is the second most common risk factor for CRVO preceded only by systemic arterial hypertension.

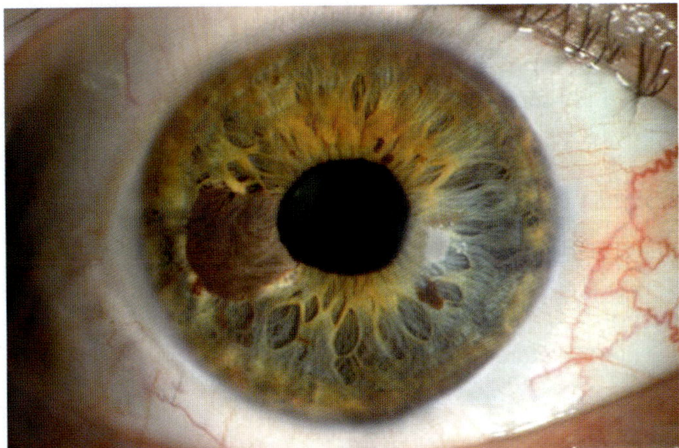

Fig. 3: Glaucoma

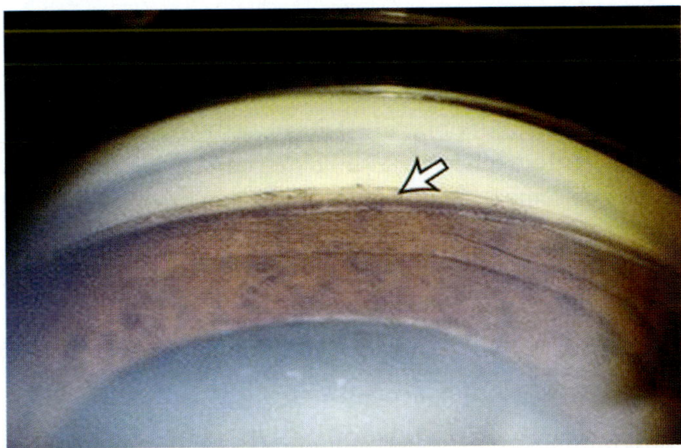

Fig. 4: Sampaolesi's line

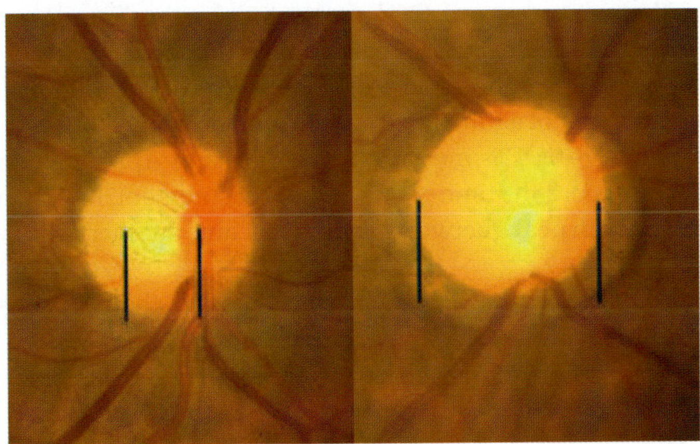

Fig. 5: Cup-to-disk-ratio

Three Definitive Signs Exist

- Elevated IOP (approximately 21 mm Hg or more)
- Enlargement of the optic cup
- Visual field loss.

Possible Signs

- Retinal nerve fiber layer loss
- Notching of the neuroretinal rim at the inferior or superior poles of the optic nerve head
- Splinter hemorrhages adjacent to the optic disc.

Work-up

- A comprehensive eye examination.
- Slit lamp examination of the anterior segment with special emphasis to:
  - — Cornea—Signs of pigment on endothelium (Krukenberg spindle) are observed in pigmentary glaucoma.
  - — Iris— Tran illumination defects - are observed in pigmentary glaucoma in the mid-periphery and in PXFG near the papillary margin.
  - — Lens—Pseudoexfoliation (PXF) material in exfoliation glaucoma.
  - — Anterior chamber—look for cells or flare to rule out uveitic glaucoma or glaucomatous Cyclitic crisis.
  - — Optic nerve/nerve fiber layer—Indirect stereoscopic examine with a +78D lens at the slit lamp will evidence optic nerve head damage and retinal nerve fiber layer damage. Look for notching or thinning of disc rim. Search for splinter hemorrhages, disc asymmetry. Document these changes with imaging of the optic nerve head (drawings; stereo fundus photographs) sophisticated imaging technologies, like the GDx VCC scanning laser polarimeter, HRT II confocal scanning laser ophthalmoscope, and OCT-Optical Coherent Tomography). These photographs and/or imaging techniques will serve for future comparison and evaluation of possible progression in optic disc damage prior to the development of a functional (visual field) damage.
  - — Tonometry—IOP is measured by Goldmann Applanation Tonometry (GAT). Record the time of day of the measurement. IOP changes during the day with peaks between 8 am and 11 am., another peak is between 2-4 am.
  - — Measure the central corneal thickness (CCT), this value is essential in differentiating ocular hypertension (OHT) from OAG, and helps determining the relative risk of progression form OHT to OAG.
  - — Gonioscopy—Shows an open angle. The presence of excessive pigment at the Schwalbe's line may suggest the diagnosis of pigmentary glaucoma or exfoliation glaucoma (Sampaolesi line).

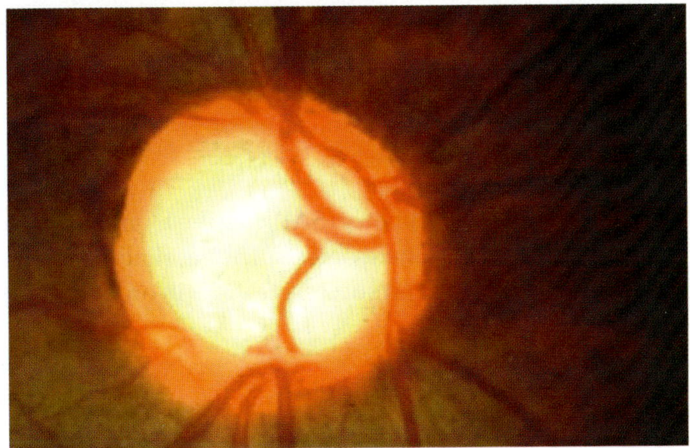

Fig. 6: Glaucoma-cupping

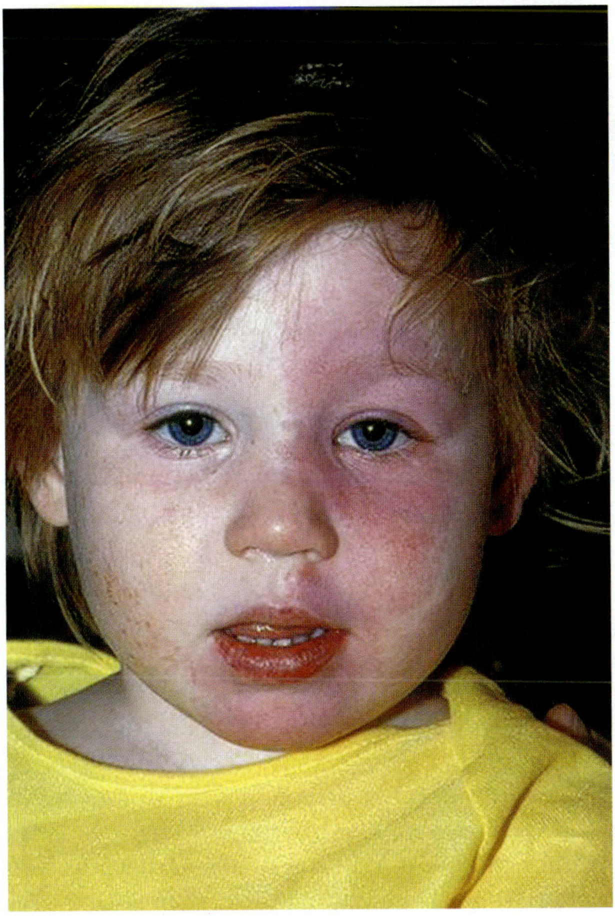

Fig. 7: Sturge-Weber-(port-wine, with hemangioma)

— Pachymetry (CCT)—Will measure corneal thickness, this will help in differentiating OAG from ocular hypertension.

Functional Tests

Visual Field Testing

Perform Standard Automated Perimetry (SAP) like the Humphrey or octopus in order to find glaucomatous visual field defects. The baseline visual field baseline needs to be repeated at least twice on successive visits in order to ensure reliable test results.

Optic Disc/Nerve Fiber Layer Imaging

Stereo Photography

In order to document cupping of the optic disc and compare it with future photographs.

Red Free Photography

Visualizes nerve fiber layer defects.

Ocular Coherence Tomography—OCT and Heidelberg Retinal Tomography—HRT

Scans both the optic nerve head and retinal nerve fiber layer, giving both quantitative and qualitative measurements.

GDx-Vcc

Scans the retinal nerve fiber layer.

DIFFERENTIAL DIAGNOSIS

The presence of an open angle will preclude all forms on closed or narrow angle glaucoma.

- Previous use of steroids (both topical and systemic), may suggest drug-induced glaucoma.
- Young age (<40 years) indicate primary juvenile open angle glaucoma.
- Unilateral manifestations of glaucoma with an open angle and mild intraocular inflammation may indicate glaucomatocyclitic crisis, (Posner-Schlossman syndrome).
- An open angle with blood in Schlemm's canal is result of an increase episcleral venous pressure, like in Sturge-Weber syndrome or carotid-cavernous sinus fistula. Sturge-Weber syndrome patients will demonstrate the typical Port-Wine Hemangioma together with hyperemia of the

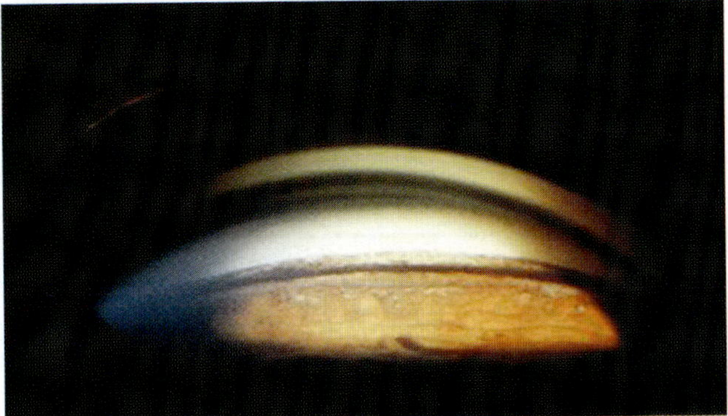

Fig. 8A: Pigment dispersion syndrome gonioscopy

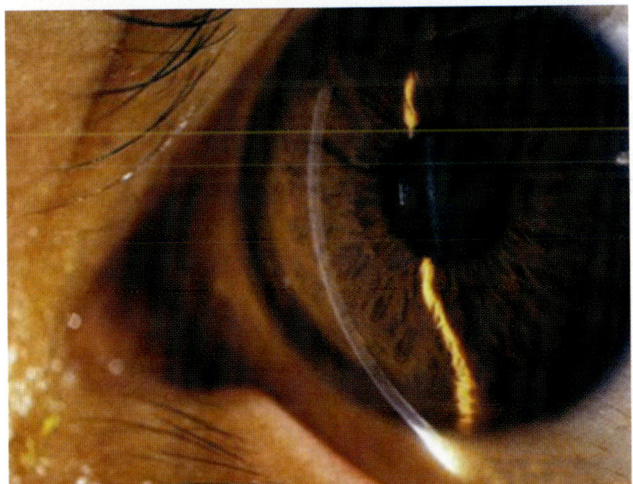

Fig. 8B: Posterior bowing of iris pigment glaucoma

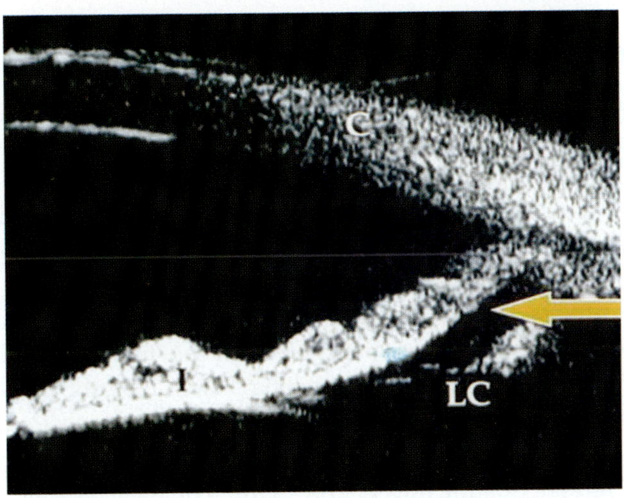

Fig. 8C: Posterior bowing of iris UBM

conjunctiva on the same side. The later may show conjunctival arterializations and chemosis, exposure keratopathy, dilation of retinal veins, optic disc swelling, intraretinal hemorrhages and other signs of ocular vasculopathy.

OAG SUBTYPES

Low Tension Glaucoma—Normal Tension Glaucoma

Low-tension glaucoma (LTG) is essentially the same diseases as primary open-angle glaucoma (POAG), without having an elevated IOP. The IOP has to be less than 22 mm Hg measure using a diurnal curve. One has to bear in mind that a single measure of IOP may miss more than half of OAG patients with IOP over 22 mmHg, and may mimic NTG; therefore it is essential to before a diurnal IOP curve before diagnosing NTG. NTG has been attributed to vascular dysregulation such as migraine, Raynaud Phenomenon, nocturnal deeps in diastolic blood pressure, systemic hypotension, Sleep apnea and vasospasm. It is estimated that as many as 20% of POAG are NTG patients. Other studies such as the Baltimore Eye Study, found that 50% OAG patients, that were diagnosed with POAG based on the presence of glaucomatous disc damage and a visual field defect had an IOP less than 21mmHg on a single visit, and 33% had an IOP of less than 21 mmHg on 2 measurements. NTG is more prevalent in Japan. NTG patients have been found to have thinner corneas. NTG is more common in females than in males, (as migraine and Raynaud Phenomenon). By definition, NTG is a diagnosis of exclusion. One has to exclude other factors such as angle recession glaucoma, previous chronic use of steroids that may have caused an elevated IOP with a secondary glaucomatous damage that persists in spite of the fact that when the use of steroids was stopped, the IOP came back to normal.

Pigment Dispersion Syndrome and Pigmentary Glaucoma

Pigment dispersion syndrome (PDS) is generally an asymptomatic disorder discovered during routine ophthalmic evaluation. PDS is a bilateral autosomal dominant disorder, with incomplete penetration; it affects males more than females, characterized by disruption of the iris pigment epithelium and deposition of pigment granules on the structures of the anterior segment. Pigment granule accumulation in the trabecular meshwork then leads to progressive trabecular dysfunction and ocular hypertension (OHT) which may lead to glaucoma. It affects young people between thirty and forty years old. Sugar and Barbour first described Pigmentary glaucoma (PG) in 1949, they describe young, myopic men with a vertical pigment deposits on the corneal endothelium - Krukenberg spindle, together with a heavy pigmented TM in the presence of an open angle. Pigment dusting may also be evident on the lens, called Zentmayer

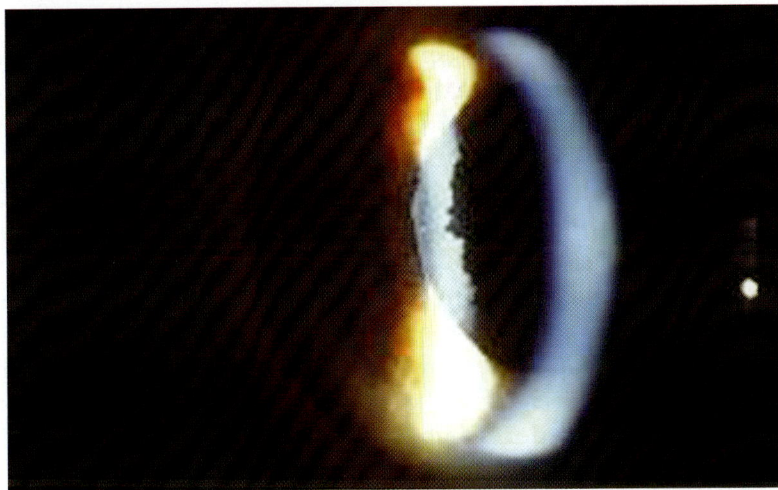

Fig. 9: Pseudoexfoliation of lens

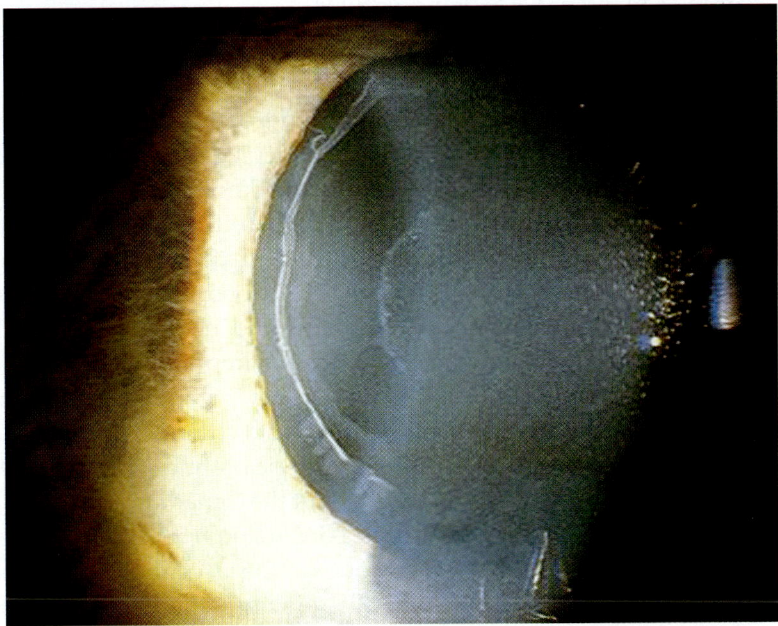

Fig. 10: Pseudoexfoliation syndrome

ring, the iris surface and Schwalbe's line. Radial, transillumination defects of the mid-peripheral of the iris are seen. Myopia is present in approximately 80% and is an important risk factor for the development of OAG. In 1979 Campbell, reported that mechanical contact between the concave posterior iris surface and anterior zonular fibers is responsible for the release of pigment granules from the IPE. Pigment dispersion results from chaffing of the posterior iris pigment epithelium ,and the zonular fibers of the lens, leading to release of pigment into the posterior chamber, which follows the flow of aqueous into the anterior chamber angle. The pigment may eventually fill the TM and obstruct the aqueous outflow and cause elevation of IOP. Recent studies using ultrasound biomicroscopy have shown that patients with PDS and PG differ in the anatomy of the chamber angle. The term "reverse pupillary block" describes a condition in which anterior chamber pressure intermittently exceeds that of the posterior chamber, enhancing this backward displacement of the iris and resulting in further pigment liberation and IOP spikes. Some advocate that a laser iridotomy may reverse this condition and prevent further release of pigment. Patients with PDS and PG are at increased risk for retinal detachment, which may occur in as many as 6-7% of individuals.

Pseudoexfoliation Syndrome and Pseudoexfoliative Glaucoma

Lindberg first described Pseudoexfoliation syndrome In 1917. He described deposits of a granular substance at the pupillary edge, and on the iris and cornea. These patients and also a form of OAG later known as Pseudoexfoliation Glaucoma,(PEXG) which is the most common identifiable form of secondary open-angle glaucoma worldwide. This is not a true exfoliation which is seen in people exposed to heat or infrared radiation like people who worked in the glass industry. Reports regarding the prevalence and incidence vary in relation to the origin of the examined population and the geographical zone. The reported prevalence is between 12% to as low as 1.8% in the Framingham eye study. In Europe the prevalence was found to be 4.7%., it is common in Scandinavian countries and is very rare among African Americans and Eskimos. PEX was never reported in the Inuit who live throughout the Canadian Arctic. It is more common in females than in males and the conversion from PEX to PEXG was reported to be 3.2% per year. PEX is considered to be an ocular manifestation of a systemic condition, and several studies have shown that PEX is linked with Alzheimer disease, senile dementia, cerebral atrophy, chronic cerebral ischemia, stroke, transient ischemic attacks, heart disease, higher homocysteine levels and hearing loss.

Signs and Symptoms

As all patients with OAG PEXG patients remains asymptomatic and usually are diagnosed on a routine eye examination or when the damage to the visual

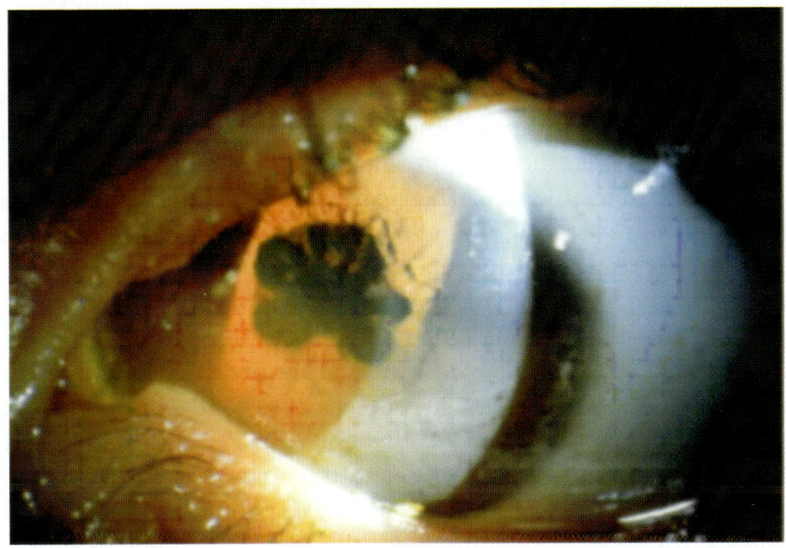

Fig. 11: Uveitic glaucoma

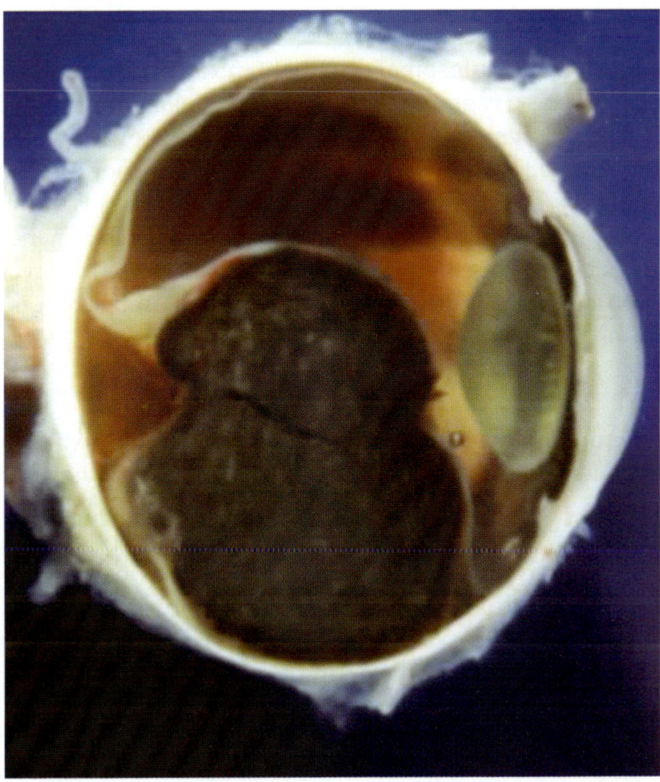

Fig. 12: Uveal melanoma

functions is advanced. PEXG is usually unilateral but may become bilateral in the course of the disease. Patients demonstrate deposits of a fibrilar/granular material on the anterior surface of the lens, the pupillary margin, the iris surface and sometimes on the corneal endothelium. It is usually seen as a 3-ring sign on the anterior lens capsule, formed by a central disk, a peripheral ring, and a clear zone, which separates the two. The clear zone varies in diameter and may exhibit curled edges. Transillumination of the iris may be seen, but unlike in Pigmentary dispersion syndrome it is seen at the pupillary margin, and not in the mid-periphery of the iris. The iris may also demonstrate atrophy usually at the pupillary margin. The angle demonstrates a pigment layer on the area anterior to Schwalbe line and on the Schwalbe line or called Sampaolesi line. At the beginning IOP is normal, but later in the course of the disease as many as 40% of patients develop elevated IOP. Patients with PEXG tend to have higher IOP values than patients with POAG and thus may develop damage to the optic nerve and the visual field faster than POAG patients. Patients with PEXG have wider fluctuations in IOP throughout the day than do patients with POAG. The highest IOP levels in patients with PEXG occur outside of normal office hours.

Pathophysiology

PEX is thought to be an autosomal dominant trait with incomplete penetrance and late onset. PEX is a type of elastosis, affecting elastic microfibrils. PEX is a single-nucleotide polymorphisms located in exon 1 of the *LOXL1* gene on chromosome 15q24.1 The product of the *LOXL1* gene modifies elastin fibers. Approximately 25% of the general population is positive for these variants. Glaucoma is caused by blockage of the TM by pseudoexfoliation material. There is also zonular laxity, causing lens donesis and an anterior movement of the iris-lens diaphragm causing a shallower anterior chamber that is some cases may result is angle closure glaucoma.

Therapy

PEXG patients are treated as all OAG patients, but one has to bear in mind that topical medications are less effective. Trabeculoplasty, whether argon (ALT) or selective laser trabeculoplasty (SLT), is very successful. Cataract surgery in PEX patients is more difficult due to the weakness of the zonular fibers, leading to lens subluxation, and phacodonesis in many cases. Surgery is associated with a higher incidence of intraoperative complications, like zonular/capsular tears leading to vitreous loss, and lens dislocation. Capsular tension rings may be used to decrease surgical stress on the zonules.

GLAUCOMA ASSOCIATED WITH OCULAR INFLAMMATION

Most intraocular inflammation (uveitis) may lead to increased IOP. The mechanism may be due to inflation mediators such as prostaglandins that are

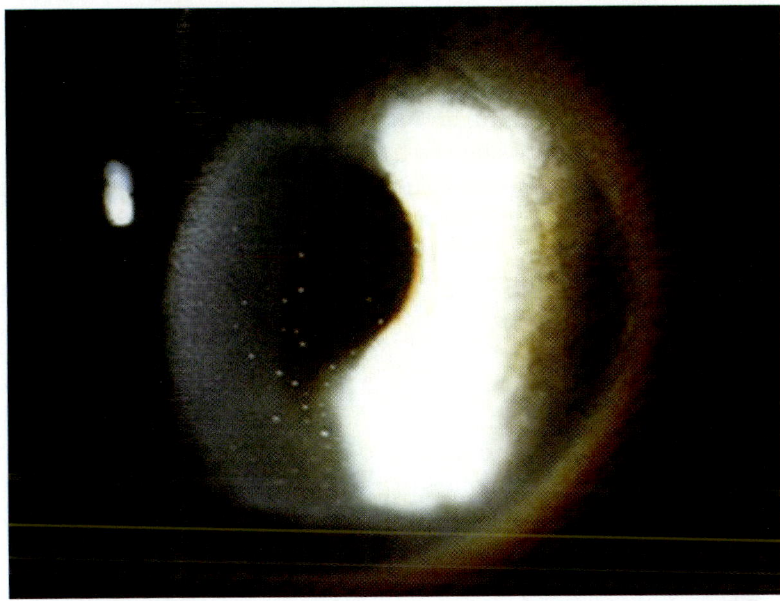

Fig. 13: Fuch's heterochromic cyclitis

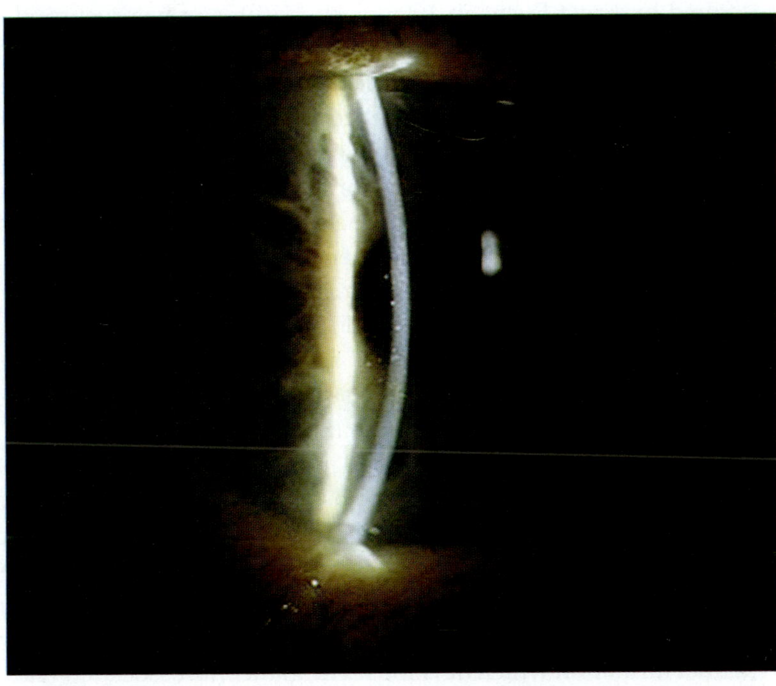

Fig. 14:Glaucomatocyclitic crisis

increased in the aqueous of eyes with uveitis, and cause elevated IOP per se , without a decrease in outflow facility, or an obstruction of the TM by inflammatory cells or fibrin , in the presence of an open angle, or the formation of peripheral synechiae causing an increased resistance to aqueous outflow with elevation of IOP by closing the anterior chamber angle, thus causing a secondary angle-closure glaucoma. Another mechanism is related to the use of corticosteroids that can result in elevated IOP. Corticosteroids increase IOP by decreasing aqueous outflow. Several theories have been proposed to explain this phenomenon, including accumulation of glycosaminoglycans in the trabecular meshwork, inhibition of phagocytosis by trabecular endothelial cells, and inhibition of synthesis of certain prostaglandins. The therapeutical challenge is to fight inflation on one hand and to treat IOP on the other hand. Topical therapy is preferred, mainly due to the fact that incisional therapy is less successful in inflammatory glaucoma. When medical therapy fails, trabeculectomy with anti metabolites or glaucoma drainage devices are used to treat IOP. There are several entities of intraocular inflammation that are directly associated with OAG , where IOP elevation is an essential part of the disease and not merely the consequence of an inflammation causing a secondary glaucoma, whether OAG or secondary angle closure glaucoma, like Fuchs' heterochromic cyclitis and herpetic uveitis.

Fuchs' Heterochromic Cyclitis (FHC)

First described by Ernst Fuchs in 1906, with features of heterochromia, low grade inflammation and an elevated IOP. It was assumed that this condition is associated with an impaired sympathetic nervous system caused by a disturbance in the iris vessel innervation, derived from the sympathetic nerve system. Later, electron microscopic studies showed that the hypochromia may result from a defective melanin production, caused by abnormal adrenergic innervation. This defective adrenergic innervation increased permeability of the blood-aqueous barrier with subsequent leaking of proteins, cells, and inflammatory mediators into the aqueous resulting in uveitis and subsequent IOP elevation which are the hallmark of FHC. Iris fluorescein angiographic studies showed leakage from iris vessels and areas of ischemia, associated with neovascularisation. Histological studies demonstrated abnormal hyalinization of the iris vessel walls, with narrowing of the vessel lumen. High incidence of cellular immunity and humoral immunity against corneal antigens were found in FHC patients, and may be associated with the typical keratic precipitates. Other possible causes were an association with ocular toxoplasmosis Horner syndrome. FHC is usually a unilateral disease that appears between the third and fourth decades with the insidious onset of mild, chronic anterior uveitis that usually is asymptomatic and is diagnoses usually due to cataract formation which develops. The glaucoma associated with FHC

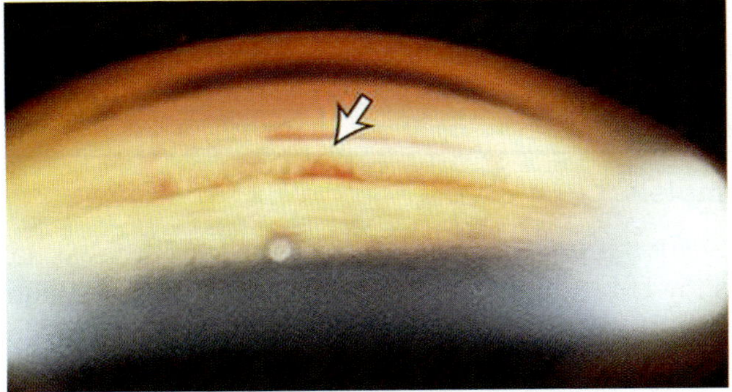

Fig. 15: Blood in Schlemm's canal SWS

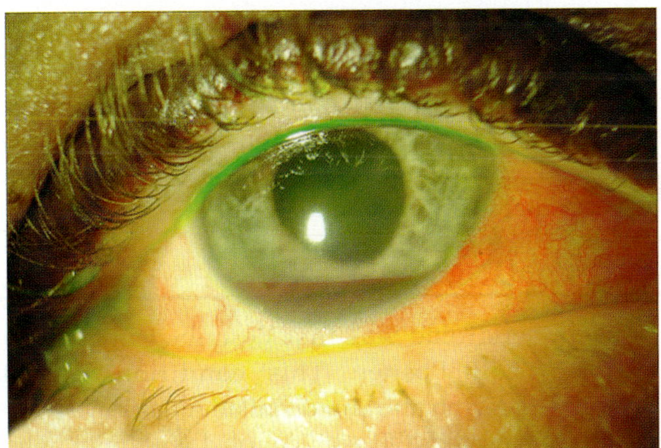

Fig. 16: Hyphema

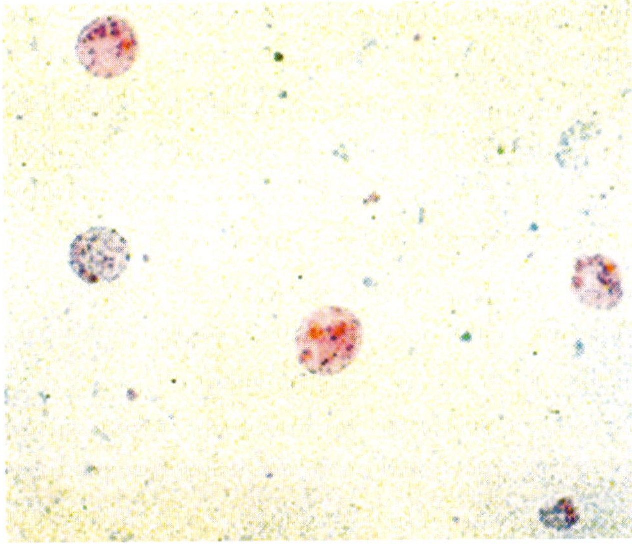

Fig. 17: Ghost cells

is OAG and is seen in 6-47% of cases. The uveitis usually does not need treatment with anti-inflammatory or immunosuppressive agents.

HERPETIC UVEITIS

Herpes Simplex

In herpetic uveitis there may be elevated IOP due to trabeculitis. Inflammatory cells obstruct the TM and cause an IOP elevation. If only trabeculitis exits, than it are an OAG, but as in all forms of chronic uveitis, eventually the inflammation will form PAS and secondary angle closure glaucoma may develop.

Varicella Zoster

Ocular involvement of cutaneous varicella zoster occurs in two thirds of patients when the ophthalmic division of the trigeminal nerve is involved. IOP elevation and glaucoma is caused by decreased outflow facility like in all cases of uveitic glaucoma, when the TM is blocked by inflammation products and trabeculitis. Treatment is directed towards the underlying cause with oral acyclovir, and reducing IOP and ocular inflammation topically.

GLAUCOMATOCYCLITIC CRISIS—POSNER AND SCHLOSSMAN

Posner-Schlossman syndrome was first described in 1948 by Abraham Schlossman and Adolf Posner. This condition, also known as Glaucomatocyclitic. Crisis is an uncommon inflammatory eye with self-limited recurrent episodes of elevated IOP with coupled with mild anterior uveitis. Glaucomatocyclitic crisis is a rare condition, although not unilateral, usually affects only one eye at a time. Patients are young to middle-aged adults aged 20-50 years. Features include uniocular recurrent episodes of mild anterior which last from days to weeks. Patients describe intermittent episodes of mild visual blurring, sign of elevated IOP like haloes around lights, and minimal pain or discomfort in one eye. Glaucomatocyclitic Crisis is usually self-limited and resolves spontaneously. Patients may present with corneal edema with mild anterior uveitis with few keratic precipitates (KP's), which are typically stellate, flat, nonpigmented, and concentrated over the inferior half of the corneal endothelium, with anisocoria, and a large pupil in the affected eye. The IOP level is out of proportion to the severity of the uveitis, it is common to measure IOP levels around 40-50 mmHg with only few cells and mild flare. The glaucoma is thought to be caused by trabeculitis and is usually self limited and in a period of days or weeks returns to normal, without any permanent damage. The inflammation never leads to the development of posterior synechiae or peripheral anterior synechiae, however, if IOP elevation persists, than typical glaucomatous damage to the optic nerve head and visual field develops. Patients

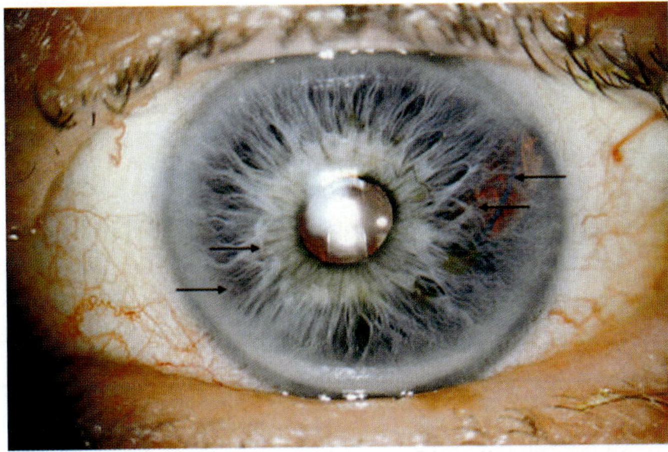

Fig. 18: UGH syndrome due to iris chaffing transillumination

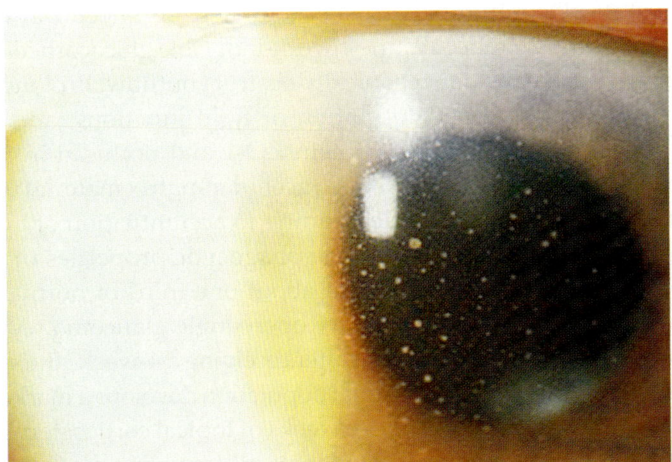

Fig. 19: Phacoanaphylactic glaucoma

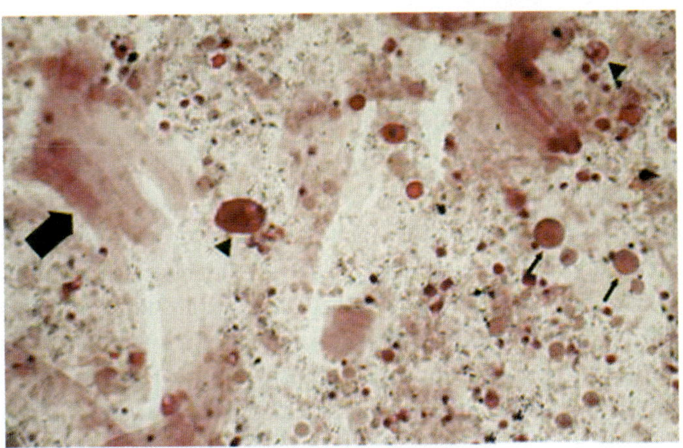

Fig. 20: Histology phacolitic glaucoma

with a 10-year or longer history of PSS are 3 times more likely to develop visual field changes and optic disc changes. These patients may be considered as steroid responders. The etiology of Glaucomatocyclitic crisis has and the underlying cause of Posner-Schlossman Syndrome is unknown. Cytomegalovirus (CMV) and Herpes simplex virus association has been suggested, but this has not been definitively proven, High levels of prostaglandins have been found during acute attacks in the aqueous humor of patients with of Posner-Schlossman Syndrome. HLA-Bw54 was found in 41% of patients.

STEROID INDUCED GLAUCOMA

The exact mechanism of steroid-induced glaucoma is unclear. We know that steroid-induced IOP elevation is secondary to increased resistance to aqueous outflow. Evidence shows that the reason for IOP elevation may lie in the accumulation of glycosaminoglycans, elastin, and fibronectin in the TM, or increased production of trabecular meshwork-inducible glucocorticoid response (TIGR) protein, which could mechanically obstruct outflow. Prolonged steroid exposure results in increased formation of tight junctions, and enhanced expression of junction-associated protein ZO-1 and occludin in Schlemm's canal. Steroids inhibit degradation of extracellular matrix material in TM, alter metabolism of mucopolysaccharides leading to accumulation of hyaluronate in the TM. Steroids may also reduce the phagocytic properties of trabecular meshwork cells. Armaly indicated that about one third of normal eyes and more than 90% of patients with primary open-angle glaucoma respond with greater than 6 mm Hg of IOP elevation after receiving a 4-week course of topical dexamethasone 0.1%. 5-6% of the normal population develops a marked increase in IOP of more than 31 mmHg after 4-6 weeks of topical corticosteroid therapy. With topical instillation, it was reported that children younger than 10 years of age were given 0.1% dexamethasone tend to have increased IOP. Following intravitreal injection of triamcinolone, over 50% of nonglaucomatous eyes will have an increase in IOP; this increase in IOP can occur as long as 6 months after the injection. After intravitreal injections triamcinolone , an IOP elevation can develop in about 50% of eyes, starting about 1-2 months after the injection. In the vast majority, IOP can be normalized by topical medication, and returns to normal values without further medication about 6 months after the injection

Patients undergoing surgery are at risk due to the use of topical steroids either preoperatively or postoperatively. In filtration surgery, even in the presence of a functioning filtering bleb, IOP may be elevated in response to topical steroids. Following photorefractive keratectomy (PRK)[1] and laser *in situ* keratomileusis (LASIK). These patients should be monitored carefully due to the difficulty to measure the IOP accurately as due to the thinning of the cornea, to corneal edema or entrapped fluid under the LASIK flap that may give a falsely low IOP reading. Treatment consists of stopping the use of topical steroids (when possible), and topical IOP lowering medication, around 15% of patients suffering from steroid induced glaucoma will need surgery. Recently it has been reported that SLT in beneficial in reducing IOP in steroid induced glaucoma.

INTRAOCULAR BLEEDING AND HYPHEMA

Intraocular bleed and hyphema are both know to cause elevated IOP, but although bleeding is the initial event the mechanism of IOP elevation differs. When vitreous hemorrhage is present, the IOP elevation is usually on a later phase when blood clears from the vitreous space and the so called "ghost cells" pass into the anterior chamber, when the bleeding is in the anterior chamber, and a hyphema is present the IOP elevation is acute. The IOP elevation is usually in direct relationship to the quantity of blood in the anterior chamber, a small microhyphema usually does not cause elevated IOP, but when a macroscopic hyphema a visible one can expect elevation of IOP. The most common cause of hyphema is trauma;, but other causes like neovascularization of the iris (Rubeosis iridis) seen in proliferative diabetic retinopathy , retinal vein or artery occlusion or in ocular ischemia. In non caucasian population one may suspect sickle cell trait. Rarely Intraocular tumors like juvenile xanthogranuloma, retinoblastoma, malignant melanoma, may cause intraocular bleeding. Iatrogenic causes include intraocular surgery. In the past ,the entity of Uveitis-Glaucoma-Hyphema (UGH) syndrome was not uncommon, nowadays, it is seen infrequently. This entity was related to some types of anterior chamber intraocular lenses (ACIOL), mostly Iris Clipped, that were implanted after cataract extraction . Chaffing of theses ACIOL's on the iris stroma led to recurrent episodes of hyphema, and uveitis, hence the term UGH syndrome. The IOP elevation is caused by red blood cells clogging the TM.

Medical Therapy

IOP can be treated with topical and oral ocular hypotensive medications to lower the IOP. Cycloplegia and topical steroids are indicated to speed up clearance of blood from the anterior chamber and to minimize

Surgical Therapy

Surgical intervention is warranted when corneal blood staining is seen, the best treatment is anterior chamber wash-out, if removing the hyphema is not effective in reducing the IOP and medical therapy has failed, a trabeculectomy is advised, but this should be done only when medical therapy has failed and the IOP level is very high for at least 72. The maximum blood clot formation is achieved 4-7 days after trauma. If clot formation has not occurred, opening the eye may simply lead to persistent hemorrhage.

GHOST-CELL GLAUCOMA

A secondary open angle glaucoma caused by blockage of the TM by erythrocytes. These red blood cells originate from a vitreous hemorrhage. After the vitreous hemorrhage absorbs, some red blood cells degenerate into ghost cell forms (smaller, khaki-colored, spherical, more rigid cells) usually within 1-3 weeks. These ghost cells contain intracellular globules consisting of denatured hemoglobin adherent to the cell membrane (Heinz bodies). The ghost-cells can remain for months in vitreous and subsequently may migrate into the anterior vitreous, and from there through a rupture of the anterior hyaloid face into the anterior chamber and then, to the TM causing an obstruction of TM, causing a secondary open-angle glaucoma. Treatment consists of paracentesis and anterior chamber lavage. If this does not control the glaucoma, then a trabeculectomy is performed. If this is unsuccessful, vitrectomy may be useful.

PHACOLYTIC GLAUCOMA

Phacolytic glaucoma is a form of an acute onset of OAG caused by a leaking mature or hypermature cataract. First described by Flocks et al in 1955, Phacolytic glaucoma is cured by cataract extraction. Patients present with sudden onset of unilateral pain and decreased vision in an eye with a prior history of poor vision due to cataract. Phacolytic glaucoma occurs in advanced cataractous lens which may be Morgagnian , with liquefied cortex and a brunescent nucleus with intact lens capsules. The chamber angle is open, but there is an obstruction of the TM by lens protein released from microscopic defects in the lens capsule that is intact clinically. Although the macrophages, may physically obstruct the TM, it seems that the obstruction is caused mostly by heavy molecular weight proteins. The anterior lens capsule may be dotted with white flecks representing collections of macrophages engulfing liberated lens material or may be wrinkled in appearance as the lens material beneath the capsule decreases in volume. Phacolytic glaucoma should be differentiated from acute angle-closure glaucoma by the open angle, uveitic glaucoma due to the absence of keratic precipitates and lens particle glaucoma, phacoanaphylactic glaucoma by the integrity of the anterior capsule. Medical therapy is only a temporary measure to reduce IOP and decrease inflammation, definite therapy is surgical with extra capsular cataract extraction and an intraocular lens implantation. Use of trypan blue dye for anterior capsular staining may greatly increase facility in creating an anterior capsulorrhexis. In some phacolytic glaucoma is caused by a dropped lens that is located in the vitreous, in this cases a pars plana vitrectomy with removal of the lens from within the vitreous cavity is necessary.

TUMOR RELATED GLAUCOMA

Intraocular tumors are rare causes of glaucoma. Tumors can cause glaucoma by several mechanisms; however, this section is focused on OAG secondary to tumors. The mechanism of TM obstruction may be from a hemorrhage, to pigment dispersion, chronic uveitis, melanomalytic (pigment-laden macrophages obstructing outflow), or from seeding of the TM by tumor cells. Depending on the primary site of the tumor the exact cause mechanism of the glaucoma may differ. For example an iris melanoma may cause IOP elevation by seeding of cells into the angle or a pigment release in the Ciliary body. Melanoma arising within the choroid may cause a secondary glaucoma by necrosis causing uveitis and or intraocular bleeding. A unique and rare 'black hypopyon' and secondary glaucoma may occur in eyes with cutaneous melanoma metastatic to the iris. Free-floating melanoma tumor cells and pigment-laden macrophages have been documented to form the 'black hypopyon'. It is postulated that these tumor cells and macrophages mechanically obstruct aqueous outflow pathways. Although individual rates vary, Shields showed a 5% incidence of increased intraocular pressure due to intraocular tumors in a series of 2704 patients with ocular tumors. Incidence of increased intraocular pressure also is dependent on location. Reports indicate a 17% incidence of glaucoma in ciliary body melanoma, 7% in iris melanoma, and 2% in choroidal melanoma. Given the relative infrequency of intraocular tumors, this condition is a rare event. Non solid tumors like lymphocytic leukemia, large cell lymphoma juvenile xanthogranuloma and Histiocytosis X despite a relative high incidence of ocular involvement in leukemia, (ranges from 50 to 80% of eyes), glaucoma is rare, and when glaucoma is present, it is most often secondary to anterior segment involvement like uveitis. Juvenile xanthogranuloma and Histiocytosis X are associated with spontaneous hyphema in children. Glaucoma results from direct obstruction of the outflow tract by histiocytes or outflow obstruction secondary to hyphema. Glaucoma secondary to tumor is usually first treated medically and an effort should be made to treat the underlying condition.

STURGE-WEBER SYNDROME (SWS)

Sturge-Weber syndrome (SWS) is a congenital disorder caused by the persistence of the transitory primordial sinusoidal plexus stage of vessel development. SWS is usually sporadic and characterized by a vascular malformation, with capillary and/or venous malformation that involve the face, choroid of the eye, and leptomeninges. The facial vascular malformation has a predilection for the distribution of the first division of the trigeminal nerve. A first-division trigeminal distribution is associated with occipital meningeal involvement; a second-division distribution, with parietal meningeal involvement; and a third-division distribution, with frontal meningeal involvement. In addition to the vascular meningeal malformation, an underlying atrophy of the cerebral hemisphere is often present. The disease process is usually unilateral. Glaucoma is present in up to 50% of cases in which the port-wine stain involves both the ophthalmic and maxillary divisions of the trigeminal nerve. Glaucoma develops before age

2 years in 60% of patients with the remainder developing by early adulthood. Ipsilateral conjunctival and episcleral vascular dilation may signal arteriovenous malformation, leading to elevated episcleral venous pressure, causing delay in the aqueous outflow. Management consists of combining medical, laser, and surgical options for late-onset glaucoma and primarily surgical intervention in infants. In one study, the median period of control was determined as the following: goniotomy (12 mo), trabeculotomy (21 mo), trabeculectomy (21 mo), argon laser trabeculoplasty (ALT) (25 mo), and medications (57 mo). However, trabeculectomy was associated with a high incidence of choroidal effusions and expulsive hemorrhage.

OAG TREATMENT

Medical Care

- Five major drug classes are used in the medical treatment of POAG:
  - Prostaglandin analogues. Reduces IOP by promoting outflow mostly through the non conventional outflow in the uveoscleral pathway.
  - Beta-blockers.
  - Alpha-agonists.
  - Carbonic anhydrase inhibitors.

  (Beta-blockers, Alpha-agonists, Carbonic anhydrase inhibitors: Reduce IOP by decreasing Aqueous Humor Section)
  - Miotic agents – Reduce IOP by increasing conventional outflow through the trabecular meshwork.

Laser Angle Surgery

- Argon laser trabeculoplasty
- Selective laser trabeculoplasty.

These laser procedures work well with all types of OAG and in particularly with pigmentary and exfoliative glaucoma. Laser trabeculoplasty may be used as a primary therapy of OAG.

Incisional Surgery

- Trabeculectomy
- Nonpenetrating drainage surgery (NPDS).

Drainage Implant (Seton/tube/shunt) Surgery

Usually used after repeated trabeculectomy have failed. , These devices consist of a tube which is placed in the anterior chamber to shunt aqueous towards the posterior conjunctiva. This area of the conjunctiva is less prone to scarring and can absorb the aqueous humor into the subconjunctival space. Types of implants include Molteno, Baerveldt, Ahmed, and Krupin. A new device currently available in the EU countries is the Gold Micro Shunt (GMS). A 24-karat gold implant that uses the eye's natural pressure differential (uveal scleral outflow) to reduce Intraocular Pressure (IOP) without a bleb. It is approximately 3 mm wide, 6 mm long; it is about the thickness of a human hair. The Gold Shunt is a flat plate designed for implantation through a single micro-incision. It contains numerous micro-tubular channels that bridge the anterior chamber and the suprachoroidal space, controlling aqueous outflow to reduce IOP. The shunt is virtually undetectable by the patient and is intended to last indefinitely. The SOLX® Gold Shunt works by increasing aqueous outflow and reducing IOP. Once inserted and positioned between the anterior chamber and suprachoroidal space, the SOLX® Gold Shunt creates a new fluid pathway by connecting these two spaces. Aqueous from the anterior chamber enters the ingress holes of the shunt (i) is directed through the internal micro-channels, (ii) exits the shunt into the suprachoroidal space and (iii) the eye's natural pressure gradient between the anterior chamber and the suprachoroidal space creates a constant flow of aqueous through the SOLX® Gold Shunt.

Ciliary Body Ablation

In order to diminish the production of aqueous humor, thus reducing the IOP the non-pigmented ciliary epithelium can be destroyed. This is usually done cyclocryotherapy, transscleral Nd:YAG or diode laser, or by an endoscopic laser device, under direct visualization.

Prognosis

Early diagnosis together with careful follow-up care and compliance with therapy, can ensure in most cases that the vast majority of patients with OAG retain useful vision throughout their lifetime.

5

Normal Tension Glaucoma

Ahmad K Khalil (Egypt)

INTRODUCTION

The young Albrecht von Graefe described in 1857 typical glaucomatous optic disc damage without elevated intraocular pressure. Few years later, facing a vigorous opposition to the concept, he abandoned his idea. By the middle of the 20th Century, the existence of "low tension glaucoma" had been firmly established. Many authors, however, considered it an uncommon entity, and referred to it as "pseudo-" and "so-called" low-tension glaucoma, with various explanations for the optic disc damage. Well into the beginning of 21st Century, normal tension glaucoma (NTG), remains to be a great source of controversy and challenge in its pathogenesis, clinical characteristics, and optimum management.

The criteria used to define NTG during the last 30 years have been highly variable. However, more recent publications generally require a maximum IOP of 21 mm Hg or lower associated with specific typical glaucomatous disc and field changes, an open angle in the absence of any contributing specific ocular or systemic disorders. The term "low-tension glaucoma" which has been commonly used in the past years, and is sometimes still used, is clearly a misnomer, as the IOP is usually within the *normal* range rather than being "*low*".

A different clinical course, and the proposition of mechanisms of damage different from those of glaucoma associated with intraocular pressures higher than statistically normal ranges led many authorities to distinguish NTG as a separate entity. Actually, with our current knowledge, it is possible that we are dealing with a collection of different disease entities. The extent to which it is a pressure-sensitive disease remains to be seen.

Recent scientific advances include elucidation of the genetic mechanism behind the disease and the study of hemodynamic and biochemical co-factors in the development of glaucomatous optic neuropathy, particularly in relation to the pathogenesis of NTG.

GENETIC PREDISPOSITION AND EPIDEMIOLOGY

Many population based studies that use optic disc and visual field changes have demonstrated that 30-70% of the patients with glaucomatous visual field loss have IOPs within normal limits. Traditionally, literature of a higher incidence of NTG among glaucoma cases comes from Japan. It is reported to

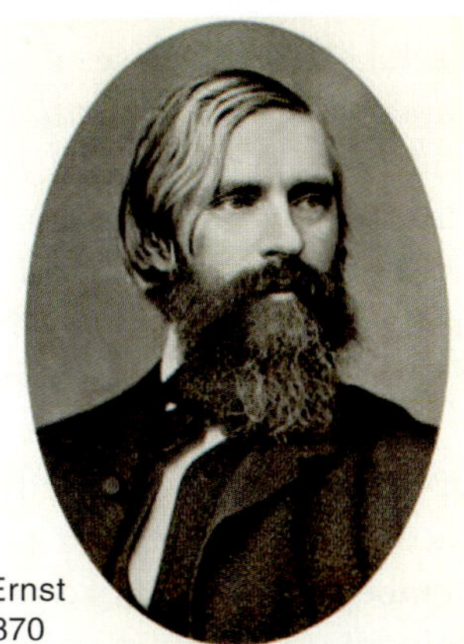

Fig. 1: Friedrich Wilhelm Ernst Albrecht von Graefe 1828-1870

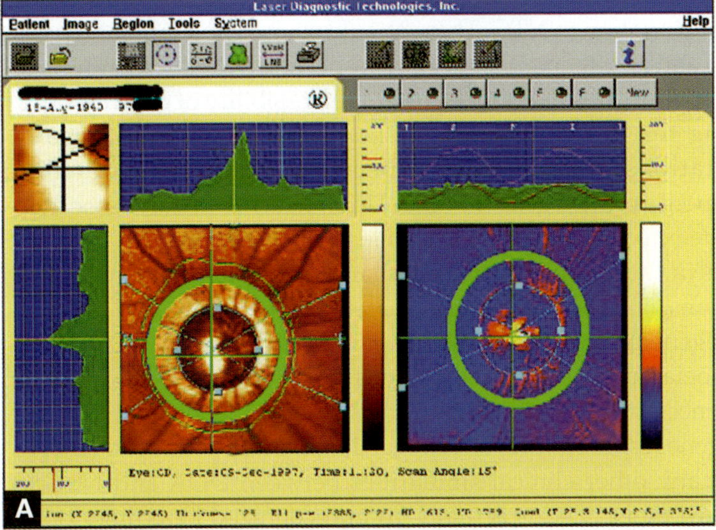

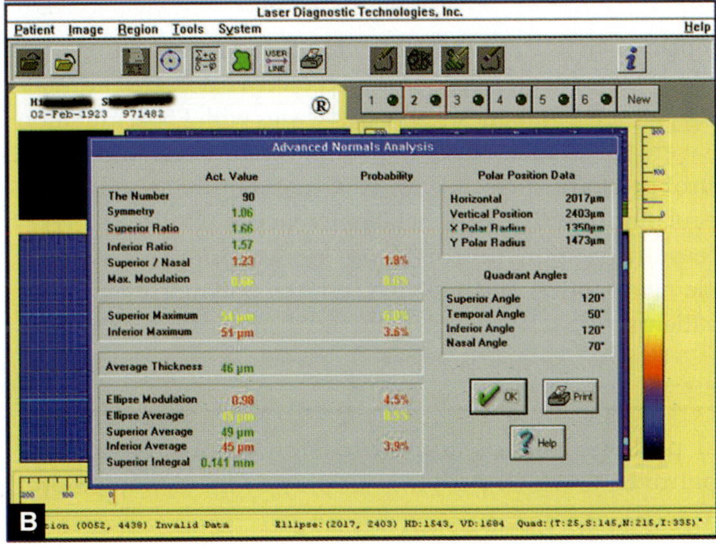

Figs 2A and B: Diffuse nerve fiber loss in a case of OAG seen by the NFA-GDx

constitute more than 60% of total glaucoma cases there. Shiose found 52 cases of high-tension glaucoma and 99 cases of normal-tension glaucoma in a population of 21,820 individuals in Japan, and in another collaborative glaucoma survey, 0.58%, of the examinees had primary open-angle glaucoma (POAG) and 2.04% had NTG. Reports in other populations vary greatly, but an incidence of 20-40% is currently accepted. Incidence in the West is much more than was previously thought. The disease appears to occur more often in women than men.

A genetic component appears to be a factor in the occurrence of NTG. A positive family history of glaucoma is often found in patients with NTG. Bennet et al detected NTG in eight members of a family of consecutive generations, and suggested an autosomal dominant trait for transmission.

In recent years more and more different gene mutations and polymorphisms are being detected in relation to NTG. These should soon supply practical basis for early detection and treatment of glaucoma in such individuals, to minimize visual loss, and hopefully in a near future offer the possibility of gene therapy.

Demonstrating the link between POAG and NTG, some potentially pathogenic mutations of **myocilin**/trabecular meshwork inducible glucocorticoid response protein gene (MYOC, TIGR) which is mainly associated with POAG were detected in NTG patients , while another study had no apparent specific mutations in the myocilin gene. **Similarly,** apolipoprotein E (Apo E) gene polymorphisms, which have been associated with cell death and survival in neurological degenerative diseases, were not linked to NTG.

NTG was associated with polymorphisms in the **OPA1 gene** without phenotypic differences in NTG patients with and without these polymorphisms. OPA1 gene is the gene responsible for autosomal dominant optic atrophy (DOA), and because of many other clinical similarities between DOA and NTG, a question arose of whether NTG is actually an unrecognized hereditary optic neuropathy.

The Glu50Lys **optineurin (OPTN)** sequence variation was associated with familial NTG. The Met98Lys change was associated with a fraction of normal-tension glaucoma in patients of Japanese ethnicity. Cases with E50K mutation in the OPTN gene were found to have NTG that appeared to be more severe than that in a control group of subjects with NTG without this mutation. A simultaneous upregulation of both matrix metalloproteinases MMP-9 and MT1-MMP gene expression (responsile for tissue remodeling involved in glaucomatous optic neuropathy) and EDNRA/C+70G polymorphism were detected in NTG patients

PATHOGENESIS

The etiology and pathogenesis of normal-tension glaucoma remains surrounded by controversy, which pertains not only to the definition and

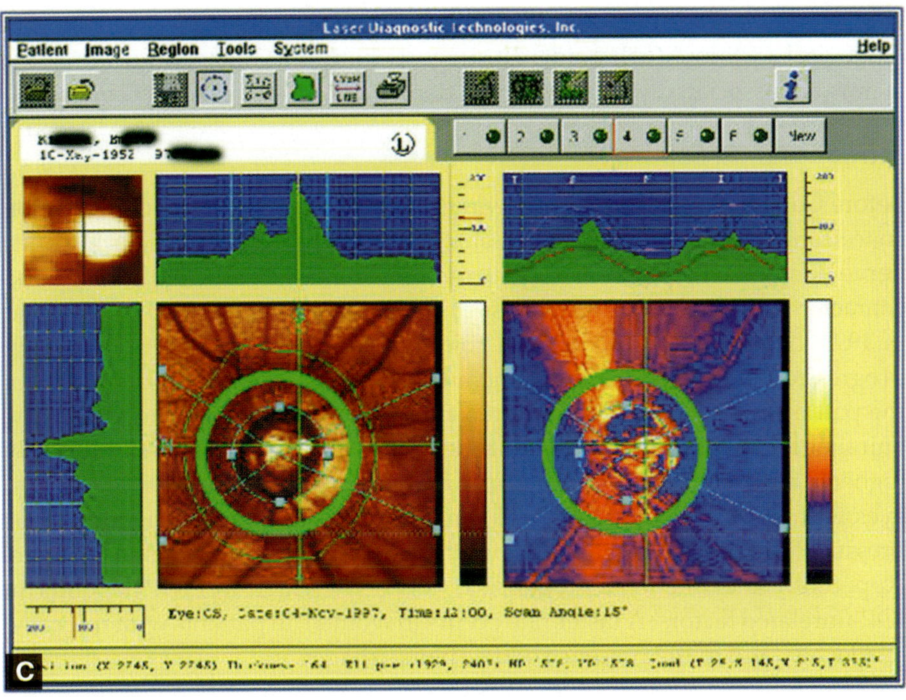

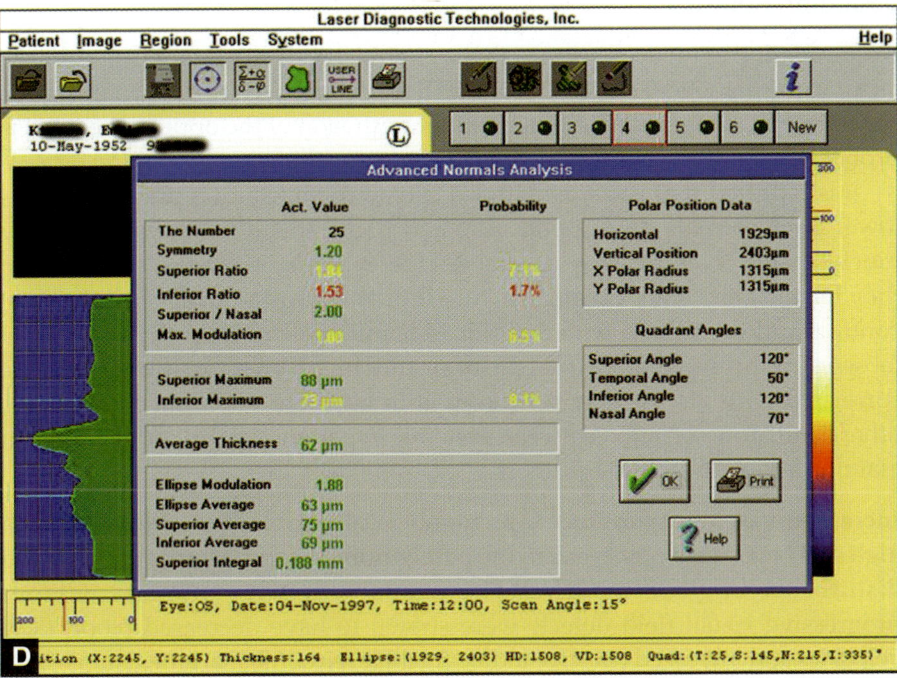

Figs 2 C and D: Localized nerve fiber loss occasionally seen in NTG cases. Readings in red show significant loss, yellow borderline, and green normal

characteristics of the entity itself, but to the possible roles played by different etiological factors. Much evidence suggests both IOP-related and unrelated factors are associated with visual field damage progression in NTG eyes.

Intraocular Pressure

Before **Collaborative NTG Study** was done, there was a difference of opinion concerning whether intraocular pressure (IOP) was involved in producing optic nerve damage when there was glaucomatous damage to the optic nerve and characteristic visual field loss in these cases. The results of this study, published in 1998, demonstrated a beneficial role for 30% IOP reduction in hindering progression of the disease, and concluded that intraocular pressure is part of the pathogenic process in normal-tension glaucoma. Even before this study, Shirai and co-workers showed that the rate of progression was significantly higher in eyes with a mean IOP equal to or higher than 15 mm Hg as opposed to eyes with pressures lower than 15 mm Hg. It is still not clear whether this pressure lowering effect may slow progression more in some cases than others. Apparently, the functional prognosis in NTG eyes with lower IOP depends on IOP-unrelated factors. A faster rate occurs in women, in patients with migraine headaches, and in the presence of disc hemorrhages.

Vascular Factors

Accumulating evidence suggests that a circulatory defect might be a primary factor in the pathogenesis of NTG. Blood flow deficits accompany, and perhaps contribute to, disease development. Hypoperfusion of the optic nerve head is probably a significant factor relating to glaucoma damage.

It is reported that patients with NTG tend to have blood pressure values lower than normals during both day and night; this difference is probably much smaller than formerly assumed. However, many studies showed that they have significantly greater nocturnal blood pressure drops than normal controls and even those with anterior ischemic optic neuropathy. Abnormal (absence or increased) nocturnal dip of systolic blood pressure was found to be correlated with disease progression in both high and NTG patients. On the other hand, no association between systemic hypertension and normal-tension glaucoma could be found by others.

Increased vascular resistance was found in all retrobulbar arteries in both high and NTG. This points out to the pathognomonic importance of perfusion disturbance in glaucoma. Eyes of patients with NTG with and without progressive visual field defects were shown to have decreased blood flow velocities and increased resistive indices in their retrobulbar arteries, suggesting that differences in ocular blood perfusion are relevant to the development of NTG and are detectable from the early stages of the disease. Furthermore, the finding of lower pulsatile ocular blood flow in NTG eyes with field loss than in the contralateral eyes with normal field suggests that hemodynamic differences between fellow eyes contribute to determine the side of onset of the disease. But may be less involved in the deterioration in glaucomatous patients with increased intraocular pressure.

The circulatory dynamics of the ophthalmic artery were different in glaucoma patients as compared to normal subjects, and the vascular resistance of the ophthalmic artery may be associated with the development of visual field defects in NTG patients. However, the prevalence of hemodynamically significant carotid stenosis, peripapillary blood flow, and serologic abnormalities were found similar in patients with normal-tension and primary open-angle glaucoma, and did not correlate with glaucoma severity. Reduced blood-flow velocities of the extraocular vessels in patients with high tension and normal tension primary glaucoma may be secondary as well as contributory to glaucomatous damage.

It was suggested that **Vasospasm** and generalized cardiovascular disease both appear to be specific risk factors for the development of particular subgroups of glaucoma and may be independent of absolute intraocular pressure levels exerting effects in patients with both "normal" or "raised" intraocular pressure. The simple assessment as to whether a glaucoma patient suffers from colder extremities than average might point to a focal ischemic type of glaucoma.

Patients with NTG were showed to have prolonged arteriovenous retinal passage time, which could cause chronic hypoxia. They also showed reduced blood flow in the peripapillary retina, a result suggesting that blood flow deficits accompany, and perhaps may contribute to, disease development in these patients. While optic nerve head ischemia induced by repeated intravitreal injection of endothelin-1 in pigmented rabbits could contribute to the enlargement and excavation of the disk cup independent of the intraocular pressure level. Decreased erythrocyte deformability was not found to be a major factor in the etiopathogenesis of either normal or HTG (HTG).

A significant decrease of **erythrocyte deformability** and increase in aggregability was found in NTG patients. These alterations seem to be inversely related to the intracytosolic calcium levels and they were not found in POAG patients and controls. Those results may suggest a possible role played by red blood cells.

Ogata found **optic nerve compression** by the internal carotid artery (ICA) in patients with NTG was 49.5%, which was significantly higher than that in control group with 34.6%, suggesting that compression of the optic nerve by ICA may be a possible causative factor or a risk factor for optic nerve damage in some patients with NTG.

Other Factors

In a study by Jamsen, six out of 25 NTG patients (24%) had thyroid disease. In the thyroid group, the mean diurnal IOP variations were significantly smaller. He suggested that thyroid disease either causes optic neuropathy mimicking glaucomatous damage or is a risk factor for glaucoma. NTG was also associated with hypothyroidism as a causative factor. The finding of higher C reactive protein (CRP) levels in NTG patients adds a vascular inflammatory process to be a possible etiological factor of this glaucoma. A higher association with one or more immune-related disease(s) as compared with ocular hypertension was found in NTG patients. Lastly, positivity for immunoproteins such as anti-Ro/SS-A and heat shock protein antibodies in patients with NTG indicate a possible involvement of an autoimmune mechanism and signify a finding associated with the glaucomatous optic neuropathy process in some patients which appears to be unrelated to intraocular pressure levels.

WORK-UP AND CLINICAL PRESENTATION

NTG is a disease often accidentally discovered by the ophthalmologist detecting a suspicious glaucomatous appearance of the optic disc, with subsequent detection of glaucomatous field changes. Less commonly, patients may present with visual disturbances resulting from extensive visual field loss. Because of the subtle onset of damage, and good central visual acuity, the disease is frequently missed. Routine careful examination of the optic disc, therefore, even when glaucoma is not suspected is invaluable for earlier detection of NTG.

Proper assessment of patients includes optic nerve head and retinal nerve-fiber layer assessment, standard static computerized visual field testing, gonioscopy, and a diurnal (24-hour) intraocular pressure evaluation. A careful history is of utmost importance. This should exclude previous phases of increased intraocular pressure, verification of present and past medication use, exposure to toxins, corticosteroid use either topically or systemically. Patient should be asked about a history of hemodynamic crisis, including blood loss, anemia, arrhythmias, and hypotensive episodes. An internal medicine check-up including 24-hour ambulatory blood pressure measurements and neurological assessment are required. Additionally, carotid artery Doppler sonography, and a computed tomography scan of the brain might prove helpful in relevant cases.

Neuroimaging

Routine head computed tomography or magnetic resonance imaging head scans are not routinely recommended. Although intracranial tumors are on the differential, it is unlikely for them to solely produce a visual field defect with absence of symptoms or other neurological signs. In a retrospective study comprising 29 patients with NTG and 28 control patients with compressive, none of the patients diagnosed with glaucoma had neuroradiologic evidence of a mass lesion involving the anterior visual pathway. Younger age, lower levels of visual acuity, vertically aligned visual field defects and neuroretinal rim pallor were recognized as predictors of the likelihood of identifying an intracranial mass lesion.

A neurological workup should probably be reserved to patients with unexplained reduction of visual acuity, color vision loss without advanced visual field loss, visual field loss out of proportion to optic nerve damage or atypical for glaucoma, including those respecting the vertical meridian, optic disc pallor more than cupping, presence of neurological symptoms or when the course is rapidly progressive despite apparently adequate treatment.

IOP

In most cases, the IOP is at or near the upper end of normal pressure range, i.e. upper teens rather than lower teens. Some studies have found that the IOP in NTG eyes does not differ significantly from that in the normal population, while others indicate that NTG patients tend to have slightly higher IOPs. Intraocular pressure might increase in NTG eyes following the initial diagnosis. A higher maximum IOP during initial 24-hour pressure curve and the development of disc hemorrhage during follow-up was significantly associated with subsequent IOP elevation in NTG patients.

Other Glaucoma Parameters

As will be seen in the following paragraphs, great controversy arose as regards the appearance of optic disc and form of cupping, pattern of field changes, peripapillary atrophy in NTG, and weather it is similar to or different from that of HTG eyes. These varying opinions probably reflect the different ways in which the 2 entities are detected. Most cases of HTG are detected because of an elevated IOP, while most cases of NTG are detected because of optic disc cupping. As it is easier to detect a suspicious IOP than a suspicious optic disc, most cases of NTG are diagnosed at a later stage of the disease process.

Optic Disc Cupping

The appearance of optic disc and form of cupping in NTG eyes, and whether it is similar to or different from that of HTG eyes had led to great controversy. Duke-Elder did not recognize any difference in the appearance of optic disc between the 2 groups. In a study by Tezel et al on 394 eyes of 197 patients with HTG, and 135 eyes of 68 patients with NTG, the final clinical appearance of optic nerve damage was similar among patients of the 2 groups, and the subgroups of NTG, regardless of their possibly different mechanisms of neuropathy. Similarly, no differences were apparent between high and NTG in morphometric parameters of optic nerve head as measured by scanning laser ophthalmoscopy. Although some other authors agreed on this similarity, they noted that disproportion between the amount of cupping and the amount of visual field loss is more common in NTG, with larger cup-disc ratios for the same amount of visual loss as compared with HTG.

On the other hand, others found larger and steeper cups in HTG patients, and paler, more sloping cups in NTG eyes. Furthermore, Caprioli and Spaeth found that the optic disc rim in NTG eyes was significantly thinner than in high-tension eyes; the largest difference occurred inferiorly and inferotemporally.

In one study reviewing the subtypes of NTG, one hundred thirty stereo photographs of optic discs were reviewed in order to identify characteristics of the three following types: focal ischemic, senile sclerotic, and generalized cup enlargement. Twenty patients in each group were selected. Focal ischemic patients were more frequently women, had a higher incidence of migraine, a relatively smaller disc size, and localized superior scotoma that often threatened fixation. Senile sclerotic patients were generally elderly, had a higher incidence of surgery under general anesthesia, more ischemic heart disease or systemic hypertension, a small rim area, and also had extensive peripapillary atrophy as well as combined diffuse and localized visual field defects. Generalized cup enlargement patients were younger, had a relatively larger disc size and a greater incidence of purely diffuse visual field loss. They suggested that the different characteristics of the groups were related to the pathogenic mechanisms specific to each group.

Visual Field

A large body of evidence suggests that NTG is different from high tension primary open-angle glaucoma not only in IOP but also in the pattern of the visual field defect, cupping and peripapillary atrophy of the optic nerve head. Many studies noted a difference in the pattern of visual field defects between the two groups. Visual field defects in NTG are noted by many as being relatively more localized and closer to fixation, especially in the superonasal quadrant and may be more predominant in the lower hemifield. Another study found that the mean eccentricity of scotomas in NTG was 4.86 degrees from fixation; and 2.96 degrees in HTG eyes. These differences were statistically significant. Koseki et al detected superonasal sectorial damage in normal and not in HTG. Another study demonstrated that the upper arcuate area was significantly more depressed in HTG and the inferior Bjerrum's area was significantly more depressed in NTG eyes. It was also shown that the lower papillomacular area was less affected in normal tension than in HTG eyes. A diffuse-type papillomacular bundle defect was also associated with NTG.

Some earlier studies pointed out that field defects in NTG tend to be deeper with steeper slopes at the edges of the defects. While no statistically significant differences were found between the slopes of the scotomas or depths of the scotomas in the two groups in other studies.

Retinal Nerve Fiber Layer (RNFL)

Early changes in the retinal nerve fiber layer may already exist even in the unaffected area of the visual field in eyes with NTG with hemifield dominant visual field defects. Similar to field changes, much controversy existed as to the damage caused to the RNFL in NTG and HTG. Some studies showed that the pattern of RNFL change is different in patients with high- and low-tension glaucoma. Using scanning laser polarimetry, the thickness of the RNFL was found to be reduced symmetrically in the superior and inferior quadrants in HTG, whereas a more localized defect on the inferior RNFL occurs in NTG. On the other hand, others denied a significant difference in the frequency of localized RNFL defects between patients with NTG and those with HTG.

Disc Hemorrhages

Over the past three decades, hemorrhages on the optic disc have been recognized as a common and significant sign of glaucomatous damage. Several studies confirmed a high prevalence of optic disc hemorrhages in NTG. They are occasionally found on the border or adjacent to the border between the retinal nerve fiber layer defect and the apparently healthy- looking retinal nerve fiber layer and associated closely with the size of peripapillary atrophy. The finding of disc hemorrhages should alert physicians that a patient might have uncontrolled glaucoma. Alternatively. They might be seen in healthy subjects, diabetic retinopathy, ischemic optic neuropathy, papillitis, central retinal vein occlusion, and posterior vitreous detachment.

Kitazawa et al. suggested that NTG eyes seem to consist of two different groups; one which develops recurrent disc hemorrhages and one which is very unlikely to bleed through its entire course. The first group probably belongs to the ischemic etiology group as some investigators believe that disc hemorrhages in glaucoma are evidence that ischemia plays a role in causing glaucomatous optic nerve damage. Their presence is a significantly negative prognostic factor in patients with NTG and may be a sign of progressive damage of the retinal nerve fiber layer, leading to functional deterioration of the visual field. Not only that, but there was a significant relationship between the location of the disk hemorrhage and the area of the progression of visual field loss in 65.4% of progressive patients with disk hemorrhage

Peripapillary atrophy was significantly associated with functional and structural optic nerve damage in NTG. The area, angular extent and location of zone beta correlated significantly with increasing visual field defects, especially localized defects, optic nerve head topography, and the location of visual field defects. However, neither zones alpha or beta differed significantly between normal and HTG in either frequency or size. Similar findings were also made by Tezel et al. Funaki, on the other hand, found that the areas of parapapillary avascular area and zone beta in NTG were significantly larger than those in HTG.

Optic Disc Size

Several studies, in recent years, showed a significantly larger optic discs in NTG as compared to HTG, and suggested that an eye with a large optic disc may be more vulnerable to glaucomatous visual field damage at statistically normal IOP readings.

CCT

It was suggested that many eyes diagnosed as having NTG have thin corneas, which would tend to lower the tonometrically recorded intraocular pressure compared with patients with primary open-angle glaucoma and normal subjects. This may lead to underestimation of intraocular pressure and misdiagnosis in some of these patients. Another study, however, concluded that for most normal-tension glaucoma patients corneal thickness is not a major factor in accounting for the lower intraocular pressure measurements when compared with primary open angle glaucoma patients.

Central corneal thickness in NTG was significantly lower than in POAG and corneas were thinner in NTG patients with vascular risk factors than in those without. Studies examining individual Asian subpopulations in isolation suggest that differences in CCT may exist among different populations, which might play a role in the racial differences of NTG. CCT does, in fact, vary among Asian subpopulations; Japanese have thinner corneas than Chinese and Filipinos. Caucasians, Chinese, Hispanics, and Filipinos have comparable CCT measurements, whereas the corneas of African Americans are significantly thinner. Central corneal thickness shows no significant difference among NTG, POAG, and normal subjects in Japan, while it is significantly greater in OH subjects. The CCT has little influence on the diagnosis of NTG in Japan.

Systemic Associations

Several systemic associations are noted in relation to normal-tension glaucoma. Patients are said to have more frequent silent myocardial ischemia. The capillary blood-cell velocity in the fingertips was found to be reduced significantly compared with control subjects. Some patients also show evident psychosomatic involvement. Women patients with collagen diseases are highly susceptible to NTG and POAG

Differential Diagnosis with Masked HTG

Early-morning IOP spikes are one of the important pathogenetic factors in patients with glaucomatous changes without other pathology. Early morning IOP measurement in supine position before rising should therefore be a mandatory part of diurnal IOP curves in patients with presumed NTG. Low scleral rigidity and thin corneas might be misleading in evaluating the IOP. Another possible confusion is damage caused by previous HTG, with subsequent lowering of IOP due to hyposecretion of aqueous in a diseased eye.

MANAGEMENT

The purpose of a clinical evaluation is to define the most important damaging factors for the individual patient. Accordingly, the therapy is directed towards the possible factors involved. Practically, this can mean: additional lowering of the intraocular pressure, increasing the blood pressure, lowering the blood viscosity and treating the vasospasms. The feasibility of lowering an already low IOP had often been questioned. The literature is full of controversy about optimum treatment protocol for NTG. Achieving sufficient IOP reduction requires topical medication, laser trabeculoplasty, or fistulizing surgery. All of these carry potential risks. As many patients show no progression when untreated, those patients destined to be non-progressive or only slowly progressive would derive no benefit from treatment. Indeed, they would have been exposed to its risks.

The favorable effect of intraocular pressure reduction on progression of visual change in normal-tension glaucoma was found when the impact of cataracts on visual field progression, produced largely by surgery, was removed. Lowering intraocular pressure without producing cataracts is optimal. Because not all untreated patients progressed, the natural history of normal- tension glaucoma must be considered before embarking on intraocular pressure reduction with therapy apt to exacerbate cataract formation unless normal-tension glaucoma threatens serious visual loss.

Medical Treatment

Beta-blockers

Many of the frequently used ocular hypotensive agents such as beta-blockers and miotics can not produce marked reductions in the IOP which is already in the teens level. A reduction of only 12% was reported in one study. In an alarming study, beta-blocker eye drops were even found to aggravate nocturnal arterial hypotension and reduce the night-time heart rate significantly. In normal-tension glaucoma, eyes receiving beta-blocker eye drops showed visual field progression significantly more often than those not receiving beta-blockers. It is also suggested that based on their mechanism of action, the beta-blockers cannot be assumed to reduce IOP during sleep.

A more beneficial effect was demonstrated with the use of **selective beta-adrenergic blockade (BETAXOLOL)**, which were shown to reduce diurnal pressure peaks, a risk factor concerning the maintenance of visual field. It also may have ocular vasorelaxant effects independent of any influence on intraocular pressure, whereas nonselective blockade (timolol) lowers intraocular pressure without apparently altering orbital hemodynamics. Similarly, carteolol hydrochloride was effective in inhibiting deterioration of the local visual field in eyes with NTG. This was attributed to increased ocular perfusion due to diminished intraocular pressure, as well as an inhibitory effect upon vasoconstriction in the optic nerve head due to intrinsic sympathomimetic activity, preventing decrease in papillary blood flow and adverse effects upon ocular circulation.

In recent years, newer agents such as the prostaglandin F2 alpha analogue, **LATANOPROST**, has been shown to reduce IOP in normal subjects and ocular hypertensive glaucoma patients by increasing uveoscleral outflow. The magnitude of this IOP reduction was found to be essentially identical during the day and at night. This mechanism should be particularly effective in the lower IOP range that is typical of NTG. Once-daily treatment with 0.005-0.006% latanoprost provides a significant and stable IOP reduction in the majority of patients after short-term treatment. This is accompanied by a significant increase in pulsatile ocular blood flow, and it is well tolerated. It appears to affect ocular perfusion pressure more favorably than timolol does in patients with NTG. Latanoprost was found also to increase the mean POBF in relation to its IOP lowering effect, while the increase in POBF noted after brimonidine was within the range of long term variation and may not be attributable to the drug effect.

These data should not go for granted on other prostaglandins-prostamides. It was found that **bimatoprost** does not influence blood flow velocities in the retrobulbar vessels. The in vitro observation of increased vascular tone in the presence of bimatoprost seems not to be relevant for ocular hemodynamics, but it could lower the IOP in NTG cases. To date, no controlled studies were made on the effect of travoprost on NTG.

DORZOLAMIDE, a topical carbonic anhydrase inhibitor (CAI), significantly reduced IOP at two and four weeks, and at the same time increased contrast sensitivity at both three and six cycles per degree. Dorzolamide also accelerated retinal arteriovenous passage time more than latanoprost. This ability to improve contrast sensitivity in persons with NTG was related to either IOP reduction or altered ocular perfusion. Though combined dorzolamide-timolol produced a favorable IOP lowering and retinal blood passage, it is probably better avoided for the effects of timolol explained earlier in this section. On the other hand, **Brinzolamide,** another topical CAI was found not to have any impact on ocular hemodynamics.

In a 30 days short term study, 0.2% **BRIMONIDINE** eye drops induced a significant 30% or more IOP decrease in eyes with NTG. However, a paradoxical effect was observed in a 70-year-old woman with bilateral NTG in whom the use of brimonidine was observed to cause IOP elevation, confirmed on rechallenge. This finding necessitates vigilance in follow-up of patients on topical brimonidine. Its high allergenicity which may increase the likelihood of allergy to subsequently used preparations can defer it as a first drug of choice in NTG.

Emerging evidence suggests that treatments designed to improve ocular blood flow may benefit glaucoma patients. **Ca^{2+} CHANNEL BLOCKADE** improves contrast sensitivity in patients with NTG and slows the progression of visual field loss. Patients show increased retrobulbar vessel flow velocities, a result supporting that visual function loss may be linked to ocular ischemia. Nilvadipine, a Ca^{2+} antagonist was found to increase blood velocity and, probably, blood flow in the optic nerve head, choroid, and retina of rabbits. It also increased blood velocity in the optic nerve head of NTG patients, and reduced vascular resistance in distal retrobulbar arteries in normal-tension glaucoma without affecting more proximal blood vessels. It also increased Ocular pulse amplitude in vasospastic type NTG patients.

Similarly, a beneficial effect has been detected for oral brovincamine, a relatively selective cerebral vasodilator in retarding further visual field deterioration in patients with NTG who have low-normal IOP, while nimodipine was found to increase ONH and choroidal blood flow in NTG patients and improves the color contrast sensitivity of these patients.

Surgical Treatment

With the current medications, marked pressure reduction can be achieved and maintained on a long-term basis by means other than fistulizing surgery in a large proportion of patients with NTG, however, surgical lowering of IOP results in a slower rate of visual field loss in the operated eye, and is worth further consideration as a potent treatment for the disease in cases with progressively deteriorating visual fields. The most effective procedure to achieve IOPs of 1 digit is probably a trabeculectomy, which can be augmented by adjunctive mitomycin C. Argon laser trabeculoplasty had neither tonometric effect nor did it affect the slope of visual field damage in NTG cases. In another study, however, when added to medications, it resulted in a further 1 mm Hg IOP drop

When embarking on treating NTG, the first choice of treatment would be using drugs for reducing IOP. In addition to these treatments a drug for increasing the blood circulation in the brain, can be beneficial in the treatment. Patients whose visual fields are shown by static perimetry to be deteriorating are indicated for filtering surgery.

6

Pigment Dispersion Syndrome and Pigmentary Glaucoma

Ashok Garg (India)

INTRODUCTION

It is secondary form of open-angle glaucoma produced by the pigment dispersion in the anterior segment of the eye. This rare condition is characterised by dispersion of pigment throughout the anterior segment typically affecting young myopic males. A strong association exists between pigmentary glaucoma and myopia. A typical patient is young myopic male in his 20s or 30s. There have been few reports of familial pigmentary glaucoma, most cases appears to be sporadic. A herediatary basis has been reported. Sugar and Barbour in 1940 reported the details of this entity which differed from other forms of pigment dispersion conditions by typical clinical and histopathological features. They referred to this condition as pigmentary glaucoma, the term pigment dispersion syndrome has been advocated.

CLINICAL SIGNS AND SYMPTOMS

Several characteristic features are helpful in making the correct diagnosis.

Iris Changes

In pigmentary glaucoma there is primary loss of pigment from the posterior surface (neuropithelium) from the midperipheral iris. The pigment granules are frequently dispersed on the stroma of the iris which may give the iris a progressively darker appearance or create heterochromia in asymmetric case.

The loss of pigment epithelium from the midperipheral iris gives rise to a series of radial spoke like (wedge-shaped) midperipheral transillumination defects. These defects can range in number from 1-2 to 65-70 and can be thin slit or coalescent areas. These defects can be seen on slit-lamp biomicroscopy by shining a small slit beam through the pupil with the light perpendicular to the plane of the iris.

A few advanced cases with severe iris atrophy may even show a mild heterochromic iridis. These pigment particles released from the pigment epithelium of iris are carried by aqueous humor convection currents and then deposited on a variety of ocular issues in the anterior segment of the eye including the corneal endothelium, trabecular meshwork, anterior iris surface, zonules and lens.

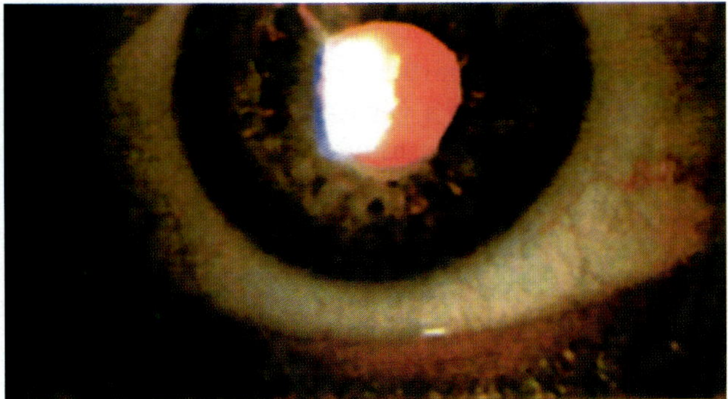

Fig. 1: Iris transillumination in pigment dispersion syndrome

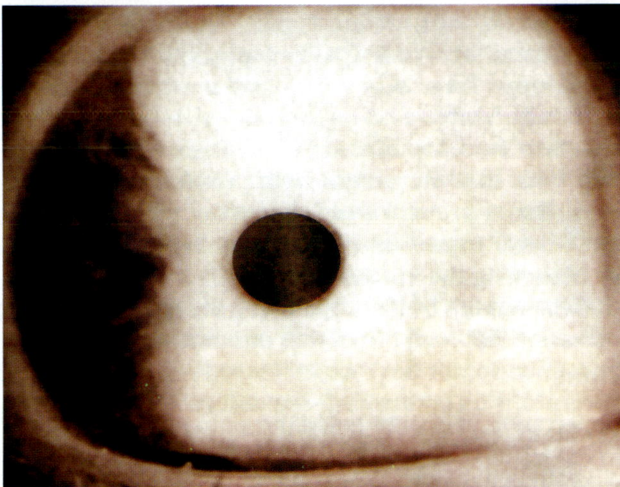

Fig. 2: Pigment deposit on corneal endothelium known as Krukenberg's spindle

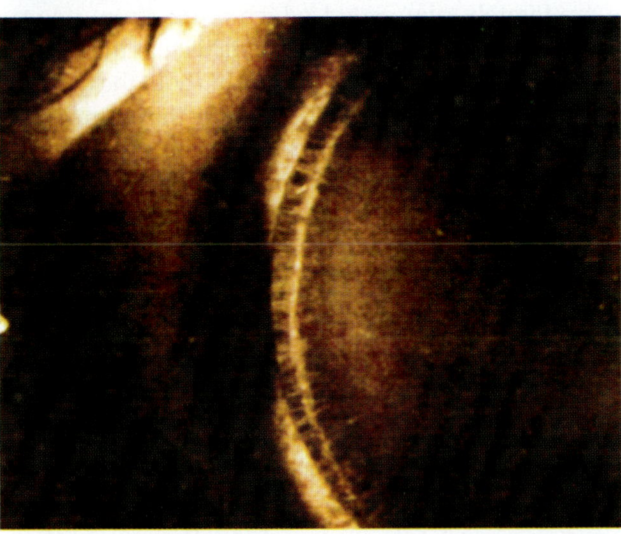

Fig. 3: Pigment deposit on zonules

Corneal Changes

There is deposition of pigment particles on the posterior surface of the central cornea (corneal endothelium) in a vertical spindle-shaped pattern known as Krukenberg's spindle. Dispersed pigment is deposited on the cornea in this pattern due to aqueous convection currents and is then phagocytosed by adjacent endothelial cells. The size and density of pigment deposition is usually proportional to the extent of associated iris atrophy. In some cases pigment is distributed more diffusely. This Krukenberg's spindle is a very useful sign of pigmentary glaucoma but not pathognomic of the disease nor it is invariably present. The spindle consists of extracellular as well as intracellular pigment granules phagocytosed by corneal endothelium.

Anterior Chamber Changes

Anterior chamber is excessively deep specially in the midperiphery where the iris tends to bow posteriorly. In fact patients of pigmentary glaucoma have a very deep anterior chamber, a concave appearance of the peripheral iris and mild iridodonesis.

Lens Changes

Pigment deposition on both lens surface and on the zonules. On posterior lens surface pigment deposition leads to Zentmayer's ring or Scheie's line.

Angle Changes

Angle is wide open and hyper pigmented through out due to pigment deposition on and within the trabeculum.

Goniscopic findings are highly typical but not absolute pathognomonic of pigmentary glaucoma. In early cases of pigmentary glaucoma the trabecular meshwork is moderately pigmented which varies from one portion of the meshwork to another. In advanced cases the trabecular meshwork appears as a dark brown, velvet band that extends uniformly about the full circumference of the trabecular meshwork. The pigment can cover the entire width of the angle from the ciliary face to the peripheral cornea creating a thin dark band that is known as Sampoelesi's line anterior to Schwalbe's line.

Pigment Deposition

In rare situations the extreme retinal periphery shows pigment deposition.

Glaucoma

About 10 percent of patients with the pigment dispersion syndrome eventually develop elevated intraocular pressure (IOP) the condition is termed pigmentary glaucoma. It is therefore very important to check the IOP in all patients with the signs suggestive of pigment dispersion. The rise in IOP in caused by pigmentary obstruction and damage to the trabeculum. Patients with asymmetrical

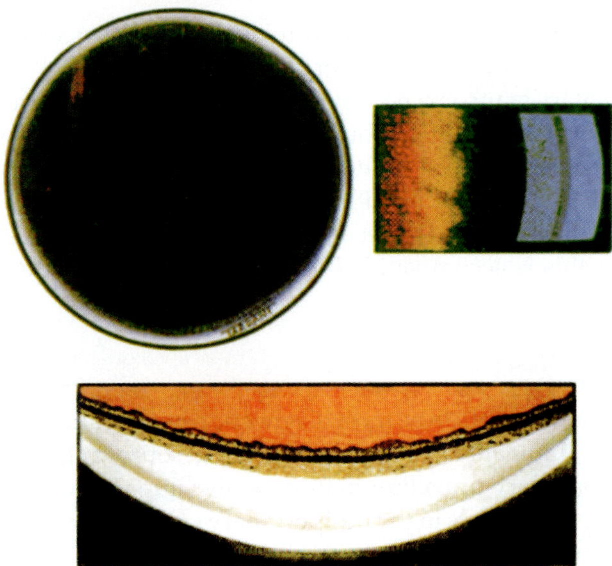

Fig. 4: Pigment dispersion syndrome
upper left: Krukenberg spindle
upper right: Iris atrophy
below: Hyperpigmentation of angle

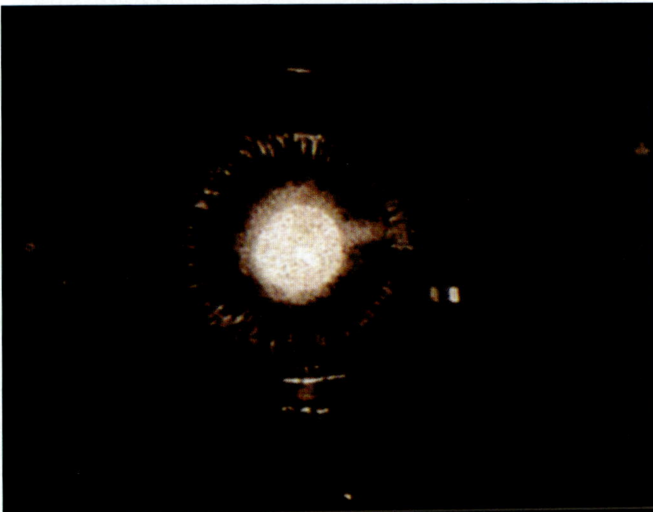

Fig. 5: Iris transillumination in pigmentary glaucoma

pigmentary glaucoma have more severe glaucoma in the eye with greater pigment dispersion. Many patients have progressive optic nerve damage and visual field loss. Pigmentary glaucoma usually resembles primary open-angle glaucoma (POAG) in most aspects including elevated IOP, decreased outflow facility, optic nerve cupping and visual field loss. Large diurnal variations of IOP are thought to occur more often in the pigmentary glaucoma and can be enough to cause corneal edema, blurring and halo vision. Patients with pigmentary glaucoma can have sudden release of pigment with severe IOP elevation after papillary dilation or exercise.

Once pigmentary glaucoma becomes established it may be somewhat more difficult to control than POAG although with increasing age there is tendency for the condition to become less severe.

Several studies have shown that pigment dispersion lessens with time so that Krukenberg's spindles and trabecular pigmentation becomes less prominent. In certain cases this is accompanied by an improvement in aqueous humor dynamics.

OCULAR EXAMINATION

Iris trasillumination appears to be most diagnostic clinical feature of pigmentary glaucoma. Transillumination using a fiberoptic light source applied to the lower lid or sclera or papillary transillumination on the slit-lamp will demonstrate typical linear slit-like defects in the midperiphery of the iris which is the key to diagnosis. In some patients with a markedly constricted pupil, it may prevent an adequate retinal reflex in which case sclera transillumination may be better technique for observing the iris defects.

Recent clinical works using the lymphocyte transformation test has shown that patients with pigmentary glaucoma do not have an increased sensitivity to corticosteroid thus confirming the secondary nature of this condition.

PATHOGENESIS OF PIGMENT DISPERSION SYNDROME AND PIGMENTARY GLAUCOMA

Mechanism of Pigment Dispersion

Ultrastructural and histopathological evaluation of the iris in eyes with the pigment dispersion syndrome or pigmentary glaucoma have shown changes in the iris pigment epithelium which include focal atrophy and hypopigmentation with an apparent delay in melanogenesis and hyperplasia of the dilator muscle. In comparison, eyes with POAG has minimal hypopigmentation of the iris epithelium and normal dilator muscle and melanogenesis. These observations lead to infer that a developmental abnormality of the iris pigment epithelium is the fundamental defect in the pigment dispersion syndrome.

Mechanisms of Intraocular Pressure Rise

- Studies have shown that pigment granules perfused in human autopsy eyes caused a significant obstruction to aqueous outflow. Subsequent histopathological studies of eyes with pigmentary glaucoma revealed excessive amount of pigment granules and cell debris in the trabecular meshwork (clogging) associated with variable degrees of trabecular endothelial cell degeneration. It is generally believed that pigment dispersion into the trabecular meshwork leads to elevation of IOP in pigmentary glaucoma.

- Another theory suggests that a primary developmental anomaly of the anterior chamber angle may lead to aqueous outflow obstruction.

INVESTIGATIONS

- Slit lamp examination
- Direct ophthalmoscopy
- Tonometry
- Gonioscopy
- Perimetry

DIFFERENTIAL DIAGNOSIS

The differential diagnosis of pigmentary glaucoma includes any condition that produces pigmentation of the trabecular meshwork. This includes nomal eyes with aging, POAG, uveitis, cyst of iris and ciliary body, pigmented intraocular tumor, previous surgery, laser surgery, trauma, angle-closure glaucoma, amyloidosis, diabetes mellitus, megalocornea, siderosis, exfoliation syndrome, ocular melanosis and melanoma. These conditions should be readily differentiated from pigmentary glaucoma by the history and physical examination. The condition most likely to confuse with pigmentary glaucoma is exfoliation syndrome. The iridial atrophy in exfoliation syndrome is more central and geographic and pigment accumulation in the trabecular meshwork consists of large particles that are unevenly distributed about the angle.

TREATMENT

Pigmentary glaucoma is managed basically the same of POAG. However, there may be an increased incidence of retinal detachment among pigmentary glaucoma patients and caution with miotics is recommended.

In pigmentary glaucoma management usual progression is from medical therapy to argon laser trebeculoplasty to filtering surgery. Beta-adrenergic antagonists like epinephrine, dipivefrin and carbonic anhydrase inhibitors are useful in the management of pigmentary glaucoma. Miotic agents reduce IOP in pigmentary glaucoma and are theoretically more useful because they increase pupillary block and lift the peripheral iris from the zonules. However, cholinergic drugs are generally poorly tolerated by the young patients.

If medical management does not control IOP, argon laser trabeculoplasty should be performed. Because of heavy pigmentation of the angle, argon laser trabeculoplasty is done with relatively low energy settings in the range of 200-600 mW.

Many patients with pigmentary glaucoma eventually require filtering surgery. Despite the young age of the patient, the results of surgery are generally successful.

7

Pseudoexfoliation Syndrome

Ashok Garg (India)

INTRODUCTION

Crystalline lens disorders are associated with several forms of glaucoma. Pseudoexfoliation syndrome (PXS) is one of the such type where causes and effect association between lens abnormality and the glaucoma is present. In fact this condition is characterized by the deposition of an amorphous gray white flake (dandruff) – like basement membrane material akin to amyloid on the papillary border, anterior lens surface, posterior surface of iris, zonules and the ciliary processes.

Pseudoexfoliation syndrome (PXS) is not associated with any known systemic disorder. The PXS and its associated glaucoma are also known by a variety of other names which include exfoliation syndrome, senile exfoliation, glaucoma capsular, senile uveal exfoliation, iridociliary exfoliation and fibrillopathia epitheliocapsularis.

Exfoliation glaucoma was first described by Lindberg in 1917 and two types of explanation have been described.

CAPSULAR DELAMINATION (TRUE EXFOLIATION)

In this condition, superificial layers of lens capsules delaminate from the deeper layers to develop scroll-like margins and sometimes float in the anterior chamber as thin clear membranes. Dvork-Theobald advocated this condition be called true exfoliation of the lens capsule to distinguish it from pseudoexfoliation. An underlying cause is usually present for capsular delamination such as exposure to intense heat as commonly seen in the glass blowers, inflammation, trauma or irradiational injury. Glaucoma in such condition is not a common feature.

EXFOLIATION SYNDROME

Vogt in 1925 described a senile form of capsular delamination which also known as senile exfoliation. This condition differs from other forms of lens capsule exfoliation in clinical picture as well as more frequent association with glaucoma (glaucoma capsulare). Devok-Theobald advocated that this condition is not a true exfoliation of lens capsule but rather precipitates of an unknown substance in the anterior ocular segment. So, this conditions is known as pseudoexfoliation of lens capsule to distinguish this condition from capsular delamination or true exfoliation. Recent ultrastructural studies have shown that exfoliative material is derived at least in part from lens capsule and it has been

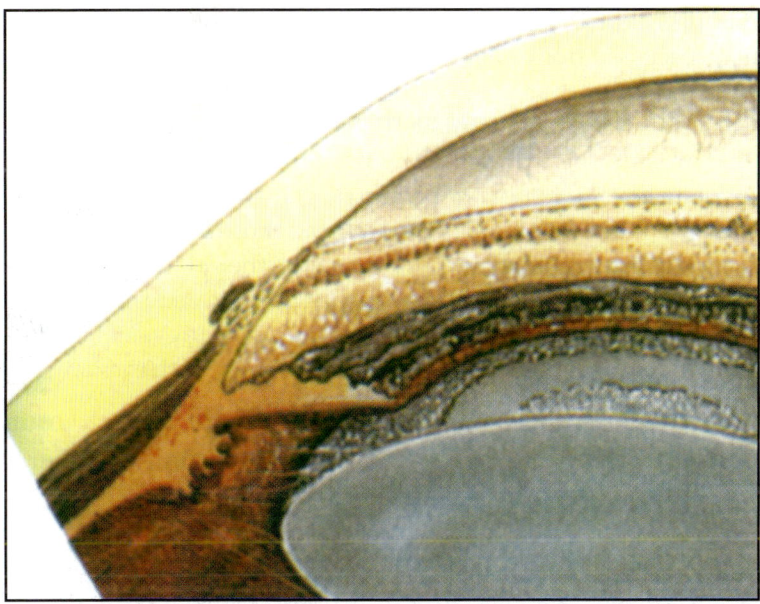

Fig. 1: Pseudoexfoliation syndrome

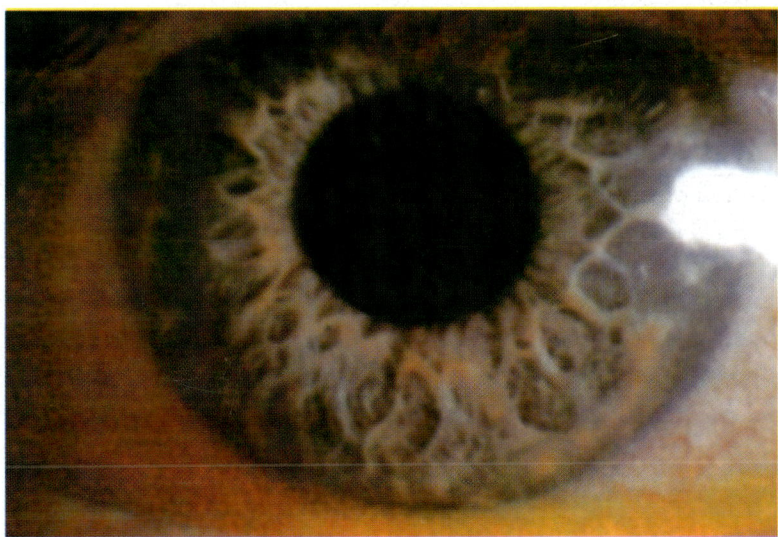

Fig. 2: Pseudoexfoliation of anterior lens capsule

recommended that this entity shall be called exfoliation syndrome and previously discussed from of lens capsule exfoliation be referred to as capsular delamination.

The pseudoexfoliation syndrome (PXS) occurs when several ocular tissues synthesize an abnormal protein. The protein may obstruct the trabecular meshwork and cause secondary open-angle glaucoma. Trabecular meshwork blockage by exfoliative material is the probable cause for glaucoma.

Pseudoexfoliation syndrome typically affects the elderly patients (geriatric population) in late sixties or early seventies. It is worldwide in prevalence and is present in all ethnic population groups. It is equally prevalent in both sexes. This condition may be unilateral or bilateral. However, both eyes are affected in 45 percent of cases.

Clinical Signs and Symptoms

Lens Changes

The characteristic exfoliation material becomes deposited on the anterior lens capsule. The constant rubbing action of pupil then scrapes the exfoliative material off the midzone of the lens giving rise to three distinct zones. (i) a translucent central disk with occasional curled-up edges, (ii) a clear zone possibly corresponding to contact with the moving iris, and (iii) a peripheral granular zone which may have radial striations. The central area of anterior lens capsule often has a dull, lusterless appearance through the undilated pupil, when the pupil is dilated, the gray membrane is seen to end in the midperiphery in a scalloped border often with curled edges.

These three zones are best demonstrated when the lens is examined with slit-lamp biomicroscopy after papillary dilatation. The central and peripheral zones can be entirely separate or can be joined by bridges of material. In some cases central disk is not present but peripheral defect is a consistent finding and pupil must be dilated before the lens changes can be seen otherwise subtle finding can be missed.

Iris Changes

The flake (dandruff)-like gray white substances becomes deposited at the pupillary margin of the iris. In addition sphincter may also show atrophic changes due to its constant rubbing action.

Iris transillumination frequently reveals loss of pigment from the posterior iris surface adjacent to the pupil in contradistinction to pigmentary dispersion syndrome where defects occur in the midperiphery. This loss of pigment from the iris may result in an abnormal accumulation of pigment in the TM (trabecular meshwork). Iris transillumination reveals a typical "moth-eaten pattern" near the pupillarly sphincter. Fluorescein angiography of the iris reveals a decreased number of vessels, neovascularization and leakage from the vessels.

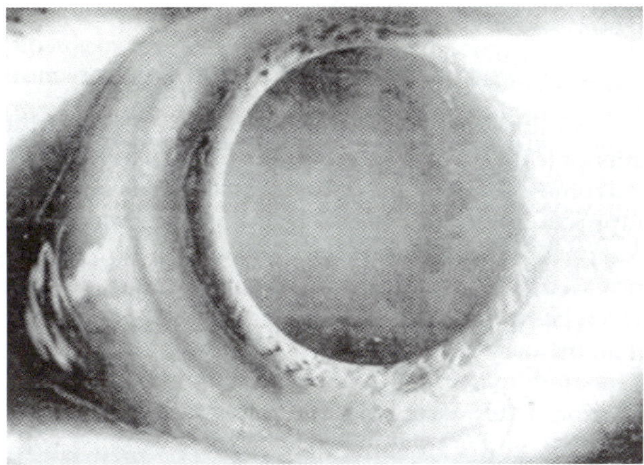

Fig. 3: Exfoliation material on the lens

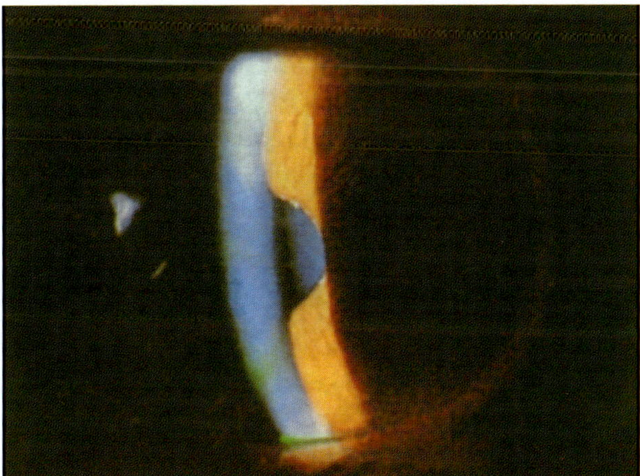

Fig. 4: Pseudoexfoliation on pupillary margin

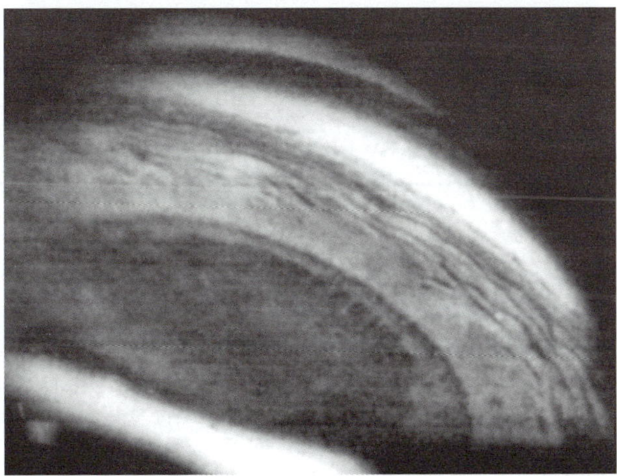

Fig. 5: Exfoliation material on the lens and in the angle

Angle Changes

The exfoliative material that has been rubbed off the anterior lens capsule by the iris than floats in the aqueous and comes to settle in the trabecular meshwork becoming trapped withing the pores. On gonioscopic examination, these deposits look like dandruff. There is increased trabecular meshwork pigmentation (moderate) which has more uneven (patchy) distribution than that of pigmentary glaucoma and is associated with flecks of exfoliative material. A wavy line of pigment extends anterior of the Schwallbe's line (Sampaolesi's line).

Course of Glaucoma

Not all patients with pseudoexfoliative syndrome (PXS) develop glaucoma and reports vary considerably regarding the frequency of secondary open-angle glaucoma with this condition. About 60 percent of the affected eyes develop open-angle glaucoma 20 percent of the fellow unaffected eyes also develop elevated IOP. The combination of glaucoma and PXS is known as glaucoma capsulare. Once glaucoma has developed in an eye with PXS is more difficult to control than cases of primary open-angle glaucoma. Acute angle closure glaucoma has also been reported in a small number of cases with exfoliation syndrome.

Other Ocular Changes

Other ocular changes noted in PXS cases are : deposition of dandruff like flecks of exfoliation material on the corneal endothelium, ciliary process, zonules, anterior hyaloids face in the aphakic eyes and adjacent four conjunctival vessels. Cataract may occur frequently in PXS eyes although this may be a function of the age of the patient.

PATHOGENESIS OF PSEUDOEXFOLIATION SYNDROME

Pathogenesis of PXS is extremely important to understand. It includes : (i) The nature and source of the exfoliative material, (ii) the mechanism of associated pigment dispersion, and (iii) mechanism of intraocular pressure elevation.

EXFOLIATIVE MATERIAL

Nature

Ultrastructural studies have shown that the exfoliative material is a fibrillar protein arranged in an irregular meshwork and sometimes coiled as spirals. This material may be mucopolysaccharide, basement membrane or protein of amyloid group. A clinical similarity has shown to occur between exfoliation syndrome and primary familial amyloidosis, and the possibility of an overlap in these two conditions exists.

Source

Lens

The exfoliative material occurs on and in the lens capsule adjacent to the lens epithelium. The soruce of material on the lens capsule is debatable.

According to some research workers it is synthesized by the subcapsular epithelial cells. Little amount of similar fibrillar protein has been seen in the aging lens capsules, and it has been shown that PXS represents excessive accumulation of this material.

Other theory argues against the lens epithelium as the source of the exfoliation material on the lens capsule since ultrastructural studies show no continuity between the capsule and the epithelial material.

Iris

The exfoliative material is also present in the iris in the anterior limiting layer, on the posterior face of pigment epithelium and the vessel walls. Iris may be the source of the exfoliation material on the lens capsule surface.

Other Sources

Other soruce of exfoliation material include non-pigmented ciliary epithelium and the conjunctiva. Conjunctiva appears to be independent source of the material rather than a secondary deposition from aqueous outflow.

It has also been suggested that lysosomal enzymes may be involved in the formation of the exfoliation material.

MECHANISM OF PIGMENT DISPERSION

Production of exfoliation material is a fundamental feature of the PXS. The associated pigment dispersion in the anterior ocular segment may have an important role in the development of secondary open angle glaucoma. The exact mechanism of the pigment dipersion is not fully known. It may be that the pigment is released from iris epithelium as a result of rubbing against the rough lens capsule. However, certain research workers show the pigment dispersion as a result from a fundamental defect of the iris.

MECHANISM OF GLAUCOMA FORMATION

Whatever, the main source of the exfoliation material and dispersed pigment may be, it is observed that these elements are responsible for secondary glaucoma formation. Ultrastructural studies of PXS eyes have revealed both fibrillar material and pigment granules in the trabecular meshwork which may lead to aqueous outflow obstruction. However, all PXS eyes have glaucoma suggesting that some additional factors may also be involved.

The additional factors responsible for secondary glaucoma may be a primary disturbance in the facility of aqueous outflow. It has been observed that glaucoma does not develop in all eyes with exfoliation and yet may develop in both eyes of patient with unilateral exfoliation. However, the increased incidence of glaucoma in PXS eyes in indicator of a causal relationship between the abnormal material and the elevated IOP.

In some cases of PXS angle-closure glaucoma develops as a result of increase in pupillary block by exfoliation materials.

DIFFERENTIAL DIAGNOSIS OF PXS

The PXS condition must be differentiated from other forms of lens exfoliation as well as other causes of pigment dispersion.

Capsular Delamination (True Exfoliation)

As already described in early part of this chapter, a group of disorders involving exfoliation of anterior lens capsules is referred as true exfoliation of the lens capsule or capsular delamination. This condition differs from pseudoexfoliation syndrome in that underlying precipitating factor is usually present such as trauma, exposure to intense heat or severe uveitis (inflammation). The nature of lens exfoliation also differs with the previously described thin, clear membranes separating from the anterior lens capsule and often curling at the margins. Glaucoma is infrequent with true exfoliation.

Primary Familial Amyloidosis

Primary familial amyloidosis is a generalized systemic disease with various ocular symptoms including glaucoma which may be associated with a white, flake-like substance on the papillary margin of the iris and an anterior lens capsule as well as pigment deposition in the anterior chamber angle.

Pigment Dispersion

A number of ocular conditions in addition to the exfoliation syndrome are characterized by increased pigmentation of trabecular meshwork. These conditions include pigment dispersion syndrome and pigmentary glaucoma, melanosis and melanoma, some forms of anterior uveitis and excessive normal pigment dispersion. This condition can be differentiated from PXS by observing the characteristic appearance of anterior lens capsule in the PXS.

INVESTIGATIONS

- Direct ophthalmoscopy.
- Tonometry
- Gonioscopy
- Perimetry.

TREATMENT

Clinically PXS behaves like primary open-angle glaucoma (POAG) so treatment is similar to POAG although IOP elevation (glaucoma) may be more difficult to treat medically in PXS cases. Trabeculectomy has been shown to the effective when medical therapy is no longer adequate. The influence of lens extraction is unclear. It has been reported that the exfoliation material diminishes and regresses after intracapsular cataract extraction (ICCE), while other research workers have observed the development of PXS years after ICCE. Nevertheless lens extraction is not indicated for primary treatment of glaucoma.

Cataract extraction in an eye with PXS in fact be complicated by synechiae between the iris pigment epithelium and peripheral anterior lens capsule which can lead to rupture of the capsule during lens removal.

The response of glaucoma to argon laser trabeculoplasty is usually good.

PROGNOSIS

Good

8

Angle-closure Glaucoma

Boris Malyugin (Russia)

INTRODUCTION

The most widespread classification of angle-closure glaucoma includes its definition as a primary or secondary. Angle-closure glaucoma (ACG) can be classified as primary when no underlying comorbidity causing IOP elevation can be identified. It is classified as being secondary if ocular or systemic disorder leading to the outflow obstruction is diagnosed.

Epidemiologic Aspects

In USA and Europe the prevalence of primary angle-closure glaucoma is estimated at approximately 0,1%. In some Arctic region populations its prevalence is much higher (upto 3-4%). ACG is relatively uncommon in blacks and its prevalence in Asian populations is varied considerably. Women usually develop ACG 3-4 times more often than men. Prevalence of the pupillary-block ACG increases with age because of the natural lens thickening. That is why between ages of 55 and 60 years acute ACG is mostly common. ACG more typically associated with hyperopia, although it may occur in eyes with any type of refraction.

Pathophysiology of Angle Closure

The most frequent cause of angle closure is the pupillary block with the forward bowing of the iris. This is the result of the impediment of the aqueous flow from the posterior chamber through the pupil. Peripheral iris bowing and apposition to the trabecular meshwork leads to the aqueous humor drainage block.

Angle closure may also occur when lens-iris diaphragm is pushed forward by the space occupying process in the posterior segment (tumor, cyst, ciliary body swelling, ciliochoroidal effusion, etc.). In some types of ACG the underlying mechanism is pulling of the iris forward by contracting fibrovascular tissue, as with neovascularization, inflammation and cells proliferation in the anterior chamber angle.

Predisposing Factors

Factors that cause pupillary dilation may induce angle-closure glaucoma. These factors include a variety of systemic and locally administered drugs, as well as emotional upset, pain or fright.

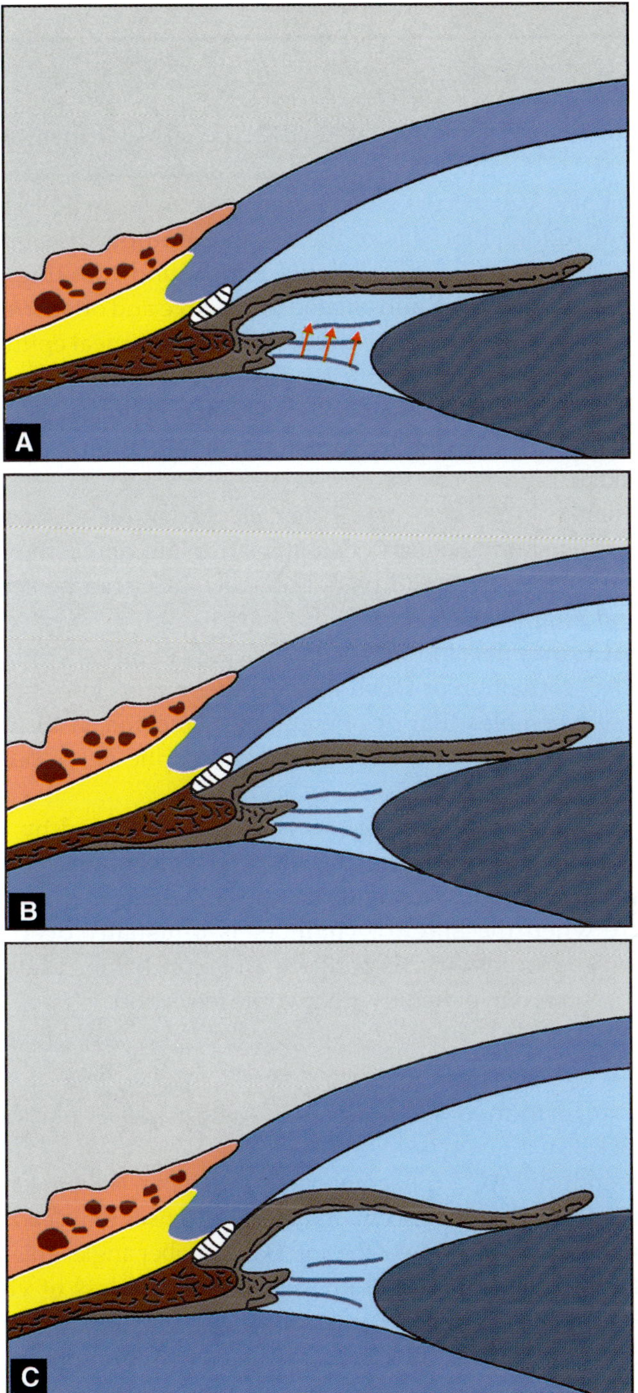

Figs 1 A to C: Pupillary block glaucoma mechanism. A functional block between the lens and the iris leads to increased pressure in posterior chamber (arrows) (A). Peripheral iris shifts forward (B) and closes the anterior chamber angle (C)

CLINICAL SIGNS AND SYMPTOMS

Primary ACG

Clinical symptoms and signs depend on the type of ACG. There are four main types of primary ACG: acute, subacute, chronic and plateau iris.

Acute primary ACG occurs when intraocular pressure (IOP) rises rapidly as the result of sudden blockage of the aqueous outflow. It is manifested by pain, blurred vision, haloes around lights, nausea and vomiting. Signs of the acute ACG include: high IOP, mid-dilated unreactive and often irregular pupil, congested episcleral and conjunctival blood vessels, corneal epithelial edema, shallow anterior chamber, mild aqueous flare and cells.

After acute ACG attacks clinical examination may reveal signs of sectoral iris atrophy, iris torsion and subcapsular whitish anterior lens opacities (glaucomflecken).

Subacute angle-closure glaucoma is characterized by the episodes of elevated IOP that resolves spontaneously. Patients complain about the intermittent blurred vision, haloes and mild pain. Subacute ACG can be confused with headaches and migraines.

Chronic ACG may develop after acute attacks leading to peripheral anterior synechiae (PAS) formation or when the chamber angle closes gradually. The clinical course resembles that of open-angle glaucoma. It includes lack of symptoms, modestly elevated IOP, progressive optic nerve head cupping, characteristic loss of visual field.

Plateau iris is a rare type of primary ACG. It is caused by the unusual anatomy of the ciliary processes that pushes peripheral iris forward and narrow the anterior chamber angle. The condition can be suspected in the patient with angle closure when the anterior chamber is unusually deep. Ultrasonic biomicroscopy is necessary to confirm this condition. Plateau iris not infrequently observed in patients with myopic refraction.

Secondary ACG

There are two main forms of secondary ACG: with pupillary block and without pupillary block.

With lens-induced ACG (phacomorphic glaucoma, ectopia lentis, aphakic or pseudophakic ACG) intumescent or dislocated lenses may lead to pupillary block, iris bombe and shallowing of the anterior chamber angle. This may present clinically as an acute event with pain, hyperemia and loss of vision or as a chronic condition with peripheral anterior synechiae (PAS) formation.

In some patients pupillary block can be caused by subretinal effusion where no retinal brakes are present. Nonrhegmatogenous retinal detachment leading to ACG can be observed in Coats disease, retinoblastoma, choroidal melanoma and some other ocular conditions.

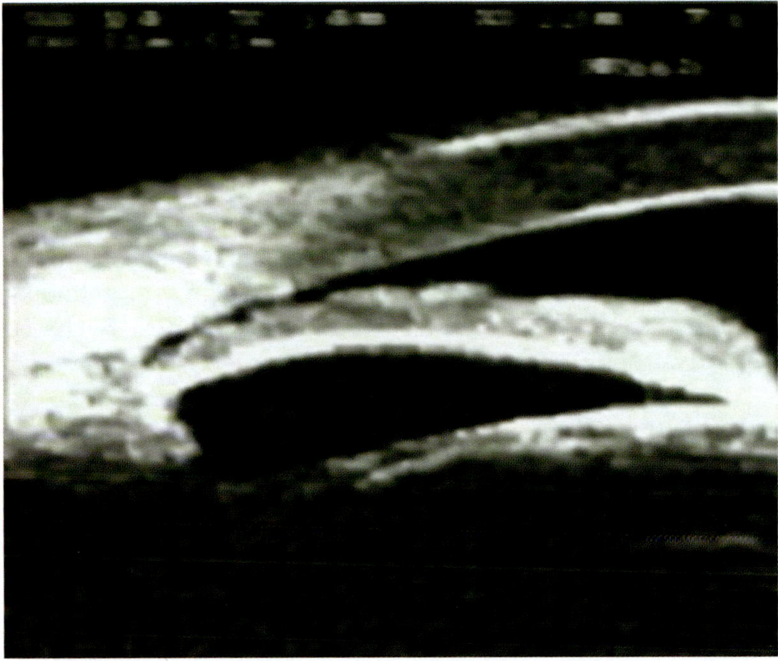

Fig. 2: Ultrasonic biomicroscopy image of a patient with angle-closure glaucoma

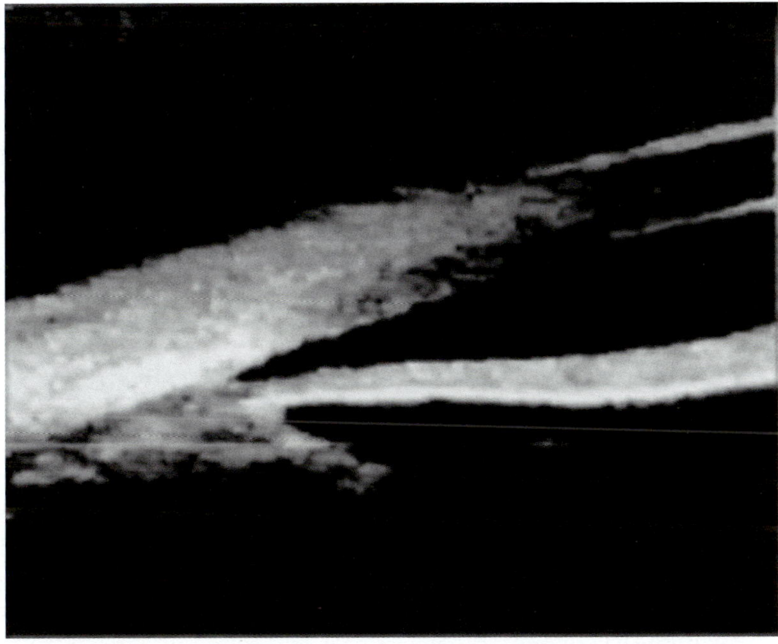

Fig. 3: Ultrasonic biomicroscopy image of a patient with plateau iris

Secondary ACG without pupillary block may occur through one of two possible mechanisms: Contraction of tissue (exudate, membrane) in the anterior chamber angle leading to PAS formation and forward displacement of lens-iris diaphragm, infrequently accompanied by swelling and anterior rotation of the ciliary body.

The most common secondary angle-closure glaucomas without pupillary block observed in patients with anterior chamber angle neovascularization, iridocorneal endothelial syndrome, tumors, inflammation, aqueous misdirection (malignant glaucoma), epithelial and fibrous downgrowth, retinopathy of prematurity, retinal vascular disease, nanophthalmos, Fuchs corneal endothelial dystrophy, after trauma and retinal surgery.

Investigations

The main examinations include: visual acuity and IOP measurement, assessment of visual fields, biomicroscopy, gonioscopy, optic nerve head examination. Gonioscopic examination is one of the most important to enable the physician to make the correct diagnosis.

In some cases with corneal edema hyperosmotic topical agents (glycerin, 20% glucose, 5% NaCl) can be helpful to enable visualization of the anterior angle structures. Corneal compression during gonioscopy may help to differentiate reversibility of the trabecular meshwork blockage (appositional vs synechial closure) by the iris and even break the attack.

Differential Diagnosis

From the therapeutical standpoint it is very important to differentiate closed-angle glaucoma from the open-angle glaucoma.

Gonioscopic appearance of a narrow chamber angle with or without peripheral anterior synechiae helps in establishing the correct diagnosis.

The next clinical decision point following the diagnosis of angle-closure glaucoma is to distinguish pupillary-block mechanism from the other mechanisms. In some cases peripheral iridectomy (PI) can be done as much for diagnostic purposes as for therapeutic ones.

Treatment

Cholinergic agents (pilocarpine 1%) can be helpful in breaking mild attacks of ACG by inducing miosos. When the IOP is high (> 40 mm Hg) the pupil can be unreactive to miotics because of ischemia. In such cases patient should be treated with combination of a topical beta-blockers, alpha$_2$-adrenergic agonists, carbonic anhydrase inhibitors (topcal, oral or intravenous) and hyperosmotic agents when necessary. The goal of the treatment is to reduce IOP to the point where miotic agent will constrict the pupil and open the angle.

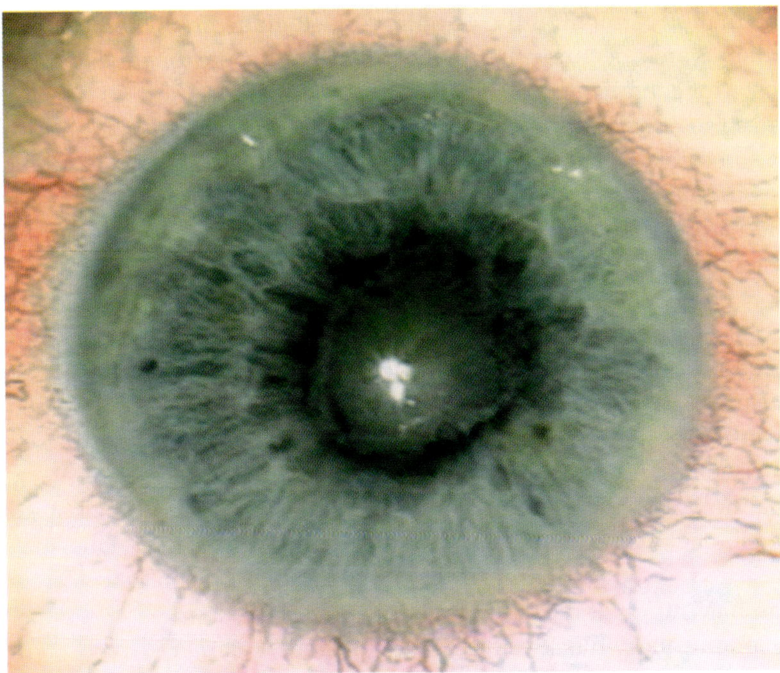

Fig. 4: Secondary angle-closure glaucoma in patient. A secluded pupil and iris bombe in a patient with long-standing uveitis

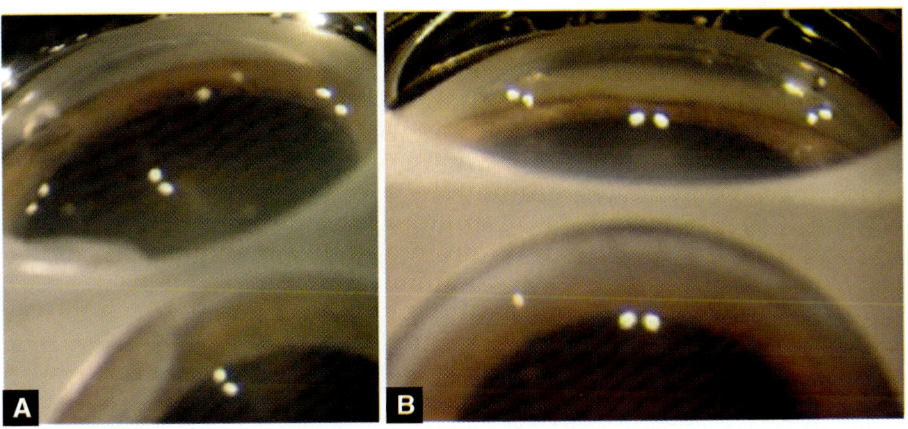

Figs 5A and B: Gonioscopic appearance of the anterior chamber angle in patient with angle-closure glaucoma

The main treatment of the pupillary-block glaucoma whether primary or secondary is an iridectomy. It provides alternative route for aqueous trapped in the posterior chamber to flow into the anterior chamber.

Once the attack is broken peripheral iridectomy should be performed as soon as possible. Laser iridectomy can be done both by Argon and Nd:YAG lasers. Surgical iridectomy is indicated when laser can not be accomplished.

After iridectomy pupillary block is relieved, pressure gradient between posterior and anterior chambers approaches to zero, iris returns to its normal position. PI can relieve pupillary block but this is ineffective in eyes with complete synechial closure as a result of neovascularization and chronic inflammation.

After successful iridectomy IOP may return to normal or may remain elevated. In the latter case the chronic use of hypotensive medications or antiglaucoma intervention are indicated.

In patients with secondary angle closure not caused by pupillary block, ophthalmologist should identify and treat underlying condition. For example, in malignant glaucoma vitrectomy is indicated, in neovascular glaucoma caused by diabetic retinopathy laser or cryo retinal ablation can lead to regress of neovascularization of the anterior chamber angle.

When pupillary block is induced by the lens, cataract extraction might be considered as a primary procedure. In some cases goniosynechialysis with viscoelastic agent, spatula or forceps may be combined with cataract extraction or performed as a separate procedure.

In some patients with extensive peripheral anterior synechiae argon laser gonioplasty, can be recommended. The other surgical procedures helpful in controlling IOP in patient with chronic ACG include trabeculectomy, tube-shunt surgery, transciliary draining of the posterior chamber and ciliary body ablation.

Prognosis

In acute primary angle-closure glaucoma high IOP lead to optic disc edema with subsequent optic nerve damage. Iris ischemia produces sector iris atrophy and peripheral anterior synechiae can form very rapidly.

Acute attack if left untreated lead to complete blindness. Subacute ACG can progress to chronic ACG or an acute attack that does not resolve without treatment.

In general primary angle-closure glaucoma is bilateral disease. That is why peripheral iridectomy is recommended in the other eye of the patient in case a similar angle configuration is present.

Patients with narrow angles should be advised of the symptoms of angle closure and the need for immediate ophthalmic examination if symptoms occur as well as the value of long-term periodic follow-up.

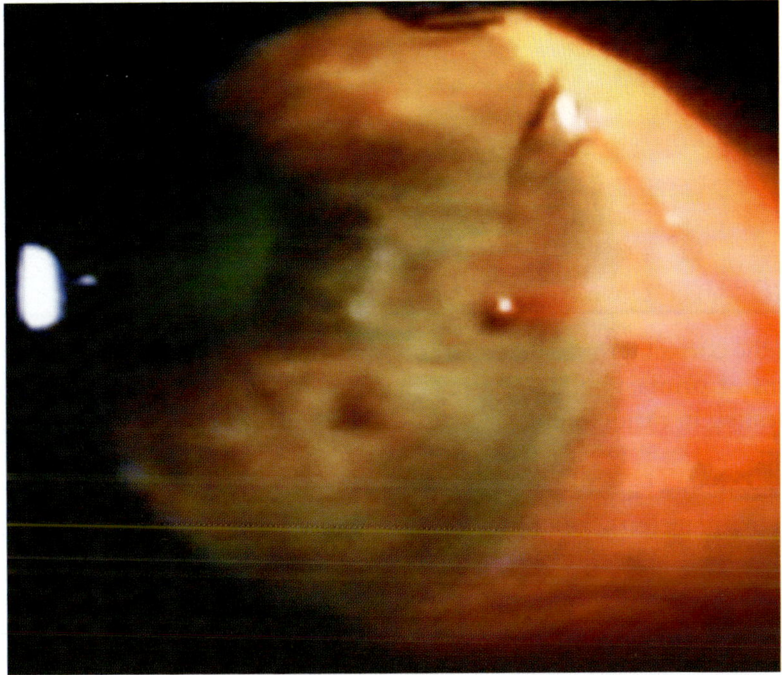

Fig. 6: Peripheral iridectomy with laser

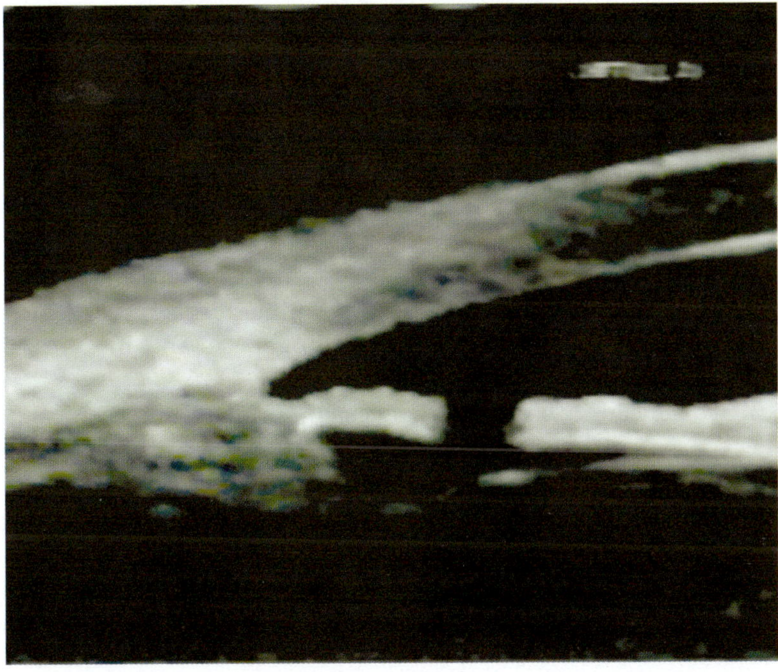

Fig. 7: Ultrasonic biomicroscopy image of a patient with angle-closure glaucoma after peripheral iridectomy

9

Primary Angle-closure Glaucoma (PACG)

G Marchini, M Marraffa, R Morbio, P Ceruti (Italy)

INTRODUCTION

Using the correct terminology is important for any clear and comprehensible account of primary angle-closure glaucoma (PACG), a disease capable of manifesting in various clinical forms, which may differ considerably one from another.

Many names have been used to define PACG: these include acute glaucoma, congestive glaucoma, irritative glaucoma, closed-angle glaucoma, narrow-angle glaucoma, and angle-block glaucoma. This terminology is imprecise and stresses only a number of the possible aspects of the disease, namely the phase of the acute attack (mistakenly regarded by many as the most frequent), the ocular congestion or irritation (absent in many cases), the closed angle (not present in the intermittent forms and in the chronic forms with partial closure), and the narrow angle (which may exist without glaucoma or which may identify eyes predisposed to closure). The term angle-block glaucoma is correct, but is not used in the international literature.

The term Primary Angle-Closure Glaucoma is the most appropriate and encompasses both the pathogenetic mechanism and the complete, partial, intermittent and potential angle closure forms. It also presents the additional advantage of being used internationally.

CLASSIFICATION

Angle-closure glaucoma is characterized by numerous clinical pictures that differ from one another both in their pathogenesis and in their clinical presentation.

The first distinction to be made in between the primary and secondary forms. The latter consist in a large number of angle closures, each of which receives its name and is characterized by the eye disease that causes it (e.g., lens displacement, inflammation of the anterior segment, irido-corneal syndrome, intraocular tumours, or in the course of systemic diseases). The secondary forms are not addressed in this chapter.

Primary angle-closure glaucoma occurs in eyes characterized by a particular anatomical and biometric constitution. This constitution is the main factor predisposing to angle closure, which manifests as a result of the effect of a

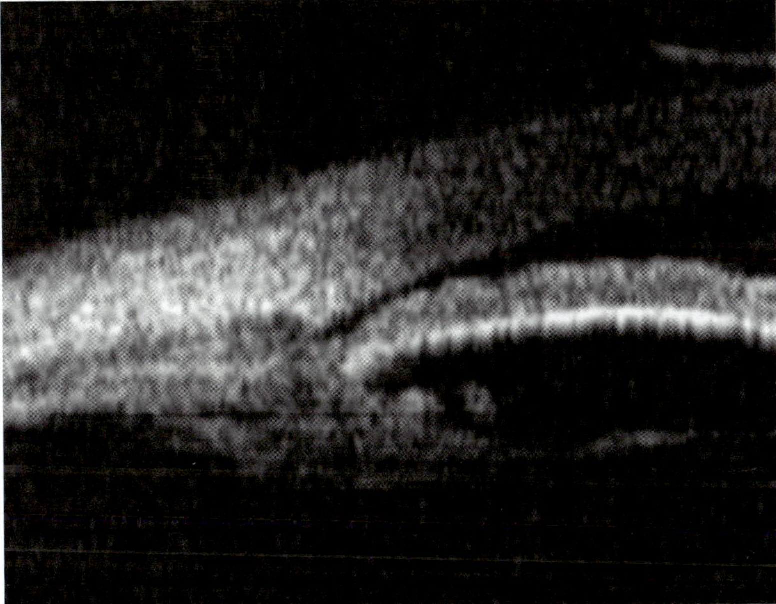

Fig. 1: UBM image. Narrow angle in the fellow eye of a patient with acute PACG in the other eye. The conformation of the iris with anterior convexity indicates the presence of a relative pupillary block

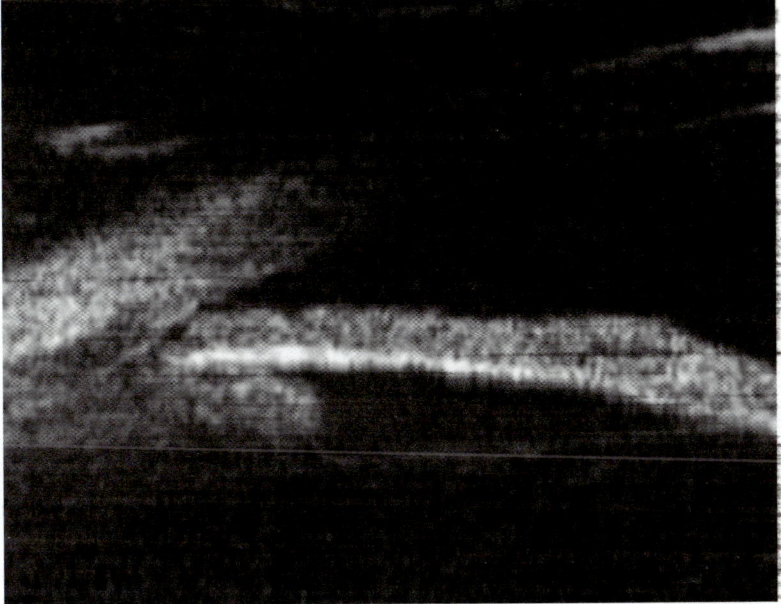

Fig. 2: UBM image. Plateau-iris conformation. The flat configuration of the iris is visible with a sharp backward bend at the level of the trabeculum and the creation of a particularly narrow angular recess. The ciliary process is positioned and rotated anteriorly and is in contact with the peripheral part of the iris

trigger factor, with different pathogenetic mechanisms, and gives rise to different clinical pictures.

CLINICAL CLASSIFICATION

PACG may present in different clinical forms.

Acute PACG

This is the well-known acute attack that constitutes an ophthalmological emergency and may occur without warning or set in subsequent to transitory episodes of angle closure.

Intermittent PACG

This is the form in which self-limited episodes of angle-closure occur, with transitory increases in intraocular pressure which usually go undetected and may be accompanied by symptoms, which may themselves also be of a transitory nature. In such cases the angle closure is functional. Between the various attacks the eye is quiescent and the intraocular pressure normal (in this case the PACG is said to be in an intercritical phase). This form may result in a classic acute attack of PACG or may give rise to the chronic form of PACG.

Chronic PACG

In this form, as a result of the transitory closure episodes, there may be residual goniosynechiae which occlude the angle in the course of time in a chronic-progressive manner, bringing about an increasingly extensive anatomical closure and a rise in intraocular pressure. The eye in this form is usually quiescent. Without gonioscopy, chronic PACG may easily be mistaken for primary open-angle glaucoma.

This form should be regarded as distinct from chronicised PACG, which is usually the result of an unresolved acute attack, and in which the angle remains completely closed; in this case, the closure is anatomical and irreversible, the intraocular pressure is stably high, and the prognosis poor.

Asymptomatic Narrow Angle (eye at risk of PACG)

In this case, the term PACG may be excessive, since, in these eyes, anatomical and biometric predisposing factors are present and the angle is narrow, but the disease is not present and the eye is normal.

Many of these eyes do not develop PACG, but are exposed to the risk of developing the disease. The problem is to identify those eyes with an unacceptable risk of developing PACG so as to submit them to appropriate prophylactic treatment.

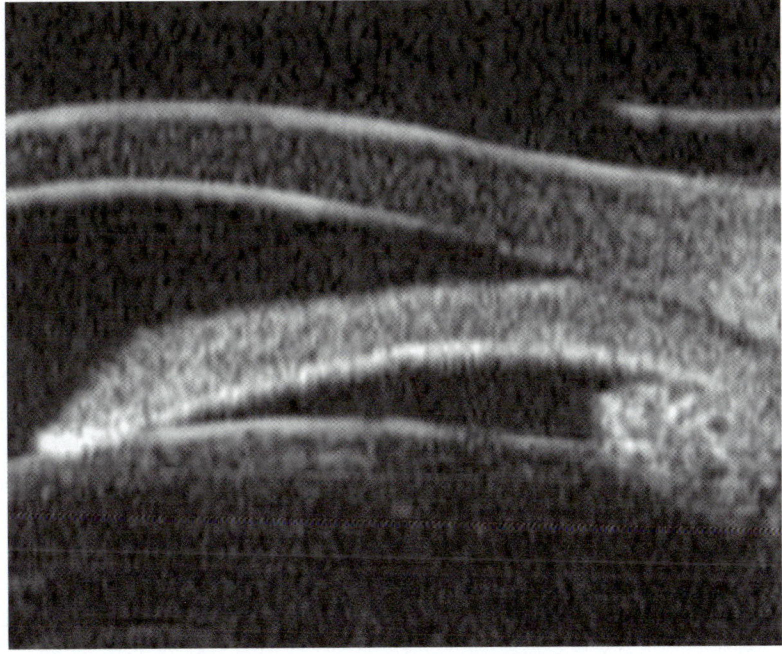

Fig. 3: UBM image. Narrow angle with intermediate iris-angle conformations between those of pupillary block and plateau iris

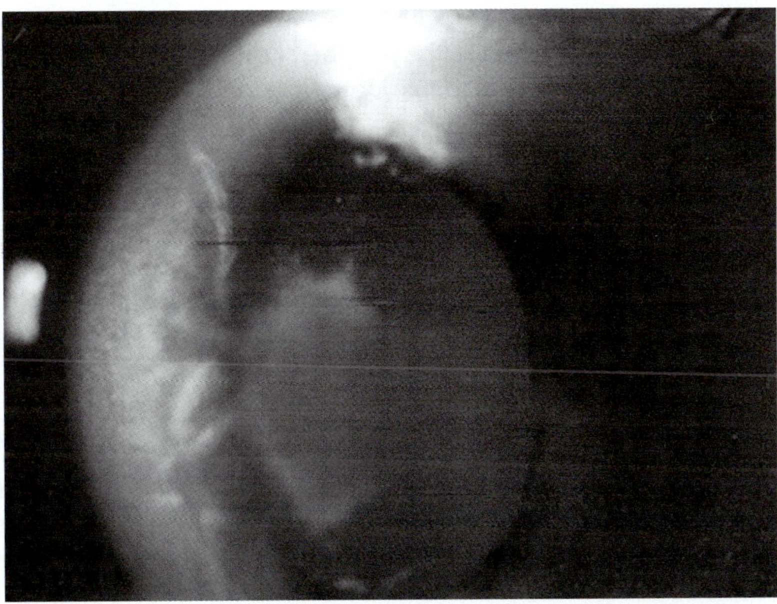

Fig. 4: Acute PACG with medium pupillary mydriasis and corneal folds

Table 1: Clinical classification of primary angle-closure glaucoma (PACG)

Clinical form	Synonyms used
1. Acute PACG	Acute, congestive, irritative glaucoma
2. Intermittent PACG	Subacute, prodromic, intermittent irritative glaucoma
3. Chronic PACG	Creeping, chronic progressive narrow-angle glaucoma
4. Chronicised PACG	Chronic irritative, chronicised irreversible subacute narrow-angle congestive glaucoma
5. Asymptomatic narrow-angle	Predisposed eye, eye at risk, pre-glaucoma

Pathogenetic Classification

PACG occurs in eyes with a particular biometric conformation which constitutes the predisposition for developing the disease. Two trigger mechanisms act upon this predisposition: pupillary block and direct crowding of the angle. From the point of view of classification, these mechanisms identify three types of glaucoma.

PACG due to Pupillary Block

This is the most frequent form, in which there is resistance to the passage of aqueous humour through the pupil. The increase in pressure in the posterior chamber pushes the base of the iris forwards occluding the trabeculum. This mechanism is resolved by iridotomy.

PACG due to Direct Crowding of the Angle

This is the rarest form, and occurs typically in the iris plateau conformation and syndrome. During mydriasis the peripheral iris collects and occupies the angle, obstructing it. In the pure form iridotomy is ineffective.

PACG due to Mixed Mechanisms

In these eyes the conformation of the angle presents intermediate characteristics between those of pupillary block and those of plateau iris. Iridotomy may not be sufficient or curative in eyes with this form of PACG.

In this classification we should also recall the pathogenetic mechanism of ciliary-block glaucoma or posterior-block glaucoma, which will be dealt in a specific section of this chapter.

Epidemiology

The prevalence of PACG varies to a considerable extent in different populations, and is greater in females and in the higher age. It is usually regarded as rare in European countries, but is more frequent in Eskimo populations and in populations of Mongolian stock in East and South-East Asia. Overall, it is the most widespread form of glaucoma in the world. An important difficulty stems

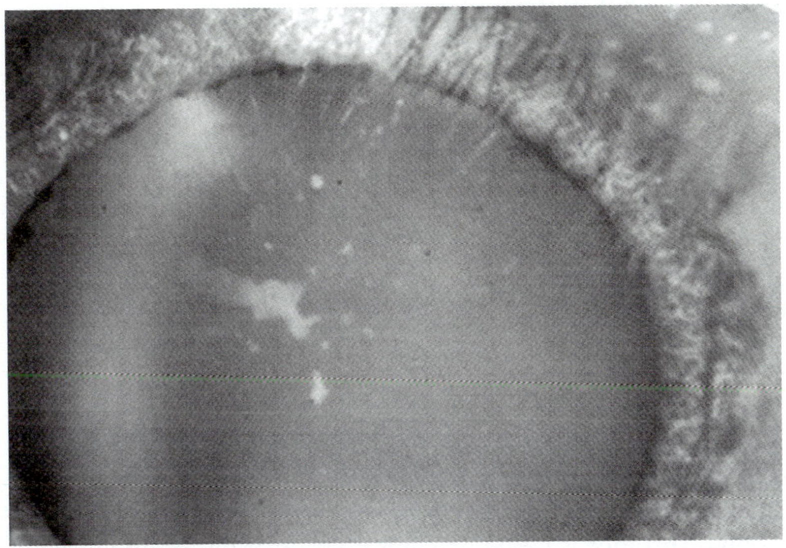

Fig. 5: Outcomes of acute PACG with fixed mydriasis, pupillary atrophy and Glaukomflecken

from the fact that in many studies the definition of the disease is unclear and a great deal of the lack of precision is due to persistence of the notion prevailing in the past whereby PACG tended to be identified essentially with the acute form, disregarding the more frequent chronic presentation. The prevalence of PACG in various different populations is shown in Table.

Table 2: Prevalence of PACG in various populations aged over 40 years

Author	*Place/Population*	*Prevalence*
Hollows and Graham (1966)	Wales	0.09%
Bankes *et al.* (1968)	Bedford	0.16%
Hyams and Keroub (1977)	Israel	0.5%
Drance (1973)	Eskimos	2.9%
Clemmesen and Alsbirk (1971)	Eskimos	5.0%
Shiose *et al.* (1991)	Japan	0.31%
Congdom *et al.* (1992)	China	1.3%
Salmon *et al.* (1993)	South Africa	1.0%

It is generally believed that the acute PACG form is more common in European populations, while the chronic-progressive form is more frequent in Asian populations. This idea is based on clinical observations or on the analysis of hospital inpatient series and might lead to selection bias errors and to incorrect epidemiological deductions.

The Egna-Neumarkt epidemiological study conducted in Italy in a district of South Tyrol on a total of 4,297 subjects has furnished important information in this regard:

- the prevalence of PACG is 0.6% as against a 3% overall prevalence of all glaucomas;
- of the various forms of PACG the most frequent is the chronic-progressive form (15/26 cases = 57%);
- the percentage distribution of PACG rises in the various age brackets, amounting to 0% in subjects from 40 to 49 years, 0.65% in those from 50 to 59 years, 0.65% in those from 60 to 69, and 1.23% in subjects above 70 years of age;
- the frequency of occludable angles is higher in women than in men and rises with age;
- the prevalence of occludable angles in the study population was almost 15%, but only 0.6% had an active form of PACG.

These data enable us to draw the following conclusions:

1. even in a Caucasian population the prevalence of PACG is greater than is generally believed, amounting to 0.6% of the population aged over 40 years;

2. eyes predisposed to angle closure are relatively frequent, but only a minimal proportion of these go on to develop PACG;
3. in Italy too, the most frequent presentation of PACG is the chronic-progressive form, which develops without an acute attack. If gonioscopy is not performed this form may be mistaken for primary open-angle glaucoma.

The likelihood that PACG will develop among consanguineous relatives is high, with a frequency ranging from 1 to 12% . The greatest risk is in first-degree relatives with a probability ranging from 2 to 5%. The risk drops to 1 to 2.5% for second-degree relatives. These data suggest the existence of a polygenic or multifactorial inheritance.

Angle-closure Mechanisms

Eyes affected by PACG present particular anatomical and biometric characteristics which distinguish them from normal eyes and constitute the predisposition to the disease. Trigger factors act upon this predisposition leading to angle closure through two fundamental pathogenetic mechanisms: pupillary block and direct crowding of the angle.

Anatomical and Biometric Predisposition to PACG

As compared to normal eyes those affected by PACG are characterized by a lower corneal diameter, a smaller corneal curvature radius, a shallower anterior chamber, both centrally and peripherally, a lower anterior chamber volume, a thicker, more curved lens in a more anterior position, and a shorter axial length.

The most important biometric characteristic predisposing to angle closure however is a shallow anterior chamber. In PACG the mean central depth of the anterior chamber, without the corneal thickness, ranges from 1.7 to 2 mm; this is equivalent to a value 0.5 to 1 mm lower than that of normal eyes of the same age. The depth of the anterior chamber depends on the position of the anterior surface of the lens and is determined by the thickness and position of the lens within the eye. In PACG the lens is 0.4 to 1 mm thicker and its position is more anterior than in normal eyes. Both these parameters increase with age, which accounts for the greater frequency of PACG after the age of 60. The use of ultrasound biomicroscopy (UBM) moreover has revealed that the ciliary processes in PACG are structurally rotated forwards, thus accounting for the more anterior position of the lens.

All these characteristics give rise to a crowding of the anterior segment, affect the narrowness of the angle, particularly in the acute form of PACG, and provide a basis for understanding the pathogenesis of the disease. It should also be noted that the simple biometric assessment of an eye with a narrow angle does not enable us to predict whether or not it will develop PACG. This would require thorough gonioscopy and assessment of the other clinical elements.

Angle Closure due to Pupillary Block

Pupillary block is the most frequent mechanism responsible for angle closure. Its presence is usually revealed by an iris conformation presenting anterior convexity.

In these eyes at the level of the pupillary margin there is contact between the iris and the anterior surface of the lens ('iris-lens contact area'), which offers a resistance to the passage of aqueous humour from the posterior chamber through the pupil. The obstacle to the passage of aqueous humour is not complete and a certain amount of pressure is brought to bear on the posterior surface of the iris which takes on the bombé conformation characterized by anterior convexity. This situation is termed relative pupillary block.

The main factors contributing to pupillary block consist in positional relationships between the iris and the lens, the iris-lens contact area, the forward displacement of the lens which occurs with ageing, and the pupillary diameter.

Trigger factors intervene in these predisposed eyes, such as emotional stress, prolonged reading, permanence in a poorly lit environment, or general anesthesia with the use of drugs with a mydriatic effect which transform the relative pupillary block into an absolute block. At this point the forward thrust of the aqueous humour brings the iris root into contact with the peripheral cornea, closing the angle and giving rise to the acute attack.

This sequence of events, however, does not always lead to acute PACG. Sometimes the attacks are self-limiting and clear up spontaneously as in intermittent PACG, or they may lead to the progressive manifestation of chronic PACG. In pupillary-block PACG, especially in the acute and intermittent forms, the main measure that interrupts the pathogenetic mechanism is the execution of a peripheral iridotomy, which creates a by-pass between the posterior and anterior chambers.

Angle Closure due to Direct Crowding of the Angle

This angle-closure mechanism occurs more rarely as a result of mydriasis in eyes that present the so-called 'iris plateau'. In these eyes the iris is characterized by a flat configuration, with a sharp bending back at the level of the trabeculum which gives rise to the creation of a particularly narrow angular recess. When the pupil dilates, the volume of iris tissue builds up in the restricted angular space and closes the angle.

The most distinctive feature of eyes with a plateau iris is clearly demonstrated by UBM and consists in the forward position and rotation of the ciliary processes, which are in contact with the peripheral portion of the iris. This causes the closure of the ciliary sulcus and the creation of a support for the iris root, which therefore cannot detach itself from the trabeculum even in the presence of an iridectomy (or YAG-laser iridotomy).

From the therapeutic standpoint, since the basic pathogenetic mechanism consists in crowding of the angle in mydriasis, the essential therapeutic measure is the constant use of miotics. In PACG due to a plateau iris, thermal laser peripheral iridoplasty or gonioplasty is also indicated, which obtains both a retraction and a thinning of the iris base with consequent broadening of the angular recess.

Angle Closure due to Mixed Mechanisms

YAG-laser iridotomy is not indicated in the typical form of iris-plateau PACG and is regarded as useless by some authors. In clinical practice however it is by no means rare to encounter intermediate iris-angle conformations between those of pupillary block and plateau iris, in which both closure mechanisms may be involved. In these cases the execution of a YAG-laser iridotomy is justified, but may not be sufficient and in any event needs the support of adjunctive miotic therapy.

Introduction to Therapy

The various different forms of PACG give rise to different clinical pictures requiring different therapeutic measures.

It is generally accepted that the aim of treatment in the various forms of angle closure is to reduce the risk of sudden, acute rises in intraocular pressure (IOP), by acting on the pathogenetic mechanisms involved, whether singly or in combination (pupillary block and direct crowding of the angle), and counteract the progressive synechial obliteration of the angle. The therapy that needs to be initiated to eliminate these angle-closure mechanisms is pharmacological and/or parasurgical with different laser treatments. Only in the case of failure of these measures does it prove mandatory to resort to surgical therapy.

The procedures used in the treatment of angle closure will be indicated distinguishing between the acute PACG attack and the other forms of PACG.

Clinical Variants of PACG

Primary angle-closure glaucoma can manifest in different clinical forms which may set in with severe, pronounced symptoms or with milder, more insidious symptoms.

Acute PACG

This form of angle-closure glaucoma is more frequent in Caucasian and Asian than in negroid subjects, sets in more often in the 50 to 70 years of age and affects women more often than men.

The acute attack comes on unexpectedly in a subject who hitherto had never complained of any kind of eye disorder. Sometimes the patient's history shows that episodes of minor importance precede the attack, with blurred vision, mild periocular pain and coloured haloes. Trigger factors may be emotional stress and reduced light levels. On other occasions the attack occurs after general or spinal anesthesia as a result of the use of mydriatic drugs, or simply as a result of the patient's emotional state, or even as a consequence of performing prolonged near-vision tasks following intense accommodation activity. Antidepressant and parasympatholytic drugs may also bring on the attack. The most frequent iatrogenic cause is the use of mydriatic eye-drops for diagnostic purposes in the course of an ophthalmological examination.

Acute PACG is generally monolateral, but may be bilateral in iatrogenic cases.

In the more typical form, the attack presents with a prodromic phase characterized by mild, though prolonged symptoms with blurred vision, mild periocular pain and mild signs of congestion. Objective findings are a medium pupillary mydriasis and moderate IOP increase.

More often there is no prodromic phase at all and the acute attack comes on in all its violence with intense pain localized in the supraorbital zone and irradiating to behind the affected eye, as well as nausea, vomiting, sweating, bradycardia, and a feeling of exhaustion. The eye appears congested with an edematous cornea and thickened Descemet's folds.

The anterior chamber presents Tyndall phenomenon due to mobilisation of iris granules and an increase in protein content. It is present, though shallow, at the centre and absent on the periphery due to contact between the posterior surface of the cornea and the iris root. The iris profile presents an anterior convexity (iris bombé appearance). Gonioscopy often does not allow visualization of the angular structures due to corneal clouding. It can however detect a completely closed angle. The IOP is very high with values often exceeding 60 mm Hg.

The lens is also altered in its transparency presenting anterior subcapsular opacities which are initially diffuse and then become more circumscribed due to restoration of lens transparency. These opacities are referred to as "Glaukomflecken" and are the result of the sharp rise in intraocular pressure causing areas of acute necrosis of the anterior epithelium of the lens.

Exploration of the fundus proves difficult in the acute phase, but, when it is possible, it can be seen that the optical disk is completely normal or edematous and rarely presents microhemorrhages. Some time after the acute attack, on the other hand, it may appear pale and atrophic, without any signs of papillary cupping.

Visual function is poor with visual acuity less than 0.2-0.3. Diffuse impairment of visual field or defects of minor clinical significance have been reported; in some cases the examination findings are entirely normal. The extent of the damage varies from case to case and depends on the level of the intraocular pressure during the acute phase and on its duration. If the acute attack is not resolved rapidly, it will evolve towards the chronicised form with severe functional defects.

In rare cases the acute PACG may regress spontaneously and the signs of the attack can be seen objectively with circumscribed areas of iris atrophy, a poorly reactive pupil with irregular mydriasis and posterior and anterior synechiae, "Glaukomflecken", and goniosynechiae.

Essential Therapy for Acute Attack of PACG

The acute attack of PACG is the most violent and dramatic form of angle closure. It is a real ophthalmological emergency in as much as the sudden, unexpected increase in intraocular pressure can cause irreversible damage to various ocular structures and seriously impair visual function. The inflammatory phenomena accompanying the attack can cause rapid adhesion between the iris and trabeculum, transforming the angle closure from appositional and reversible to anatomical and irreversible, characterized by definitive synechial fusion.

The fundamental aim of therapy must be to reopen the angle, eliminating iris-trabeculum contact and resolving the pathogenetic mechanism responsible for the pupillary block. To achieve this, the ophthalmologist has a number of pharmacological, parasurgical and surgical options which have to be used, bearing in mind both the patient's clinical and systemic situation.

The initial therapeutic approach is pharmacological. In the case of episodes without congestive phenomena or episodes of an acute attack in the initial stage, with IOP values that are not particularly high (< 40 mm Hg), cholinergic drugs such as pilocarpine can be used to induce miosis and separate the iris root from the trabeculum. This measure alone may be capable of resolving the attack.

On the other hand, if the IOP value is higher than the pressure of the arterial system of the iris, ischemia of the pupillary sphincter occurs, so that the pupil does not respond to the drug and fails to contract. In these cases the reiterated administration of pilocarpine may potentiate the systemic toxic effects of the drug without achieving the desired miotic effect. A different therapeutic approach is therefore necessary, at least initially, aimed at achieving a lowering of IOP with different mechanisms such as inhibition of the production of aqueous humour and reduction of the vitreal volume.

Reduction of the vitreal volume is achieved by means of the use of osmotic agents and is usually the most effective measure. Osmotic agents such as intravenous mannitol, and oral glycerol and isosorbide, are substances that increase the osmolarity of the plasma and thereby create a concentration gradient that recalls liquids from the tissues to the vessels, thus giving rise to dehydration of the vitreal body. This makes it possible to achieve a substantial, rapid IOP-lowering effect. It should be stressed that these substances are used to control acute episodes of increased IOP, in that their effects are momentary owing to the rapid restoration of the equilibrium of the osmotic gradient. To be effective they must be administered rapidly and at an adequate concentration. The most commonly used osmotic agent is mannitol, which is administered by rapid oral infusion (not more than 20 minutes) in 20% solution at the dose of 2 g (10 ml) per kg body weight. It is worth recalling that, on account of the imbalance induced (hypervolaemia and tissue dehydration), mannitol may be dangerous in cardiopathic or hypertensive subjects, or in subjects with severe kidney problems.

Owing to the hyperglycemia it induces and its disagreeable taste glycerol (administered in syrup form at the dose of 1.5 g/kg) may be dangerous in diabetics and is currently not used.

Inhibition of aqueous humour is achieved by means of the systemic administration of the carbonic anhydrase inhibitors (CAIs) acetazolamide and dichlorphenamide. CAIs administered orally (250 mg, 4 times daily) or parenterally (500 mg, i.v.) reach high concentrations in the eye thus permitting total inhibition of the enzyme at the level of the ciliary body whereas the activity of the enzyme persists partially at a more general level (this limits the systemic effects). The IOP-lowering effect initiate on average half an hour after administration and last up to 6 hours.

With this approach the attack is generally resolved within 3 hours. When IOP has been lowered to a reasonable extent, blood supply to the iris resumes and pilocarpine efficacy is restored.

In the presence of marked congestion with disruption of the blood-eye barrier, the effect of osmotic agents is reduced. For this reason the combination of osmotics with drugs capable of reducing the production of aqueous humour is indicated. To this end topical beta-blockers and CAIs dorzolamide and brinzolamide are used. The administration of alpha-2-agonists such as brimonidine may also be useful in the acute phase.

The patient with an acute attack is in a state of great distress and is also often frightened. Antiemetics should be administered to reduce the nausea and vomiting that may accompany the acute attack, while a sedative may additionally be given to relieve the patient's anxiety. When the pain is severe it is also useful to administer analgesics. Systemic non-steroidal anti-inflammatory drugs (NSAIDs) such as diclofenac may be used for relieving pain and for blocking the production of inflammatory mediators.

Laser Iridotomy

After the emergency measures it is necessary to prevent the mechanisms responsible for the acute attack from re-establishing themselves either in the affected eye or in the fellow eye. To prevent the pupillary block direct communication must therefore be created between the anterior and posterior chambers by means of a laser iridotomy or a surgical iridectomy. Laser iridotomy is currently the operation of choice: it has been shown to be as effective as surgical iridectomy, but with fewer complications. It can be performed with an argon or Nd:YAG laser. The latter is the type of laser more commonly used owing to its characteristics of comfort and relative harmlessness.

The preferred site of treatment is the upper peripheral area, so that the iridotomy can be covered by the upper eyelid and monocular diplopia and dazzle phenomena can be avoided. Locating the iridotomy in a crypt where the iris is thinner makes it easier to perform the procedure. The treatment is also facilitated by preparation with 2% pilocarpine eye-drops to stretch the iris.

It has been calculated that to prevent pupillary block effectively the iridotomy should have a diameter of at least 150-200 mm. In patients with light-coloured irises 1 to 3 laser pulses with a power of 1-2 mJ will usually be sufficient. With dark irises and/or irises with thick stroma, 2-5 Ng-YAG pulse trains may be necessary up to a total energy of 150 mJ. By eliminating the pupillary block the iridotomy give rise to a widening of the angle and an increase in the peripheral depth of the anterior chamber, but does not substantially alter the central depth of the anterior chamber.

Laser iridotomy often produces a short-lasting increase in IOP due to the release of prostaglandins and other mediators, to disruption of the blood-eye barrier and to the release of iris pigment. The hypertensive peak may be important and even dangerous in those eyes characterised by severe anatomico-functional damage. To prevent this, treatment with 1% apraclonidine eye-drops, administered one hour before and immediately after the laser procedure, has proved effective. Apraclonidine also presents the advantage of being a vasoconstrictor and thus it may reduce the risk of iris bleeding. For the purposes of inhibiting the release of prostaglandins and the rise in IOP, topical NSAIDs (diclofenac) and oral acetazolamide 500 mg, respectively, have been used.

The most frequent complications of Nd-YAG iridotomy are not severe, consisting in microhaemorrhages, iritis, and lens and corneal lesions. Over the long term progressive myopisation and cataract have been demonstrated.

Various studies have demonstrated the short- and long-term efficacy of this parasurgical therapy.

A number of authors prefer to use a a sequential Argon/Nd-YAG laser technique. The aim of this procedure is to reduce bleeding through an initial photocoagulation. A crater is created in the iris stroma with a series of 20 to 80 argon laser spots (power 700-1200 mW, duration 0.1 sec., diameter 50 mm) which can later be easily perforated with a few 1- to 2-mJ Nd-YAG laser pulses. In these cases steroid eye-drops should be used at hourly intervals on the treatment day and four times daily over the following week.

Surgical iridectomy which historically was the first successful surgical intervention performed by von Graefe in 1857 to cure angle-closure glaucoma, may still be necessary in the acute attack phase whenever corneal edema and the condition of the iris make it difficult to perform a laser iridotomy.

Other measures

Alongside the classic treatment described here above, other types of therapy for acute attacks of PACG have been tried.

Corneal Indentation

In patients with thin, flexible irises such as those of Caucasian subjects, corneal indentation with the tip of a cotton-stick applicator or a gonioscopic lens has been proposed to resolve the acute attack. With this mechanical technique, the aqueous humour is pushed into the periphery of the anterior chamber and the pupillary block is reduced by balancing the differential pressure across the iris. Corneal indentation is thus supposed to release the trabeculum and increase the hydrostatic pressure which pushes the aqueous humour outside the eye. In subjects with very dark irises such as those of Asians or in cases of plateau iris corneal indentation is of very limited use. What is more, in the days following the procedure clinically significant corneal edema and marked Descemet membrane folds may be observed in the indentation area, suggesting that this technique may contribute to the damage of the endothelium.

Paracentesis of the Anterior Chamber

During the acute attack a number of authors implemented paracentesis of the anterior chamber when medical treatment may have proved risky, as is the case with the use of mannitol in cardiopathic subjects or in situations of emergency. The procedure proved effective, causing a sharp decrease in IOP which rapidly relieved the patients' symptoms, and was associated with not many risks, similar to those of iridectomy (infections, hemorrhages). According to the authors immediate paracentesis of the anterior chamber would allow earlier execution of Nd-YAG laser iridotomy by reducing the corneal edema.

LASER PERIPHERAL IRIDOPLASTY

Other studies have demonstrated the usefulness of laser peripheral iridoplasty (or gonioplasty) in cases in which the IOP is not controlled after four hours of medical therapy or even as emergency treatment of the acute PACG attack. The aim of this operation is to contract the iris stroma (both peripherally and at the level of the sphincter), which causes it to separate from the trabeculum with consequent opening of the angle. The technique entails the use of an argon laser, which by means of a series of 5 to 10 spots (diameter 500 microns, duration 0.5 sec, power 200-400 mW) in each quadrant, induces a cicatricial iris-retracting reaction. The laser treatment must be preceded by the instillation of 4%

pilocarpine to achieve maximal stretching of the iris and must be followed by the use of topical corticosteroids (1% prednisolone) at hourly intervals on the day of the operation and four times daily over the following 5 to 7 days.

FILTERING SURGERY

The performance of trabeculectomy has proved to be of limited efficacy in the management of acute attacks of PACG unresponsive to pharmacological therapy, owing both to the high operative risk in inflamed and congested eyes and to its possible postoperative complications such as athalamia, hyphema, and early transitory IOP elevation. In a retrospective study conducted in Singapore, only 56.2% of subjects had achieved satisfactory control of IOP without medical therapy after a 22-month follow-up.

Phacoemulsification of the Lens

A number of authors have proposed lens extraction by phacoemulsification for the management of an acute PACG attack. The rationale consists in the fact that by replacing the natural lens with a smaller-sized artificial intraocular lens it is possible to obtain a deepening of the anterior chamber, increased opening of the angle, and the impossibility of pupillary block. To date however no adequate follow-up data are available for this procedure.

Intermittent PACG

Intermittent PACG comprises those forms in which eyes with a narrow angle suffer brief self-limiting episodes of angle closure. The ocular hypertension is generally variable and the subjective and objective symptoms are only moderately severe. After the hypertensive phase has cleared up the eye is completely normal, presenting only its anatomical and biometric characteristics. It is referred to as intermittent PACG precisely because the most typical aspect is angle closure which occurs on an occasional, casual basis.

During the acute phase an angle closure occurs which is only functional and appositional, and therefore reversible, due mainly to pupillary block. However one should not rule out the possibility that other mechanisms may be superimposed such as direct crowding of the angle in cases of plateau iris. During the crisis IOP values may be variable, ranging from a slight increase in pressure to values of above 60 mm Hg. The more extensive the closure of the circumference of the angle the greater will be the IOP level.

The acute intermittent phase manifests itself preferably in poorly lit environments, during the performance of near-vision tasks, and as a result of intense emotional states. In most cases it goes entirely unnoticed. Sometimes an above-normal IOP value may be detected in the course of an eye examination. In less frequent cases, intermittent angle-closure glaucoma presents with more marked, but equally mild subjective symptoms, with transitory blurred vision, coloured haloes, and tenderness of the supraciliary area. The picture lasts only a few hours and clears up spontaneously. The transitory attacks may also repeat themselves over long periods without any residual consequences, but with the major risk of developing into an acute PACG attack. The optic disk cupping encountered in a number of acute attacks is a sign that these were preceded by episodes of intermittent angle closure.

In the intercritical periods, the eye may be entirely normal with normal IOP and well conserved visual acuity. Gonioscopy reveals a narrow but open angle or an angle with goniosynechiae. Perimetry mainly shows mild defects, which are not easy to interpret, or entirely normal findings.

Therapy of intermittent PACG

After a history-taking and clinical assessment based above all on dynamic gonioscopy which detects the pupillary block, the therapy to be advised in these eyes is an Nd-YAG laser iridotomy.

In some patients the closure mechanism is due to episodes of direct crowding of the angle or is of the mixed type. In these cases it is important to add miotic therapy with 0.5% dapiprazole three times daily or with 0.5-1% pilocarpine four times daily so as to prevent potentially dangerous episodes of mydriasis. For these eyes a thermal laser gonioplasty may also be indicated for the purposes of thinning the iris base and widening the angular recess.

We should not forget the possibility that intermittent PACG may develop into the chronic-progressive form, which requires the measures described in the following section.

Chronic PACG

Chronic PACG has a progressive trend. It is due to gradual obliteration of the angle which develops without any very marked symptoms and for this reason may remain undetected or misdiagnosed for a long time. On account of its particular clinical course it is also referred to as creeping glaucoma.

It simulates the course of open-angle glaucoma with which it is often confused if gonioscopy is not performed. It is the most frequent clinical entity in the Asian population and in negroid ethnic groups. Epidemiological studies have revealed that the chronic form is the most frequent among the different variants of PACG.

It generally sets in without presenting any very pronounced signs and with pressure values that are not very high but progressively reach higher levels. In the frank stage, a degree of moderate ocular hypertension sets in, though this tends to be stable and poorly responsive to therapy, with the occasional development of brief hypertensive episodes of greater severity. As time passes, the ocular hypertension persists for longer periods, and the visual field and optic disk deteriorate to a more marked extent, taking on the typical progressive characteristics of closed-angle glaucoma.

This typical trend is the result of the formation of goniosynechiae which spread more extensively, involving the angle to a greater extent. The goniosynechiae generally begin in the narrowest portion of the angle, the upper part, and progress both nasally and temporally. They tend to be fairly continuous and uninterrupted, as can be observed after an acute attack. The pressure increases more markedly when over half the circumference of the angle is occupied. In its natural evolution may be detectable an organic closure of the angle as a result of anatomical fusion and partly a functional closure due to apposition of the iris root to the trabeculum. How one type of closure may predominate over the other can be evaluated by dynamic gonioscopy, which reveals an angle that opens if the closure is predominantly of the appositional type, whereas it reveals an angle that remains closed if the closure is predominantly of the cicatricial type. From the clinical standpoint this form of glaucoma may evolve in two different ways: there may be a superimposed acute attack or a progressive obliteration of the angle with a slow, insidious trend that leads to definitive angle closure.

The diagnosis is based on the subjective symptoms with transitory blurred vision, and episodes of supraciliary headache, or, in the absence of these, evidence of ocular hypertension proves to be the most important finding associated with the typical biometric characteristics and gonioscopic appearances. Without gonioscopy, chronic PACG may easily be mistaken for primary open-angle glaucoma.

Therapy of Chronic PACG

The initial pathogenetic mechanism of chronic PACG is often pupillary block, and therefore it is important to perform an Nd-YAG laser iridotomy in these patients, too. In addition it makes sense to combine this with the continuous administration of a miotic as pilocarpine or to resort to an argon laser iridoplasty in an attempt to stretch the iris and counteract the formation of goniosynechiae. However this therapy is only capable of preventing the pupillary block and the appositional closure of the angle. In chronic PACG, the outflow is usually obstructed by synechiae at the level of the trabeculum, and the measures described here are almost always insufficient to guarantee good pressure control. They should thus be combined with pharmacological therapy that reduces the production of aqueous humour by means of the use of beta-blockers, CAIs and brimonidine, or that increases uveoscleral outflow by means of the use of prostaglandins. In recent years both latanoprost and bimatoprost have proved effective also in this type of glaucoma.

When medical therapy is no longer capable of controlling IOP, surgery must be resorted according to the therapeutic progression habitually adopted in glaucoma: trabeculectomy possibly with antimetabolites, and, should the latter fail, valve implants and cyclophotoablative procedures. In PACG, particularly in the chronic form with diffuse angular synechiae, non-perforating trabecular surgery such as deep sclerectomy and viscocanalostomy is not indicated.

When medical therapy was no longer sufficient, the surgical intervention known as goniosynechialysis was also used combined with phacoemulsification and/or laser peripheral iridoplasty for the purposes of re-opening the aqueous humour outflow route. All these procedures proved useful, with success rates even higher than 90%, but no significant difference in efficacy emerged between them. Lastly, it should be recalled that we must distinguish between chronic PACG, with a progressive development, and so-called chronicised PACG. The latter form of the disease usually follows an unresolved acute attack in which the angle remains completely closed; in this case the closure is irreversible and the IOP stably high. Chronicised PACG requires surgical measures (filtering operations with antimetabolites and possibly subsequent valve implants and cyclophotoablative treatments), though it generally remains a disease characterized by a poor prognosis,.

Chronicized PACG

This is the phase that follows an unresolved acute attack of PACG, which leads to complete closure of the angle owing to the presence of goniosynechiae.

In cases of partially regressed acute angle closure large goniosynechiae are usually formed mainly in both the upper and lower sectors and are characteristically associated with the symptom triad consisting of Glaukomflecken, areas of iris atrophy and deposition of pigment on the surfaces that delimit the anterior chamber. The ocular hypertension is stable, the visual field is damaged and the optic nerve shows the cupping of the chronic form.

Sometimes after an iridotomy may persist residual hypertension due to the slow progression of the goniosynechiae which extend the angle closure.

In the most unfavourable cases the acute attack does not regress, but develops towards the phase with stable hypertension due to an angle which is completely closed. IOP values are above 30 mmHg, conjunctival hyperemia persists for a long time, the cornea is clouded due to the bullous epitheliopathy, the iris shows areas of atrophy, the pupil is in medium mydriasis, the pupillary synechiae are well established and the lens opacities rapidly develop into a frank cataract. The patient complains about periocular pain which may be continuous and severe. This picture, if not treated, inevitably evolves towards absolute glaucoma characterized by the lack of perception of light and by a congested eye.

Therapy of Chronicized PACG

The therapy based on iridotomy (if one has not already been performed) and on usual medical agents (miotic, CAIs, beta-blocker, alfa-2-agonist and prostaglandins) is very often insufficient. It proves necessary to resort to surgical therapy with a filtering operation, usually combined with lens extraction. In cases of absolute glaucoma, in which there is no residual function, cyclodestruction techniques are implemented or alcohol injection of the ciliary ganglion to reduce the pain.

Asymptomatic Narrow Angle (Eye at Risk of PACG)

Asymptomatic narrow angle is referred to as "eye at risk" and consists in a situation presenting a narrow angle in the absence of any signs of glaucoma. Rather than denoting an objective finding, it indicates the risk that the angle may close on the basis of the assessment made by the ophthalmologist, who has to decide whether to implement therapy or not.

The eye at risk is characterized by: i) absence of disease with normal ocular functions; ii) biometric factors characteristic of PACG with a shallow anterior chamber and a narrow angle.

The assessment of the occludability of the angle may vary from one observer to another. The angles that are most likely to close are those with an amplitude of less than 20°, and therefore are angles 0, 1 and 2 according to Shaffer classification, angles IV, III and II according to Scheie classification and the narrow and closed angles according to Spaeth. Another method for identifying narrow angles is the Van Herick method, whereby grade 0, 1 and 2 angles are assessed as occludable.

Asymptomatic narrow angle is a frequent finding in the normal population, but only a minimal proportion of people with this condition will develop a form of angle-closure glaucoma. Epidemiological studies have revealed that the prevalence of grade 0, 1, and 2 angles is 19% and grade 0 and 1 angles is 3% according to Van Herick. Contrasting with these relatively high percentages is the finding that the prevalence of PACG in the population is only 0.6%.

Therapy of Asymptomatic Narrow Angle

In cases of narrow angle which are asymptomatic, but potentially occludable and without any sign of anatomico-functional damage, the decision whether to implement treatment or not is difficult. In these cases dynamic gonioscopy proves to be a method for identifying eyes at risk. According to Mapstone, therapy is not necessary since the likelihood that a narrow angle will give rise to angle-closure glaucoma is very low. Spaeth on the other hand suggests that it is right to implement antiglaucoma therapy in patients with a long life expectancy, in those who are distinctly unreliable, and in those who are unable to attend regularly for check-ups.

It is not regarded as sound practice to use provocation tests results as a basis for obtaining indications as to the advisability of initiating therapy. These tests are dangerous and create situations which are not easily controllable and not sufficiently predictive to justify the therapeutic decision. It has been established that 40% of subjects with negative phenylephrine-pilocarpine tests develop a form of angle-closure glaucoma within 10 years.

To obtain reliable information regarding the advisability of implementing antiglaucoma therapy we can base the decision on practical indicators that emerge during examination of the patient. These indicators are clinical and biometric criteria.

These indicators, if present in combination, may condition the ophthalmologist's clinical and therapeutic judgement. Nevertheless it is still no clear in what percentage and with what probability these eyes will develop a form of PACG and this subject remains a source of controversy. Iridotomy is capable of reducing the onset of PACG, but not of eliminating it, whereas we should bear in mind the potential risks it involves and its cataractogenic effect. A number of authors believe that the risks - low but well established - and the costs of prophylactic treatment are not acceptable, in view of the fact that the potential benefits are still not clearly quantifiable.

The problem remains as to what approach to adopt in cases of asymptomatic narrow angle. However in cases of transitory, repeated episodes of possible angle closure marked by tenderness of the eye and supraciliary area, blurred vision, coloured haloes, significant biometric predisposition (anterior chamber depth £ 1.5 mm, high lens/axial length factor) and positive familiarity for PACG, it is important to implement prophylactic measure based essentially on Nd-YAG laser iridotomy and follow-up.

PACG without Pupillary Block

As mentioned earlier in the section on pathogenetic mechanisms, the most common form of PACG is due to pupillary block, which is resolved with Nd-YAG laser iridotomy. There are however eyes in which the angle closes as the result of different mechanisms. The most typical form of PACG without pupillary block is due to direct crowding of the chamber angle, as occurring characteristically in plateau iris. In the pure form of plateau iris, iridotomy is ineffective and is not indicated. In these eyes the peripheral iris collects during mydriasis and occupies the angle obstructing it. The aim of therapy in such cases is therefore to prevent mydriasis, for which less potent miotics can be used such as 0.5% dapiprazole three times daily, 0.5-1% pilocarpine four times daily, or 2% aceclidine three times daily.

Aceclidine is a direct activator of the muscarinic receptors, induces less accommodation spasm than pilocarpine and may be therefore better tolerated in young subjects.

Table 3: Clinical criteria indicating possible closure of the angle
• History: positive familiarity, supraciliary tenderness, blurred vision, coloured haloes
• Objective findings: dystrophy of the iris, lens opacities
• Fellow eye assessment
• Gonioscopy: angle amplitude, goniosynechiae, dynamic gonioscopy

Table 4: Biometric criteria indicating possible closure of the chamber angle
• Central anterior chamber depth < 1.5 mm
• Central anterior chamber depth < 2 mm + Van Herick grade 0-1
• Increased lens thickness (> 5 mm)
• Increased lens/axial length factor (> 2.1 mm)

Dapiprazole is an alpha-blocker and, unlike pilocarpine, has no effect on accommodation; it does not reduce the depth of the anterior chamber and does not give rise to vasoconstriction. Dapiprazole induces miosis indirectly by blocking the iris dilator muscle and causing the iris constrictor muscle to prevail; the miosis is thus less marked than that induced by the parasympathicomimetics which directly activate the iris constrictor muscle.

As an alternative to miotic drugs, or in combination with them, an argon laser peripheral iridoplasty can be performed in eyes with a plateau iris so as to produce a thinning of the iris root and widen the angular recess.

However in clinical practice it is not so rare to encounter iris-angle configurations with characteristics which are intermediate between those of pupillary block and those of a plateau iris, and in which both closure mechanisms may be operative. In these eyes, the execution of an Nd-YAG laser iridotomy is justified, but cannot be sufficient and curative and requires the support of miotic therapy and follow-up. Lastly, it should be recalled that PACG without pupillary block can also present clinically in the form of intermittent episodes and/or develop into the chronic-progressive form.

10

Malignant Glaucoma

V Velayutham (India)

INTRODUCTION

Malignant glaucoma is a rare but a serious glaucoma responsible for the loss of one or both the eyes. This was first described by von Graefe in 1969.

Malignant glaucoma occurs immediately after glaucoma surgery especially in primary angle-closure glaucoma (PACG) with flat anterior chamber, also can occur after cataract or any intraocular surgery or anterior segment laser surgery or even rarely in nonoperated eyes, also it can occur either in phakic, aphakic or pseudophakic.

Synonyms

Ciliary block glaucoma, direct lens block, aqueous misdirection syndrome and ciliovitreolenticular block.

Definition

The term malignant glaucoma is used here as von Graefe used it to identify a specific type of glaucoma which is a postoperative shallowing or flattening of anterior chamber with increased IOP and not responding to conventional treatment. The term "malignant" glaucoma indicates the difficulty with which it responds to conventional therapy and does not imply malignancy in sense of neoplastic disease, hence Welss and Shaffer have suggested the term ciliary block glaucoma in order to direct the attention of the clinician to the region of ciliary body.

The present concept has been expanded to include several clinical conditions that share the following features (i) shallow/flat anterior chamber (AC) – both at the center and periphery (ii) raised IOP (iii) therapeutic response to mydriatic-cycloplegic and (iv) non/adverse response to miotics.

So, malignant glaucoma is not a single disease entity.

Clinical Importance

Malignant glaucoma poses the following problems :

- Difficulty in early recognition.
- Maximum medical therapy for the affected eye is not often instituted early enough or effective.
- Difficulty in starting prompt prophylaxis for fellow eye.
- Difficulty in surgical management.

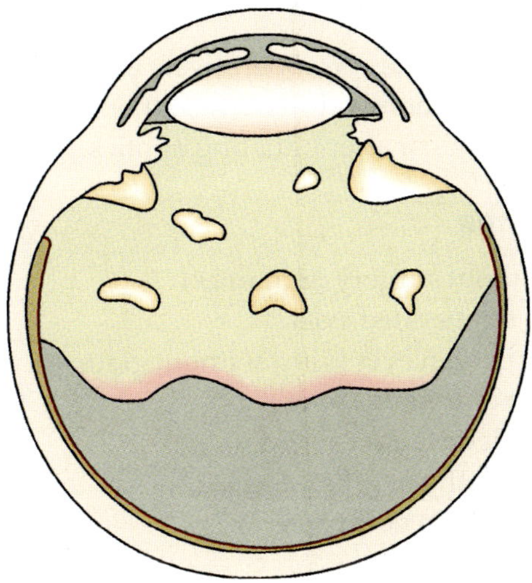

Fig. 1: Malignant glaucoma in phakic eye (Fluid is trapped in or behind the vitreous body)

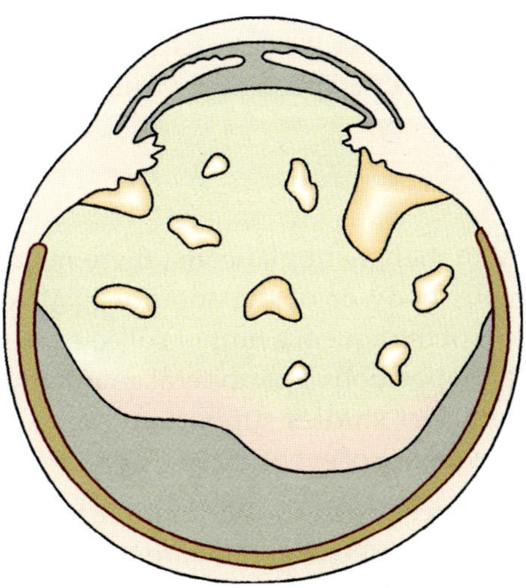

Fig. 2: Malignant glaucoma in an aphakic eye

Onset

Malignant glaucoma can occur intraoperatively or any time following surgery (days, weeks, sometimes months to year) – either occurs after discontinuing postoperative cycloplegics or after initiating miotics.

Other Clinical Forms

- Spontaneous (without surgery or miotics)
- Use of miotics in unoperated eyes
- After cataract surgery in eyes with/without glaucoma
- Following trauma or inflammation
- Following retinal detachment surgery
- In eyes with retinopathy of prematurity
- After central retinal vein occlusion.

Pathophysiology

Shaffer's Hypothesis

According to this hypothesis aqueous humor is diverted posteriorly into, behind or beside the vitreous cavity. Relative block to the anterior movement of aqueous humor near the junction of ciliary process, lens equator, and anterior vitreous face causes aqueous to be diverted posteriorly. This is supported by the success of Chandler's vitreous surgery.

Grant's Hypothesis

Grant speculated that in malignant glaucoma there may be a decrease in the permeability to vitreous body or of the anterior hyaloids membrane cause decreased anterior flow of the aqueous humor collected besides and behind the vitreous gel leading to opposition of peripheral anterior hyaloids to the ciliary body. Epstein et al and Flat studies supported grant's speculation. Angley postulated following sequence of events.

- An event occurs that increase the posterior force to the vitreous gel.
- Fluid flow through the vitreous gel towards AC at an increased rate but some compaction of gel occurs.
- Because of dehydration of gel fluid conductivity is decreased.
- The compressed vitreous gel moves forwards leading to shallow AC.

Certain anatomical features have been regularly observed in the region of ciliary processes,lens equator, the anterior face.

- The tips of the ciliary processes may touch the lens.
- The ciliary processes are frequently rotated anteriorly.
- Their tips are flattened against the lens.
- Ciliary processes may get firmly adherent to the lens
- Vitreous face is abnormally forward.

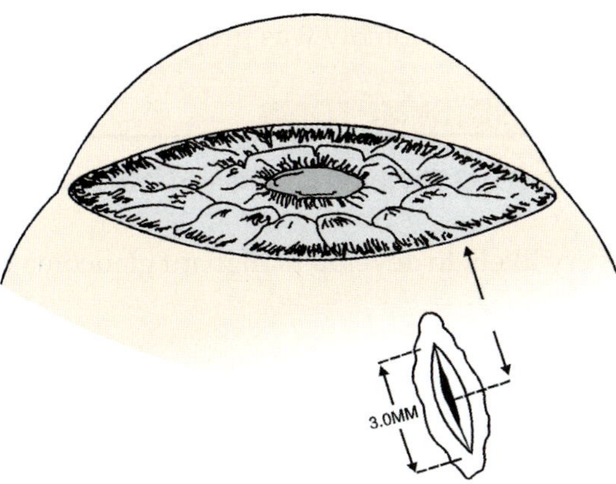

Fig. 3: Size of the Sclerotomy incision and its distance from the limbus

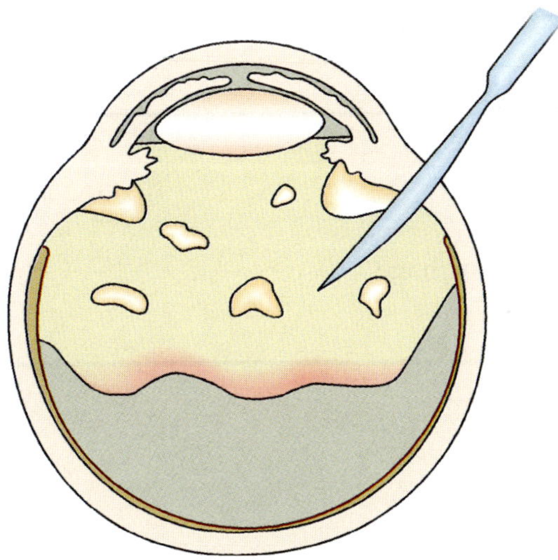

Fig. 4: Sclerotomy technique

Thus a congenital structural anomaly was proposed to cause the condition.

CLINICAL SIGNS AND SYMPTOMS

- Flat AC in the presence of patent PI with raised IOP resistant to conventional therapy.
- Fellow eye is very likely to develop malignant glaucoma following similar surgery.

Predisposition

Malignant glaucoma is likely to occur in

- Eyes whose AC becomes markedly shallow with miotics application and deeper with cycloplegics
- Eyes with chronic angle-closure glaucoma.

Malignant glaucoma is unlikely to occur.

- If IOP can be normalized with miotics before surgery
- If the eye is normotensive at the time of surgery.

DIFFERENTIAL DIAGNOSIS

- Choroidal separation
- Pupillary block
- Iridovitreal block
- Suprachoroidal hemorrhage.

INVESTIGATIONS

- Direct ophthalmoscopy.
- Tonometry
- Gonioscopy
- Perimetry

MANAGEMENT

Medical Therapy

- Argon laser treatment of ciliary processes.
- Nd : YAG laser hyaloidotomy.

Surgical Therapy

- Manual technique Chandler's three step (surgical confirmation procedure).
- Automated technique.

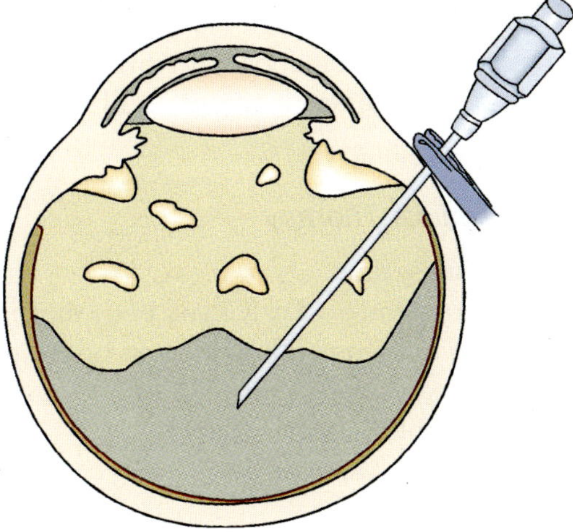

Fig. 5: Sclerotomy Technique: An 18 gauge needle with a hemostate gaurd is inserted 12 mm from the needle point. 1.0 – 1.5 ml of vitreous is aspirated

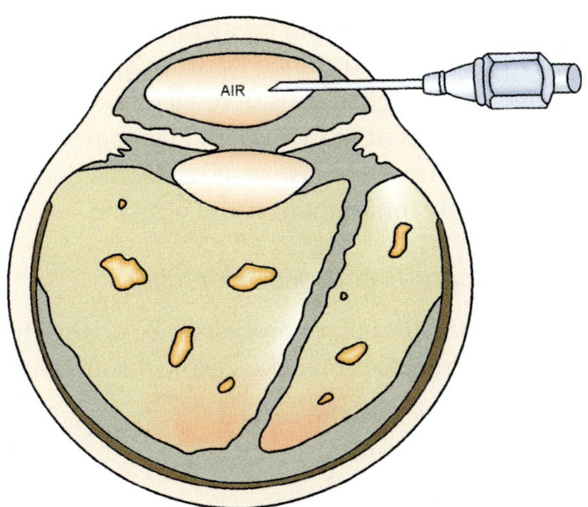

Fig. 6: Sclerotomy technique air bubble is placed in the anterior chamber to deepen it

Medical Therapy

Mydriatic cycloplegic drugs in combination with carbonic anhydrase inhibitors, hyperosmotic agents, beta adrenergic agents will help in decreasing the intraocular pressure.

Optimal Regimen of Medical Therapy

- 1 percent Atropine 4 times/day
- 10 percent phenylephrine 4 times/day (Ciliary body moves posteriorly away from the angle, zonules tightens pulling the lens posteriorly)
- 0.5 percent Timolol maleate drops 2 times/day.
- Acetazolamide 500 mg tablets 2 times/day.
- Hypersmotic agents every 12 hours.
- Oral glycerol 50 percent, and
- Intravenous 20 percent Mannitol 2 gm (10 ml) / kg.

Any one of the medication should be reduced in concentration or discontinued if the patient shows intolerance. When no contraindication exists the entire regimen is given for five days.

If the condition is relieved, the regimen is gradually tapered and discontinued over several days. Hypersmotic agents are discontinued first and then carbonic anhydrase inhibitors, mydriatic (phenylepinephrine) and and timolol drugs are stopped, but the cycloplegic (atropine 1%) drops are continued indefinitely. This treatment regimen must not be considered a failure until it has been tried for 4 to 5 days. About 50 percent of malignant glaucomas are relieved within this interval. To prevent recurrences, use of oral prednisolone 30 mg qid is also useful to relieve ciliary body inflammation and effusion.

Argon Treatment of Ciliary Processes (Herscher)

Argon laser is used to shrink the ciliary processes. To do this the media must be clear and visible. Ciliary processes must be visible through iridectomy.

- Laser beam is applied through the cornea.
- Topical glycerin may be required.
- The power used is 100 to 300 mW
- The duration of radiation is 0.1 to 0.25 second
- Spot size varies from 50 to 100 mm.

Laser shrinkage of two or four processes is usually required. Pre and Post-laser medical regimen is required.

Nd: YAG Laser Hyaloidotomy (Epstien)

Nd : YAG laser hyaloidotomy is to disrupt the anterior vitreous face in malignant glaucoma in aphakia and pseudophakia – which relieves the entrapment of aqueous within the vitreous.

Incisional Surgery

In 1964 Chandler devised a simple technique involving puncture and aspiration of the vitreous with removal of the lens.

CHANDLER'S THREE-STEP SURGICAL CONFIRMATION PROCEDURE

Manual Technique

Step 1: Confirmation of Communication between

Posterior and Anterior Chamber

The anterior segment is examined carefully for the presence of a patent iridectomy. If it is doubtful a laser iridectomy is performed failing which an incisional peripheral iridectomy should be done to rule out pupillary block. If there is a pupillary block aqueous will be released from posterior chamber to anterior chamber after this procedure. So, anterior chamber deepens and the procedure is terminated. If anterior chamber remains flat the surgeon must proceed with the steps below.

Step 2: Sclerotomy to Confirm Absence of Suprachoroidal Fluid or Blood

With the modern ultrasound suprachoroidal fluid can be documented. However when this is not possible or when in doubt the following confirmation is considered.

A beveled incision is made in the peripheral cornea with a Wheeler's knife or a similar instrument to allow access to the anterior chamber for later injection of fluid and air. The incision is made in the periphery of the cornea roughly parallel to the limbus. This incision should be tested to ensure that easy access with a cannula can be obtained. Later, access to the anterior chamber through the wound will be more difficult, when the eye is hypotonus.

At the sites chosen for sclerotomies, conjunctiva and Tenon's capsule should be incised with a radial incision, which is less traumatic and more convenient than a circumferential one. Usually a site away from the area of the previous ocular surgery is chosen (i.e. both the lower quadrants). A radial incision through the sclera to the suprachoroidal space, about 3 mm in length behind the external limbus is then made in both quadrants. The incision should not be placed more posteriorly. The center of the incision must be 3.5 mm from the limbus.

When sclerotomies are made in case of malignant glaucoma, no fluid will be present in the suprachoroidal space. If straw colored fluid is found in the suprachoroidal space, the diagnosis suprachoroidal separation for which the fluid should be drained completely from the suprachoroidal space. The anterior chamber is deepened through the corneal incision with balanced salt solution (BSS), viscoelastic or air. The conjunctival incision is closed. The sclerotomy wounds are not sutured, hoping that any future fluid in the suprachoroidal space will drain spontaneously.

If suprachoroidal hemorrhage is present, blood (or) blood mixed with suprachoroidal fluid will be found and is drained. Anterior chamber reformed with saline and conjunctival incision closed. The sclerotomy wounds should not be sutured.

If no fluid flows through the sclerotomies, a smooth spatula (cyclodialysis spatula) should be passed circumferentially through the lips of the sclerotomy into the suprachoroidal space parallel to the limbus. Sometimes, loculated fluid (or) blood present does not flow freely until this maneuver is performed.

If an iridectomy has been done and yet the anterior chamber remains shallow (or) flat, and if the sclerotomies into the suprachoroidal space did not show fluid (or) blood, the diagnosis of malignant glaucoma is established.

The operation of choice for malignant glaucoma is Chandler's deep vitreous surgery. This is performed using the paracentesis entry into the anterior chamber and sclerotomies made for suprachoroidal drainage without making additional incisions on the globe.

Next a Wheeler's knife (or) a long, thin vitreous blade is plunged into the vitreous cavity to a depth of about 10 mm through the ciliary body. The knife is aimed towards the optic nerve to avoid damage to the lens. The wound in the uvea is enlarged slightly anteriorly and posteriorly to a length, in radial direction of about 3 mm with its center 3.5 mm behind the external limbus.

A hemostat is placed around the shaft of an 18-G needle 12 mm behind the tip of prevent excessively deep penetration into the globe. The needle is passed into the vitreous cavity towards the optic nerve. The tip of needle is moved back and forth in an area of about 4 mm to allow slight separation of the vitreous membranes in its path. Then a syringe is attached to the base of the needle (5 mm Leur-Lock syringe) and maintaining the position of the needle in one hand, 1 to 1.5 ml of fluid is aspirated using the other hand. The material obtained may be water-like fluid, fluid vitreous (or) vitreous.

Before the needle is withdrawn from the eye 0.25 ml of aspirated fluid is reinjected into the eye to clear the tip of the needle of any vitreous strand engaged within its lumen.

The needle is then carefully withdrawn from the eye exactly along its path of entry. At this point the eye will be hypotonus markedly. A small amount of BSS is injected into anterior chamber to partially restore the shape of configuration of the globe. It is important that the eye should not be completely filled with BSS because in some cases the fluid will flow posteriorly into and behind the vitreous cavity and recreate the original malignant glaucoma. A large air- bubble is injected into the anterior chamber to force the iris and lens posteriorly.

Automated Technique

In this modified approach instead of needle aspiration, an automated vitreous suction cutter is used to remove fluid and vitreous. Then needle is removed and a suction cutter without infusion is inserted through needle track into the vitreous cavity to remove fluid and / or formed vitreous.

PARS PLANA VITRECTOMY WITH AUTOMATED INFUSION SUCTION INSTRUMENTATION

The above vitrectomy is not necessary to relieve malignant glaucoma and can be more traumatic to the external ocular tissues, existing filtration blebs and conjunctiva. Since the eyes often have hazy anterior segments, the visualization for vitrectomy will be poor. If the malignant glaucoma does not respond after two trials of medical therapy and two trials of Chandler's procedure, the use of pars plana vitrectomy should be strongly considered.

FELLOW EYE

- Miotics to be avoided
- Full thickness peripheral iridectomy by laser is preferred.
- Postlaser mydriatics with cycloplegics to be used.
- Avoid surgery if possible
- Deliberate cut in the anterior hyloid face and aspiration of vitreous during filtering procedure.
- In very shallow-chambered eye primary lens extraction with anterior vitrectomy is the safest procedure.

11

Traumatic Glaucoma

V Velayutham (India)

INTRODUCTION

Trauma to the eye leads a chain of various complications, of this one dreadful but often overlooked complication is raised intraocular pressure (IOP).

ETIOPATHOGENESIS

Glaucoma in traumatic eyes can occur in the early post-traumatic period or late depending on the cause of raised IOP. Glaucoma may be either open angle or closed angle. The onset may be acute or insidious

Mechanisms of Raised IOP in Penetrating Injuries

Penetrating injuries can include elevated IOP through various mechanisms, these include:

- Flat anterior chamber with formation of peripheral anterior synechiae
- Inflammation
- Intraocular hemorrhage including hyphema and ghost cell glaucoma
- Lens swelling with pupillary block
- Lens subluxation with pupillary block
- Lens-particle glaucoma
- Vitreous filling anterior chamber
- Phaco anaphylaxis
- Posterior synechiae with pupillary block
- Epithelial downgrowth
- Fibrous ingrowth
- Retained intraocular foreign body
  (a) Organic - Inflammatory Glaucoma
  (b) Iron - Siderosis
  (c) Copper - Chalcosis

Mechanisms of Raised IOP in Contusion Injuries

- Trauma to the trabecular meshwork
- Inflammation
- Hyphema
- Lens swelling with pupillary block
- Lens subluxation with pupillary block

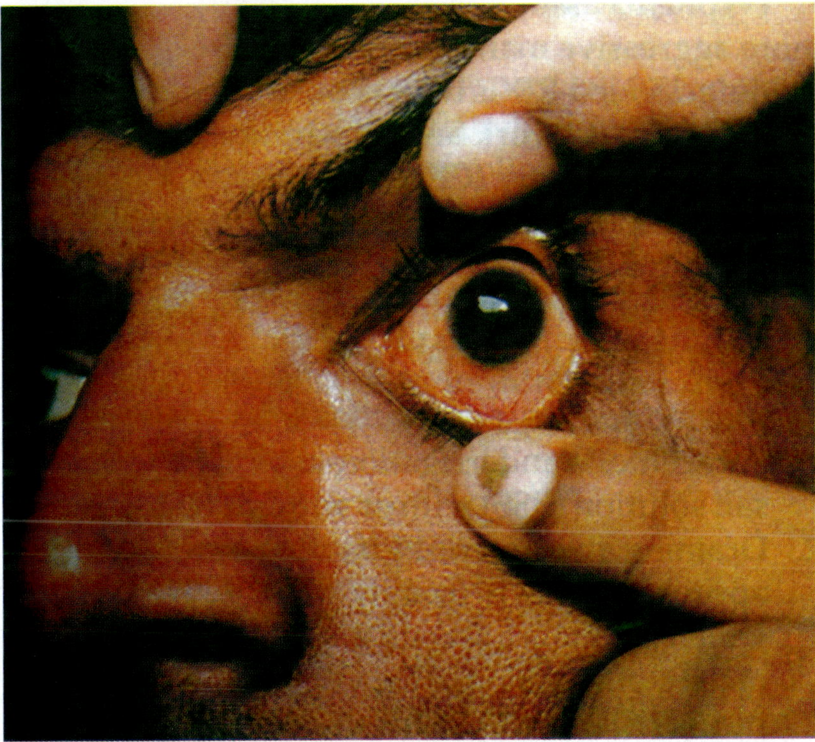

Fig. 1: Traumatic hyphema

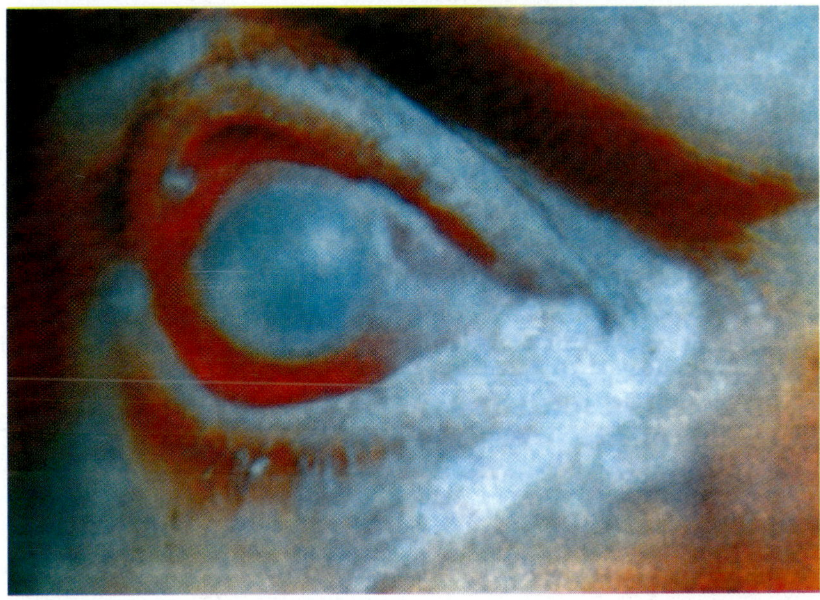

Fig. 2: Anterior dislocation of cataractous lens

- Angle recession
- Ghost cell glaucoma and hemolytic glaucoma
- Peripheral anterior synechiae following trabecular tear
- Posterior synechiae with pupillary block
- Vitreous filling the anterior chamber
- Uveal effusion and angle closure (rarely)
- Neovascular glaucoma.

Mechanism of Raised IOP Following Chemical Injuries

Early phase : IOP elevation in the early phase is caused by scleral shrinkage and release of active substance including prostaglandins which increase the uveal blood flow.

Intermediate Phase : IOP elevation is usually caused by inflammation, pupillary block by posterior synechiae or acute swelling of the lens which may also cause rise in IOP.

Late phase : IOP elevation is usually cused by trabecular damage and formation of peripheral anterior synechiae.

ELECTRIC SHOCK

Transient elevation of IOP is noted after electrical injury, cardioversion and electrical shock therapy. It is due to venous dilation and contraction of extraocular muscles and pigment dispersion.

RADIATION

Radiation can cause elevated IOP through a variety of mechanisms, including neovascularization, open-angle glaucoma (OAG) associated with diffuse conjunctival telangiectasia, and ghost cell glaucoma associated with radiation retinopathy and vitreous hemorrhage.

THERMAL BURNS

Rarely produce rise in IOP by orbital congestion and massive periorbital swelling.

CAUSES OF OPEN ANGLE GLAUCOMA FOLLOWING TRAUMA

Early Causes

Hyphema "Blood in AC"

Blunt trauma to the eye can be associated with anterior segment injuries, including hyphema, iris sphincter tear, iridodialysis, cyclodialysis, trabecular tear, inflammation and zonular rupture and lens subluxation.

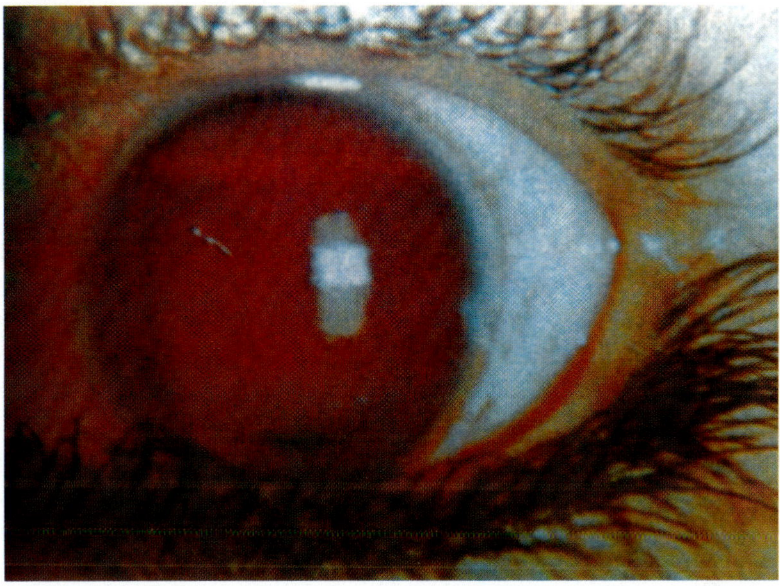

Fig. 3: Total hyphema

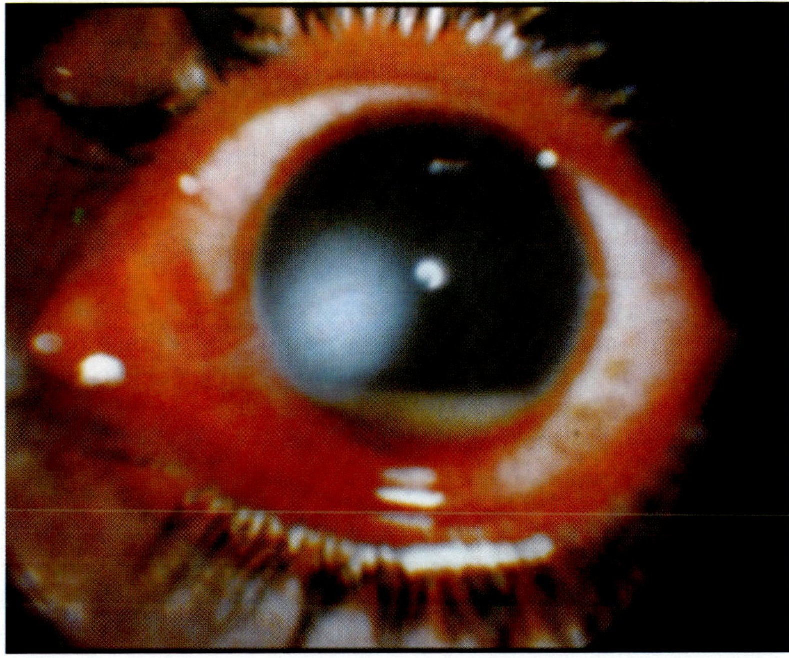

Fig. 4: Anterior Uveitis with hypopyon

PATHOPHYSIOLOGY OF BLUNT INJURY

Blunt injury caused by object small enough or sufficiently deformable to fit inside in the rim of the orbit in order to strike the globe and indent the anterior surface of the eye. This causes stretching of the limbal tissue, equatorial scleral expansion, posterior and peripheral movement of the aqueous, posterior displacement of the lens, iris, diaphragm, and acute rise in IOP.

All these cause tearing of the tissues near AC angle, 90 percent of hyphema is from tear in the anterior phase of the ciliary body.

The usual source of bleeding is a tear in the phase of the ciliary body between the longitudinal and circular fibers which leads to disruption of branches of major arterial circle causing bleeding into the AC (also from recurrent choroidal arteries or ciliary body vein's).

In small percentage of causes the bleeding is from rupture iris vessels, cyclodialysis or iridodialysis. As the IOP rises bleeding diminishes and a clot forms. Clot lysis and retraction occur 1 to 2 days after the injury and maximal incidence of rebleeding from the injured vessels occurs at this time. The rebleed is often more severe than the initial episode can lead to a total hyphema, also known as "a black ball" or eight ball hyphema. Unlike the typical initial bleeding episode total hyphema is initially associated with extreme pain, nausea and other symptoms related to acute glaucoma.

PATHOPHYSIOLOGY IN PENETRATING INJURY

Direct damage to the vessels or rarely to sudden chop in IOP.

The mechanism of raised IOP is mechanical obstruction of the trabecular meshwork by red blood cells, blood products and some time pupillary block may occur. Typical black appearance of the anterior chamber is probably caused by the deoxygenated hemoglobin.

Late raise in IOP is due to descemetization and fibrosis of angle, hemosiderosis, ghost cell glaucoma and angle recession. It can develop weeks to year after the initial insult. Patient with sickling hemoglobinopathies develop glaucoma following a small hyphema. Since obstruction in the outflow is increased by sickling of RBCs. At least 50 percent of the patient who have rebleeding have glaucoma.

COURSE OF HYPHEMA

Bleeding stops by IOP tamponade, vascular spasm, formation of fibrin or platelet clot. Maximum integrity of the clot occurs between 4-7 days. Main pathway out of anterior chamber is trabecular meshwork for degraded products. Incidence of secondary hemorrhage or rebleeding is 3.8 to 38 percent mostly occurs in 2 to 5 days, nearly all occur before 7th day.

Pathology of rebleeding is fibrinolysis and clot retraction or bleeding from fragile new capillaries.

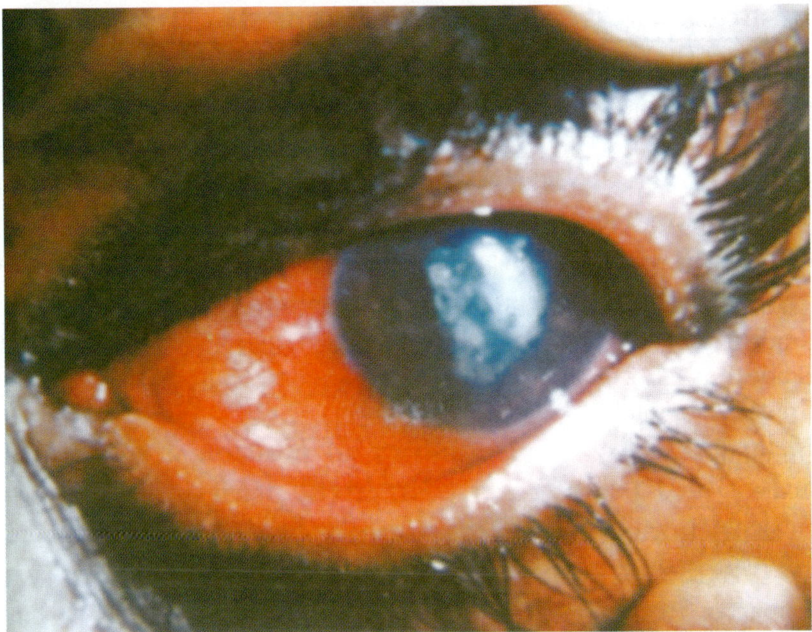

Fig. 5: Lens particle glaucoma

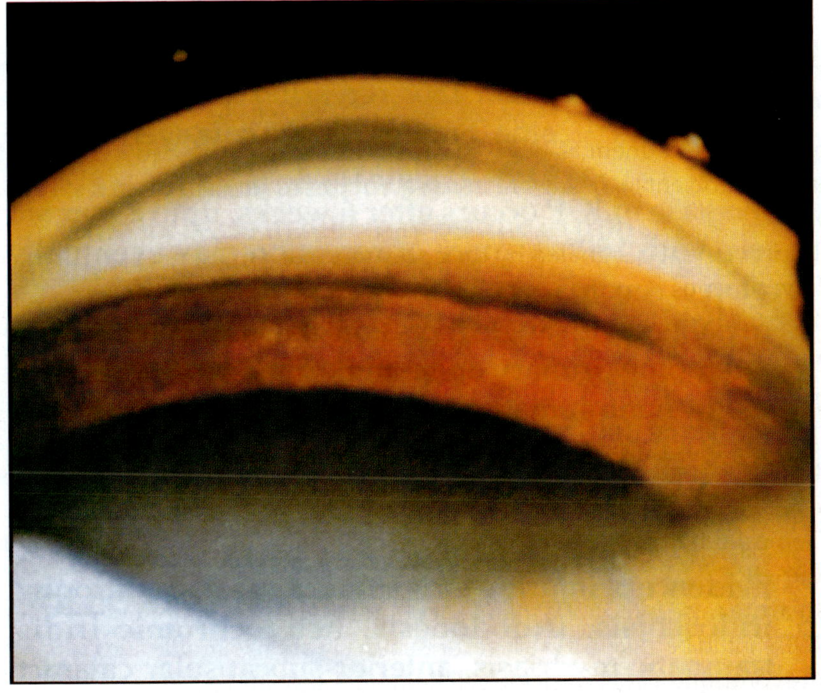

Fig. 6: Angle recession

CLASSIFICATION OF TRAUMATIC HYPHEMA

According to

Type of hemorrhage:

- Primary
- Secondary
- Continuous
- Volume (Microscopic) - No layered blood, only circulating RBC.

Grade I - < 1/3 of the anterior chamber
Grade II - 1/3 – 1/2 of anterior chamber
Grade III - 1/2 of anterior chamber
Grade IV - total

Duration

Acute - 1-7 days
Subacute - 7-14 days
Chronic - 14 days

Character

Liquid - Red
Clotted - Brown or black or mixed
Organized - Tan gray or white.

Management

Medical Management

Conservative treatment of elevated IOP- drugs that reduce aqueous formation resulting sufficient lowering of the pressure so as to allow gradual resorption of hyphema.

Improvement is signaled by the appearance of a mixture of brighter blood and the aqueous near the upper limbus.

If no further rebleeding occurs, total resorption of the residual blood usually occurs in 5 to 7 days.

1. Pad and bandage to protect from further injury.
2. Topical cycloplegics to relieve ciliary spasm prevent posterior synechia and to view the posterior segment. Topical steroids to reduce significant anterior chamber inflammation.
3. Topical β-blockers, and systemic carbonic anhydrase inhibitors to reduce the IOP.
4. In acute raise in IOP, IV mannitol or oral glycerol monitor every 12 hours. IOP should be lowered to a level of 24 mm Hg acetazolamide and epinephrine are contraindicated in sickle cell hemoglobinopathies.
5. Aspirin and other nonsteroidal anti-inflammatory drugs (NSAIDs) are avoided.

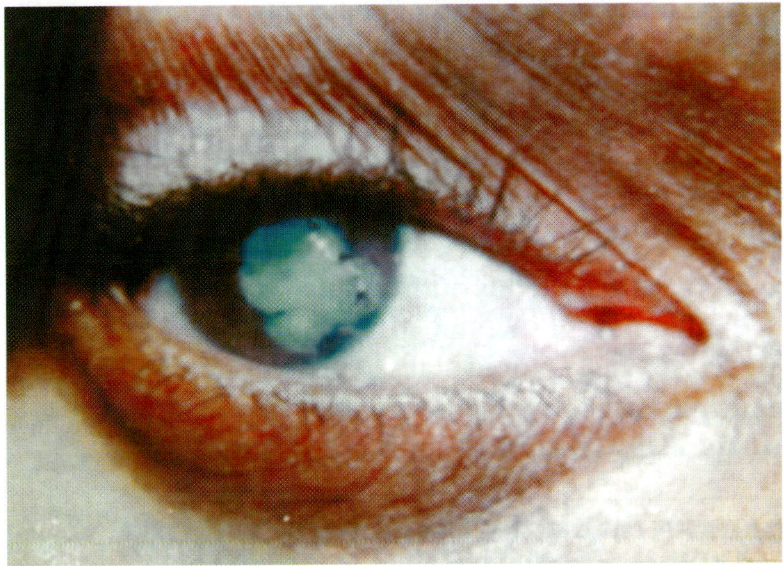

Fig. 7: Traumatic cataract

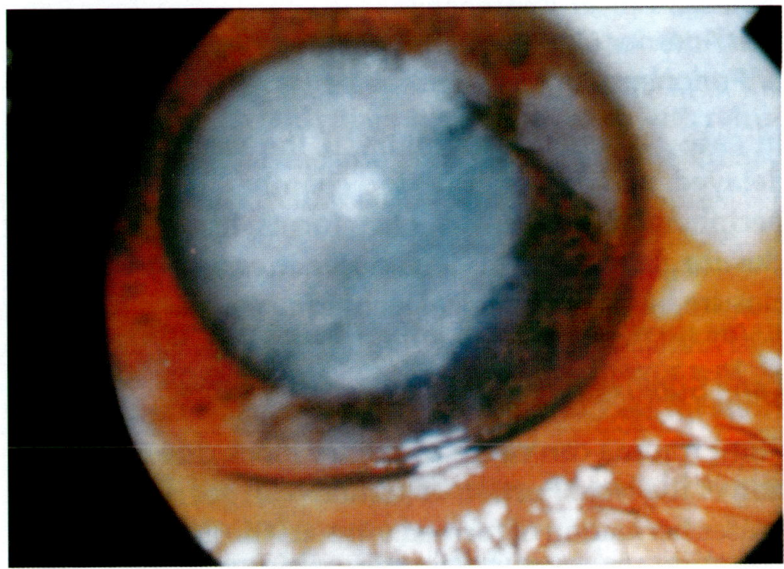

Fig. 8: Corneal tear with lens matter in AC

6. Aminocarproic acid : Oral antifibrinolytic agent dose 50 mg/kg body weight every 4 hours for 5 days upto 30 gm per day (or) tranexamic acid—oral antifibrinolytic agent.
7. Intracameral tissue plasminogen activator.

Surgical Management

The optimal time and method of surgical intervention for medically unresponsive cases is often debated subject. For fear of rebleeding early intervention should be avoided. A significant number of cases will resolve spontaneously in 3 to 5 days.

Total removal of the clot is unnecessary for resolution of glaucoma and also exposes increased risk of rehemorrhage and loss of uveal tissue which may adhere to the clot.

Hyphema associated with sickle cell disease requires more aggressive management, because of sludging and sickling, sickled RBCs have more difficulty in trevarsing trabecular meshwork and in addition increased risk of central retinal artery (CRA) occlusion.

Severe and unremitting pain and early blood staining of the cornea warrant surgical intervention, similarly uncontrolled IOP large or total hyphema of more than 10 days require surgical intervention.

Suggested Surgical Approaches

1. Paracentesis and irrigation-aspiration with balanced salt solution (BSS) with or without fibrinolytic agents.
2. Draining the anterior chamber via trabeculectomy approach. This is usually done with a paracentesis which facilitate a second entry site for later irrigation of the clot, injection of the viscoelastic agent to extrude the resistant clot. This trabeculectomy approach achieves the goal of reduction in IOP and clot removal and no recurrence of hemorrhage.
3. Automated hyphemectomy "aspiration with emulsification or vitrectomy type of instrument". If indicated a filtering procedure may be combined.

INFLAMMATION

Inflammation by trauma can produce glaucoma through a variety of mechanisms including :

- Increased viscosity of aqueous humor.
- Obstruction of the trabecular meshwork by inflammatory cells and debris.
- Swelling and dysfunction of the trabecular meshwork.
- Liberation of active substances such as prostaglandins and substance P.

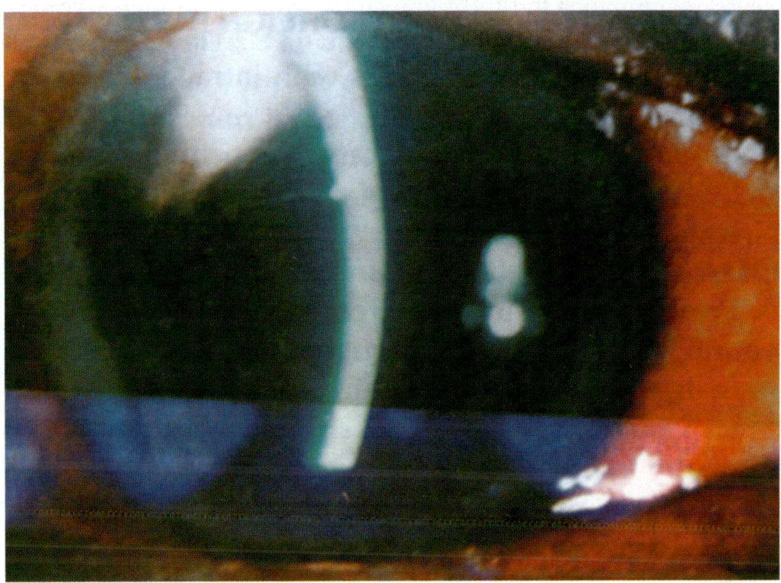

Fig. 9: Epithelial in growth

In acute inflammation the IOP is low due to reduction in aqueous production, but later the production normalizes but the outflow facility remains low thereby increasing the IOP.

Treatment with topical cycloplegics and steroids, usually helps to resolve the inflammation and decrease the IOP. Systemic steroids employed with possible adverse side affects must be accepted. Rarely a retinal detachment related to traumatic retinal dialysis causes inflammatory changes in the anterior segment leading on to increased IOP after several months. Though rare it is an important consideration in differential diagnosis since surgical treatment can cure this rare type of glaucoma.

LENS PARTICLE GLAUCOMA

Disruption of the lens capsule by penetrating trauma liberates lens material which can obstruct the trabecular meshwork. The resulting glaucoma depends on the amount of lens material liberated, the inflammatory response of the eye and the ability of the trabecular meshwork to clear the foreign matter.

If tension is not relieved, surgical intervention should be considered.

Late Causes

Angle recession glaucoma.

Pathogenesis

At the movement of impact aqueous is forced laterally and posteriorly against the iris and angle. These hydrodynamic forces cause a tear between the longitudinal and the connecting circular and oblique muscle. This may disrupt branches of anterior or posterior ciliary arteries resulting in bleeding into the anterior chamber.

Eyes with unusual wide angle may be more prone to develop angle recession that eyes with narrow angle.

In years following trauma the inner circular radial muscle may atrophy, on microscopic examination the trabecular meshwork undergoes degenerative changes with resultant scarring. There is fibrosis and obliteration of the intertrabecular spaces and Schlemm's canal. This leads to decrease outflow facility.

Damage to the ciliary muscle disrupts the tension exerted on the trabecular meshwork and may reduce the functional capacity of the meshwork.

CLASSIFICATION OF ANGLE RECESSION

Shallow

Shallow angle recession consists of a separation of the iris processes from the meshwork such that the ciliary body band and scleral spur are more visible as compared to the fellow eye. Here no actual traumatic cleft in the ciliary body occurs.

Moderate Tear

A cleft appears in the ciliary body corresponding to the separation of the longitudinal and circular muscle fibers.

Deep Tear

A fissure extends deeper into the ciliary body. Moderate and deep tears can be visualized with anterior segment ultrasound biomicroscopy. Patients with moderate to severe tears often proceed to sealing of these clefts with formation of peripheral anterior synechiae and fibrosis in the angle, obscuring the evidence of angle recession later.

Eyes with less than 180° recession are unlikely to develop later glaucoma. But this is not a rule even smaller recession may give rise to glaucoma.

Increase in IOP occurs after 6 week, upto 8 percent of eyes with 180° or more of recession may eventually develop glaucoma.

In patient with angle recession glaucoma lifetime risk of developing primary open-angle glaucoma (POAG) in the fellow nontraumatized eye may be high as 50 percent.

CLINICAL FEATURES

- Anterior chamber deep.
- Evidence of injuries—Iris sphincter tear, iris atrophy, iridoschisis, iridodonesis, heterochromic iridis, traumatic mydriasis, anterior subcapsular cataract, vossious ring, phacodonesis, etc.
- Gonioscopy : Asymmetry of the angle of the both eyes or in different portions of the angle in the involved eyes. Broad ciliary body band seen with retro-displacement of the iris root, including the ciliary processes and circular ciliary muscle.

TREATMENT

Initial therapy is medical-effective in eyes with small degree of angle recession. Surgical management is difficult. Laser trabeculoplasty – limited success for short-term.

Nd : YAG laser trabeculopuncture is an additional modality for selected cases.

Trabeculectomy bleb fibrosis in more common. So antifibrotic agents are coupled with the conventional surgery.

In failed cases – implant surgery can be done.

GHOST CELL GLAUCOMA

Ghost cell glaucoma occurs in association with intraocular hemorrhage with vitreous hemorrhage.

HISTORY AND TERMINOLOGY

In 1960 Vannus discussed the role of hemosiderosis in eyes with intraocular hemorrhage as a mechanism of IOP elevation, often occurring years after the initial bleed.

In 1963, Fenton and Zimmerman emphasized the role of macrophages as a mechanism of blood induced glaucoma. They noted that degenerated blood products originated in the vitreous and passed into the anterior chamber to obstruct the trabecular meshwork and termed it as hemolytic glaucoma.

In 1975, Campbell and Grant and in 1976 Campbell, Simmons and Grant described a secondary glaucoma associated with vitreous hemorrhage that they thought was caused primarily by degenerated red blood cell (ghost cells, erythrocyte ghost). Light and electron microscopic studies of anterior chamber aspirates showed little or no debris and few to more macrophages. They named this condition "ghost cell glaucoma" and defined it as a transient secondary glaucoma resulting from obstruction of the trabecular meshwork by degenerated erythrocytes. The ghost cells develop within the vitreous cavity after several types of hemorrhage. Then they enter the anterior chamber though a disruption in the anterior hyaloids face.

PATHOGENESIS

Red blood cell degeneration within the vitreous cavity.

An understanding of ghost cell glaucoma requires knowledge of the fate of blood within the vitreous cavity after vitreous hemorrhage.

After the erythrocytes reach the vitreous cavity, they undergo morphologic, calorimetric, rheologic changes. The RBCs degenerate from red, biconcave, pliable cells to tan or khaki colord, spherical and hollow, less pliable "Ghost cells". Within one to three weeks, the changes occur and remain in the vitreous cavity for months. The intracellular Hb is lost presumably through leaky membranes into the extracellular vitreous space, during the conversion the hemoglobin that remains within the cell, denatures and forms clumps called Heinz bodies, which adhere to the inner surface of the plasma membrane. The extracellular hemoglobin forms clumps or large accumulations that tend to adhere to vitreous strands. In contrast, the ghost cells do not adhere to each other or to the strands and free to move anteriorly. The ghost cells are 4 to 7 m in size. The anterior hyaloids face severs as a natural boundary for the products of the hemorrhage. In trauma disruption in the anterior hyaloids face, allows the ghost cells to come into the anterior chamber, which in turn obstruct the trabecular meshwork causing glaucoma (the ghost cells are less pliable and cannot pass through human trabecular meshwork with ease).

CLINICAL FEATURES

Patient usually gives history of trauma 2 to 3 weeks earlier, with poor vision, pain, in the presence of inflamed or uninflamed eye. Occassionally an 8-ball hyphema is complicated by ghost cell glaucoma in association with vitreous hemorrhage. Conjunctiva is generally white, unless the IOP is very high. Cornea may be normal or edematous or may have collections of khaki-colored cells at its back. Anterior chamber- the aqueous humor is typically filled with a multitude of tiny, tan colored cells, often circulating slowly. If fresh blood also co-exists, a double layer precipitate of light, khaki on top of red is present called "candy" – "stripe" sign- pathognomonic of ghost cell glaucoma.

Gonioscopically angle is wide open, discolored trabecular meshwork due to the presence of fine layer of khaki-colored cells, sometimes pseudohypopyon in the inferior angle.

DIFFERENTIAL DIAGNOSIS

Neovascular glaucoma, hemosiderosis, siderosis.

Management

Vitreous examination shows khaki-hue of degenerated hemorrhage and aqueous tap examined under magnification shows Heinz bodies. In milder cases, standard medical therapy including B-blockers and carbonic anhydrase inhibitors will suffice to lower the IOP. In few cases, repeated irrigating of anterior chamber to remove the ghost cells and in turn to lower the IOP. If the vitreous hemorrhage is large, vitrectomy with special attention to remove all ghost cells including at the base, otherwise vitrectomy itself will further increrae the IOP. Since ghost cell glaucoma is not inflammatory, topical steroids are effective.

Prognosis

Ghost cell glaucoma is typically transient. No permanent damage to the trabecular meshwork, prognosis is fairly good.

ANGLE CLOSURE GLAUCOMA FOLLOWING TRAUMA

Early Causes

Flat Anterior Chamber Leading to Formation of Peripheral Anterior Synechiae

In case of penetrating injury if the wound closure is delayed and if the anterior chamber is not formed, peripheral anterior synechia forms leading to angle closure glaucoma. This is also seen in case of poor wound closure by a poor surgical technique.

Lens Subluxation

Blunt trauma can cause pupillary block due to subluxation of the lens. Portion of zonules can get ruptured that causes herniation of formed vitreous through the equator of lens, or lens itself may get incarcerated in the pupil thereby causing obstruction to the flow of aqueous from PC to AC leading to bulging of peripheral iris causing angle-closure glaucoma.

Mydriatics may allow more vitreous to move forwards, miotics aggravates and problem and thus angle closure attacks may be alleviated in the manner. Iridectomy on lens extraction may be needed. Treatment need to be vigorous and timely to prevent the formation of peripheral anterior synechiae.

A dislocated lens may fall into vitreous cavity and remain silent posing no problem. But if it is a hypermature cataract it may cause phacolytic glaucoma. A total dislocation of lens into the anterior chamber will cause papillary block and angle-closure glaucoma which is a surgical emergency in order to prevent corneal decompensation due to lens endothelial touch.

Forward movement of the lens-iris diaphragm can cause angle-closure glaucoma. It is difficult to differentiate from pupillary block due to subluxation. The mechanism though not clear it appears to be due to ciliary block, usually resolve within 3 to 5 days with cycloplegic and steroids. Iridectomy is not necessary as a rule.

Lens Swelling

A blunt trauma can cause traumatic cataract, sudden swelling of the lens causing papillary block or a sudden increase in intraocular content may lead to glaucoma. Treatment is removal of the lens.

Uveal Effusion

Uveal effusion may lead to angle-closure glaucoma in small eyes also a post-traumatic uveal inflammation causes obstruction to outflow by inflammatory cells, debris, protein. Topical steroids will settle the problem.

Late Causes

Posterior Synechiae with Pupillary Block

Following chronic inflammation due to injury or retained foreign body, dense posterior synechiae forms, leading to seclusio pupillae, iris bombe and peripheral anterior synechiae resulting in secondary angle-closure glaucoma.

Peripheral Anterior Synechiae

This follows healing of trabeculitis, trabecular tear, retained foreign body, angle recession, iridodialysis, peripheral iridocorneal touch due to penetrating injury, etc.

Epithelial Ingrowth following Penetrating Injury

Complicated and difficult surgery or faulty surgical techniques resulting in incarceration of tissue serving as a wick and facilitating postoperative wound gape.

Mechanism : Obstruction of trabecular meshwork by epithelial sheet which later contracts and produce peripheral anterior synechiae and secondary glaucoma.

Prevention : The separate closure of conjunctival and corneoscleral wound,finer suture material, attention to good wound opposition and use of microscope can prevent and development of this complication.

Fibrovascular Downgrowth

This is due to difficult surgery, incarceration of material in the wound, poor wound closure and chronic inflammation.

Fibrous membrane located adjacent to the wound extends on the posterior corneal surface and extend over the angle, iris and vitreous seen as a thick enveloping membrane.

In the angle fibrovascular tissue contract to form peripheral anterior synechiae.

Causes of Glaucoma

- Pretrabecular block by membrane
- Peripheral anterior synechiae.

Neovascular Glaucoma

Following injury is rare and is usually due to chronic inflammation.

12

Pediatric Glaucomas

Nicola Freeman (South Africa)

INTRODUCTION

The pediatric glaucomas are a heterogeneous group of conditions. Primary maldevelopment of the aqueous outflow system may be named ***primary congenital glaucoma*** when presenting at birth, ***primary infantile glaucoma*** when presenting at birth to three years of age or ***primary juvenile glaucoma*** when presenting at three to sixteen years old. The secondary pediatric glaucomas include the ***secondary developmental glaucomas***, e.g. aniridia, Sturge-Weber/ periorbital port wine stain, neurofibromatosis, hyperplastic primary vitreous, Peter's anomaly and the ***secondary pediatric glaucomas***, e.g. aphakic, uveitic, traumatic, cicatricial ROP, ectopia lentis, intraocular neoplasm and steroid induced glaucomas.

CLINICAL PRESENTATION

Primary congenital glaucoma (PCG) and primary infantile glaucoma (PIG):

- Epiphora, photophobia, blepharospasm = clinical triad of PCG
- Corneal clouding, corneal enlargement, corneal edema
- Haab's striae (curvilinear breaks in Descemet's membrane)
- Optic disk cupping (stretching of optic canal in young patients; may be reversible)
- Raised intraocular pressure on tonometry (Tonopen, Perkins or Goldman tonometry).

Secondary developmental glaucomas and Secondary pediatric glaucomas:

- Seldom present with the above mentioned symptoms
- Diligent follow-up and IOP monitoring essential in conditions such as aphakia, uveitis, trauma, ROP, intraocular neoplasm, aniridia, periorbital port wine stain, neurofibromatosis, hyperplastic primary vitreous and Peter's anomaly.
- Up to 1/3 of pediatric aphakic and pseudophakic eyes develop glaucoma. There are usually no clinical symptoms and long-term vigilance is necessary to make the diagnosis early.

DIFFERENTIAL DIAGNOSIS

Of Epiphora:

- Nasolacrimal duct obstruction

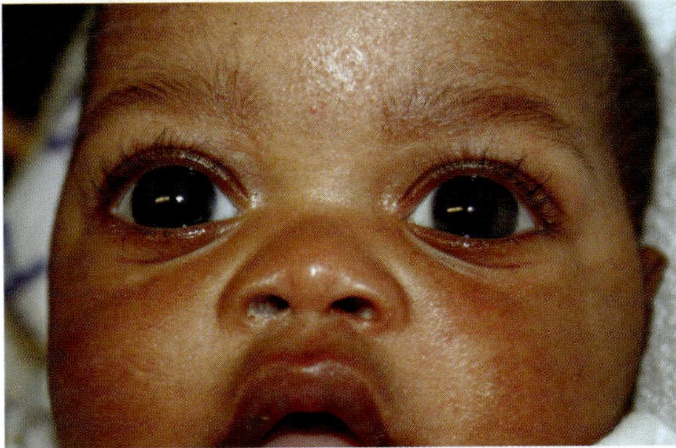

Fig. 1: Bilateral buphthalmos with corneal enlargement and scarring

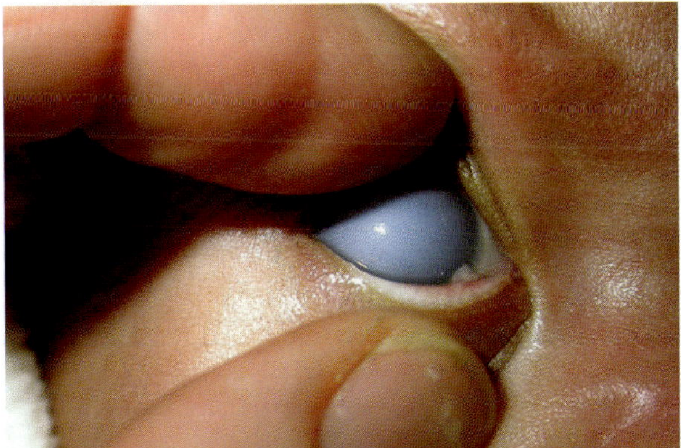

Fig. 2: Differential diagnosis: The cloudy Cornea of Rubella keratitis

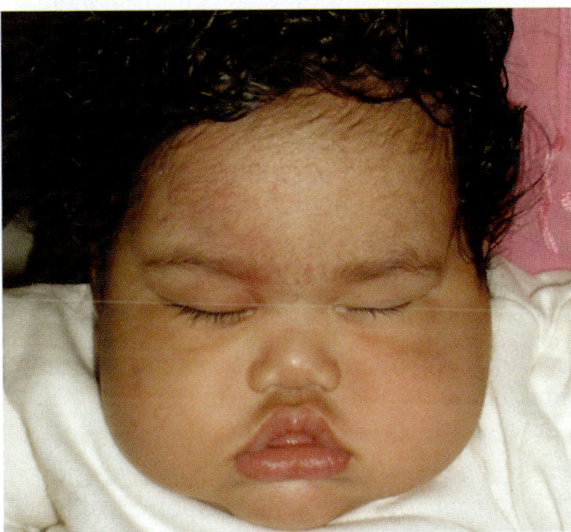

Fig. 3: Right periorbital port wine stain or cutaneous hemangioma in Sturge Weber can be subtle in infancy. This child was born with right buphthalmos and had a diffuse choroidal hemangioma of the right eye with leptomeningeal changes on CT scan

- Conjunctivitis
- Corneal epithelial defect or abrasion
- Ocular inflammation

Of corneal edema or opacification:

- Rubella keratitis – Rubella also causes microphthalmos and congenital glaucoma
- Birth trauma – forceps delivery causing Descemet's tear
- Congenital anomalies – Sclerocornea, Peter's anomaly
- Storage diseases – Mucopolysaccharidoses, Cystinosis
- Corneal dystrophies – congenital hereditary endothelial and posterior polymorphous dystrophy.

Of enlarged cornea:

- Megalocornea
- Axial myopia.

Of enlarged optic nerve cupping:

- Optic nerve coloboma or malformations
- Optic nerve hypoplasia or atrophy.

MANAGEMENT

General

- Examination under anesthesia (EUA): Ketamine hydrochloride IVI using local anesthetic patch. Atropine and midazolam pre-med. NB Inhalation anesthetics all decrease IOP unpredictably and substantially.
- Examination: IOP, corneal diameters and corneal changes, corneal thickness, anterior segment, angle gonioscopy, optic disks, retina and vitreous, refraction, axial lengths and AC depth with ultrasound if possible.
- *Primary congenital and infantile glaucomas*: Surgical intervention—treatment of choice with medical used preoperatively and as adjunct to surgery.
- *Secondary developmental and secondary pediatric glaucomas*: Medical treatment first-line. Surgical intervention only when medical fails.

Surgical Intervention Options

- Goniotomy: corneal clarity required, angle surgery under direct visualization with goniotomy lens and goniotomy blade
- Trabeculotomy: corneal clarity not required, trabeculotome inserted into canal of Schlemm and swept into anterior chamber rupturing the trabecular meshwork. A temporal approach spares superior conjunctiva
- Trabeculectomy: antimetabolite modification usually necessary

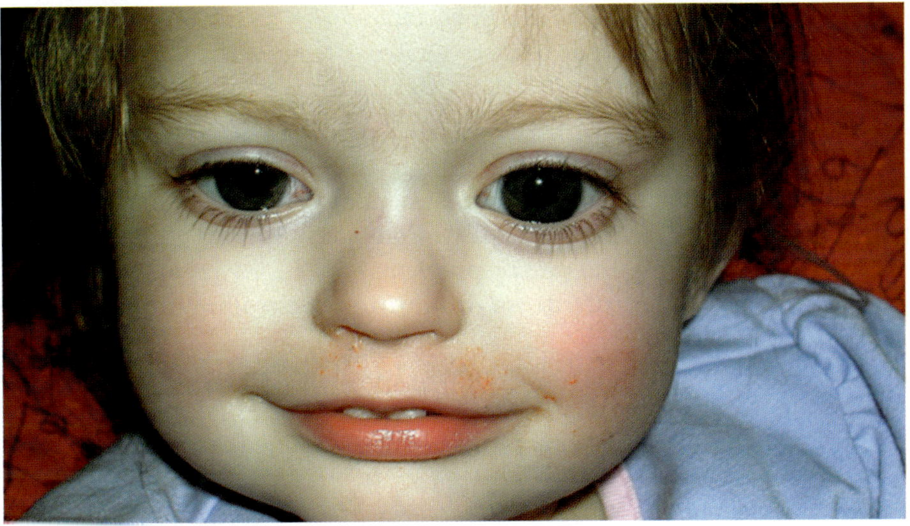

Fig. 4: Left buphthalmos. The right eye is receiving atropine penalization for amblyopia management

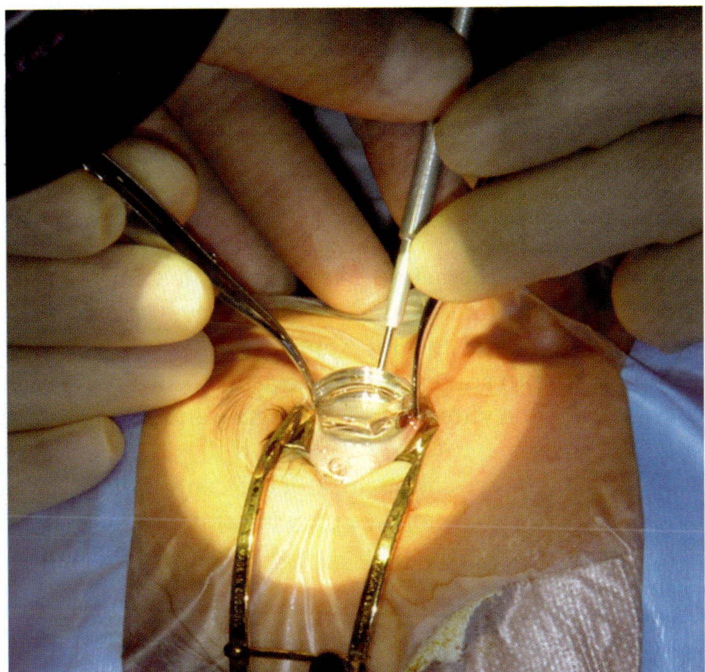

Fig. 5: Goniotomy lens and locking forceps held by assistant in goniotomy procedure

- Combined Trabeculectomy and trabeculotomy
- Artificial drainage shunts: refractory cases
- Cyclodiode laser: usually in last resort refractory cases.

Medical Treatment Options

- Punctal occlusion for 5 min reduces systemic effects.
- Topical beta-blocker: Betaxolol 0.25% (Betoptic S), Timolol 0.25% (Timoptic XE) (Beware asthma and cardiac problems)
- Topical carbonic anhydrase inhibitors: Dorzolamide (Trusopt), Brinzolomide (Azopt)
- Prostaglandin derivatives : Travaprost (Travatan), Bimatoprost (Lumigan), (Latanoprost (Xalatan)
- Oral carbonic anhydrase inhibitors : Acetazolamide (Diamox) 10-30 mg/ kg/ day; qid
  (Beware metabolic acidosis. Use short term preoperatively only)
- Alpha- agonists: may cause apnea, bradycardia, hypotension.

Follow up

- Regular EUA's required when uncooperative age
- Monitor IOP, Corneal diameters, axial lengths, refraction
- Early detection and treatment of amblyopia.

PROGNOSIS

Visual loss in childhood glaucoma is multifactorial. It may result from corneal scarring, optic nerve damage or amblyopia secondary to myopia, astigmatism or anisometropia.

Onset at birth, corneal diameter >14 mm and failed angle surgery are all poor prognostic indicators for *Primary congenital and primary infantile glaucoma..*

The poor prognostic indicators for Aphakic and Pseudophakic glaucomas are younger age at cataract surgery and pre-existing ocular abnormalities. The role of preservation of the vitreous face at surgery and IOL placement is still uncertain.

Even in poor prognosis eyes, all attempts at IOP control should be continued. Any amount of vision preservation in a growing child is important for neural integration development.

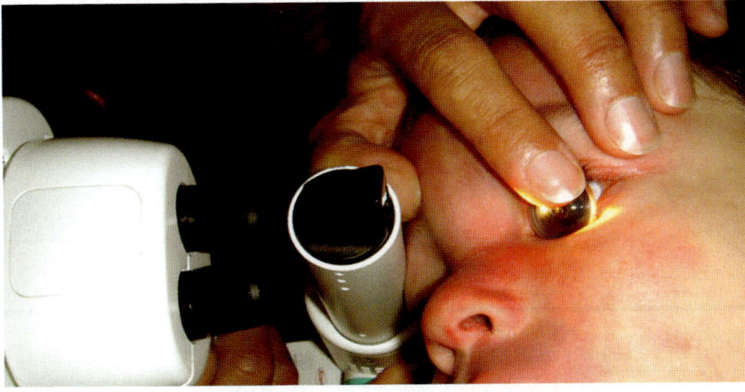

Fig. 6: Slit lamp examination with the Koeppe lens in a child with Sturge Weber glaucoma

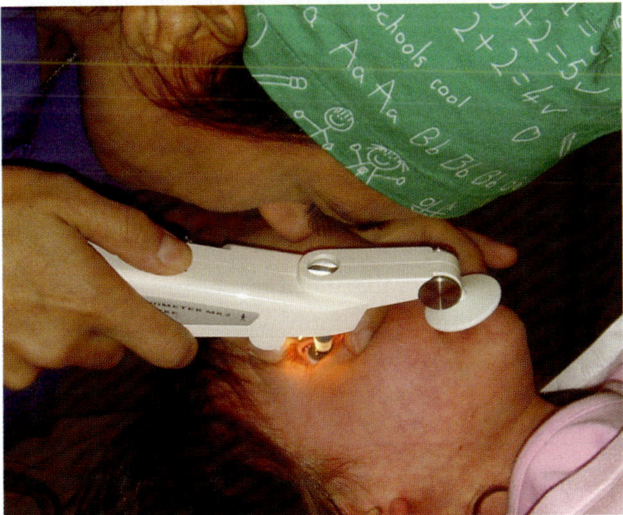

Fig. 7: Perkins tonometer used in the examination under anesthesia

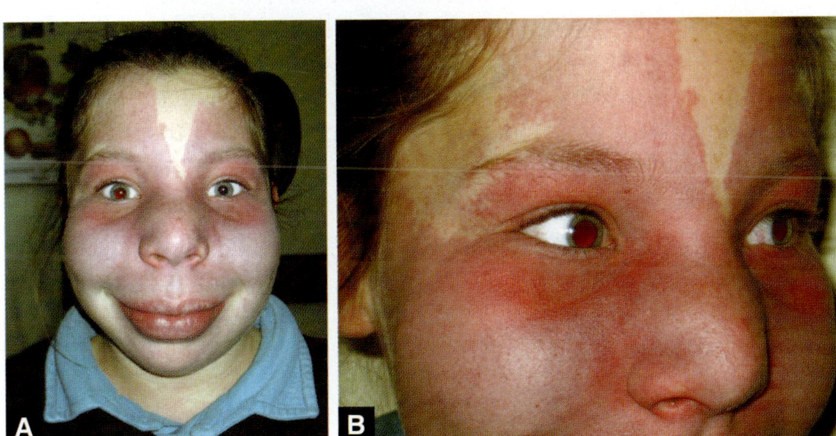

Figs 8A and B: Bilateral Sturge Weber syndrome

13

Glaucoma Implants in the Treatment of Pediatric Glaucoma

Peter WT de Waard (Netherlands)

INTRODUCTION

Management of primary congenital glaucomas is primarily surgical. Goniotomy or trabeculotomy each have success rates of 40-90% in the management of primary congenital glaucoma. In case of secondary glaucoma's associated with, e.g. aphakia, aniridia, anterior segment dysgenesis and Sturge-Weber syndrome, goniotomy or trabeculotomy success rates are low. When goniotomy or trabeculotomy fail or are inappropriate to control intraocular pressure (IOP) in pediatric patients, alternatives include filtering surgery or drainage implants.

Beck found that aqueous shunt implantation (Ahmed or Baerveldt) offers a significantly greater chance of successful IOP control compared with trabeculectomy with Mitomycine-C in infants up to 24 months of age. They found cumulative probabilities of success at 12 months of 87% for the aqueous shunt group and 36% in the trabeculectomy group. In pediatric patients in whom goniotomy, and/or trabeculectomy with or without antimetabolites have failed, success rates of 56-95% have been reported with these glaucoma implants.

CHOICE OF IMPLANT

As the normal IOP in children is the same as in adults, we may assume that the aqueous production at least equals that of adults. Studies showed that glaucoma implants with a large surface, like the Baerveldt 350 (mm^2), have higher success rates then the ones with smaller surfaces, like the Baerveldt 250 (mm^2) and the Ahmed (184 and 96 mm^2). So it seems justified to implant the Baerveldt 350 in children without a compromized aqueous production. The latter can be found in uveitic glaucoma or after cyclodestructive procedures. In these cases one should choose a smaller implant to reduce the risk of hypotony. In case one needs immediate lowering of the IOP, e.g. very high IOP unresponsive to maximal tolerable medical therapy, the valved Ahmed implant is the best choice.

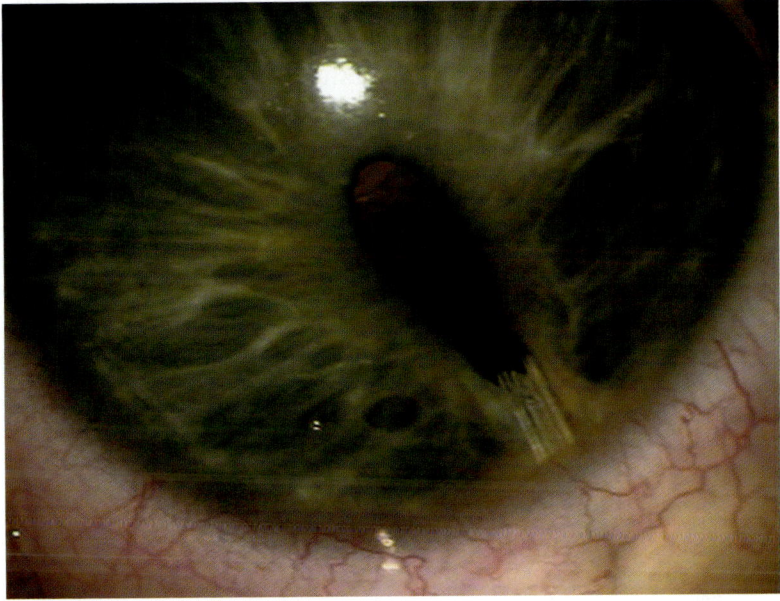

Fig. 1: Dyscoria in buphthalmic eye with BGI

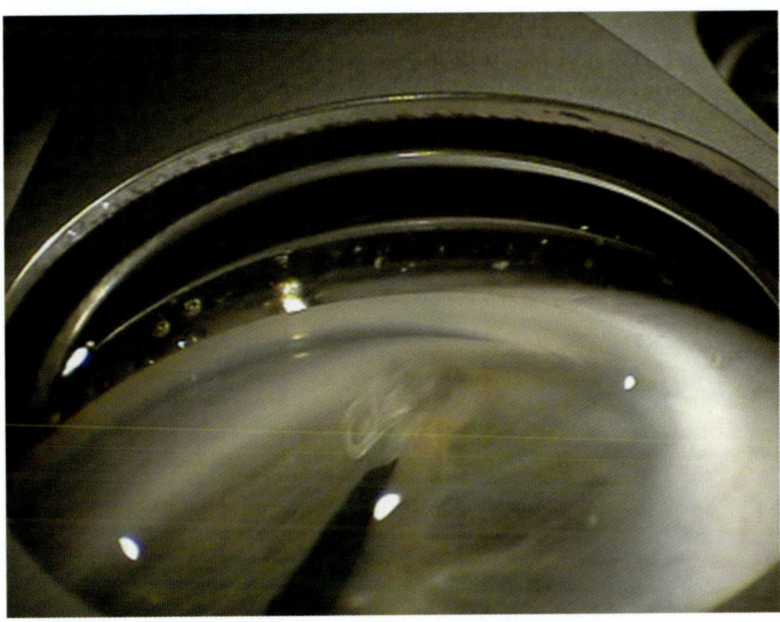

Fig. 2: Gonioscopic view of dyscoria of figure 1. Entrapment of peripheral iris in tube-track can be seen

OPERATION TECHNIQUE OF BAERVELDT IMPLANT

The sclera in the superior temporal quadrant is exposed with a limbus-based conjunctival flap, and the superior and lateral rectus muscles are identified and isolated with muscle hooks. The wings of the implant are positioned under the insertions of the muscles. The plate is secured 1-2 mm posterior to the insertions with 2 interrupted 9-0 nylon sutures. The tube is trimmed so that it would extend 1-2 mm beyond the posterior surgical limbus with the bevel toward the corneal endothelium. A stent (3-0 prolene), 1-2 mm in length, is passed into and down the tube and positioned ± 7 mm behind the limbus. The tube is ligated with 7-0 vicryl around the stent. This stent is used for easy constriction of the tube and ensures a watertight closure, preventing early postoperative hypotony. The stent itself hardly affects the flow through the tube (personal measurements with donor eyes). The tube will opened after 5-7 weeks. A paracentesis track through the cornea into the anterior chamber is made to control the IOP and the anterior chamber depth intraoperatively. A 23-gauge needle is used to create an opening for insertion of the tube into the anterior chamber. Glycerin-preserved donor sclera is used to cover the tube near the limbus and secured with interrupted 9-0 vicryl sutures. Finally tenon and conjunctiva are reapposed with running 9-0 vicryl sutures. A subconjunctival injection of corticosteroids is administered before the eye is patched. Postoperatively, topical steroids are tapered slowly and glaucoma medications are removed or added as IOP and clinical status requires. Many but not all steps apply to the other glaucoma implants as well.

Preoperative and postoperative examinations must include slit-lamp examination, ophthalmoscopy, IOP measurement with a pneumatonometer (Model 30 classic, Mentor O and O, Norwell, MA, USA), and measurement of axial length by ultrasound A-scan (A-5500 A-scan system, Sonomed, Lake Success, NY, USA). Most examinations are performed under general anesthesia in patients younger than 6 years. Older patients may be able to undergo examinations in the office.

Complications

Early postoperative high IOP can be medically treated. Early postoperative hypotony does not require treatment as long as the anterior chamber (AC) is not flat. Logically, IOP lowering medication can be stopped. This hypotony can be caused by a little flow of aqueous through the needle-track round the tube or more serious by inadequate closure of the tube. The latter will very often lead to a flat anterior chamber needing reclosure of the tube with 7-0 vicryl under general anesthesia as soon as possible.

The tube will open 5-7 weeks postoperatively. A relatively large volume of aqueous will flow through the tube from the anterior chamber to the filtration bleb formed around the plate of the BGI. Consequently, a transient shallow anterior chamber and hypotony can be seen until the bleb is filled with aqueous and an equilibrium is reached between the IOP and the counterpressure in the bleb.

After opening of the tube the IOP depends on the diffusion of aqueous through the wall of the bleb. In its turn, this diffusion depends on the surface and the thickness of the blebwall. The surface is controlled by the choice of platesize (e.g. Baerveldt 350 or 250 mm^2). The thickness depends on the reaction of Tenon´s to the silicon implant before and to aqueous humour after opening of the tube. As the active reaction to aqueous continues for life, slow changes in the thickness of the blebwall will lead to IOP changes. In this way, late hypotony can not only be caused by compromized aqueous production but also by thinning of the blebwall due to inhibition of the mitotic activity of fibroblasts (e.g. methotrexate in the treatment of juvenile idiopathic arthritis). The latter cause of hypotony can be treated by temporary occlusion of the tube (vicryl 7-0) and injection of autologous blood in the bleb to increase the thickness of the blebwall. Antimetabolites should be reduced or stopped if possible.

In case the blebwall becomes to thick and the resulting high IOP can not be medically controlled, a second glaucoma implant should be placed because the thickness of the blebwall can only be controlled (thinning) with a ,probably non-acceptable, longlasting treatment with antimetabolites.

The most frequent complication of the BGI is tube related, varying from mild dyscoria to tube exposure. Studies reported 6.5-39.1% tube related complications. The variability in the published incidence of tube related complications after BGI, may be partly due to inclusion of differing proportions of buphthalmic eyes in these studies. The thin elastic sclera in buphthalmic eyes gives little support to the implanted tube and predisposes these eyes to changes in size and shape when the IOP is reduced, leading in turn to tube related complications.

In our study dyscoria was observed, only in buphthalmic eyes, shortly after opening of the tube caused by entrapment of a tuft of peripheral iris tissue in the needle-track. The entrapment could be a result of a shallow anterior chamber during the period of hypotony after opening of the tube, in combination with movement of the tube in the needle-track creating space next to the tube due to thin elastic sclera. It seems likely that movement of the tube is induced by movement of the eyelids over a hypotonous eye. In combination with the dycoria we often see an anterior movement of the tube, eroding through the thin sclera, frequently coming in close contact with the cornea endothelium. These eyes need to be reoperated by opening the conjunctiva/tenon at the limbus, removing the tube from the anterior chamber, closing the tube-track and replacing the tube in the AC through a new track. The latter must be made as long as possible, the sclera giving more support to the tube. Future adjustments to the tube and avoiding the hypotonous period with valves could diminish or even prevent these tube related problems.

In case of tube exposure immediate re-covering of the tube with donor sclera, tenon and conjunctiva is required because of the high risk of endophthalmitis.

Tube retraction asks for extension of the tube. This is best performed in the fornix near the connection of tube and plate. The tenon and conjunctiva overlying the tube is opened (± 6 mm) and the soft fibrous capsule encircling the tube is incised. The exposed tube is cut (± 5 mm proximal to the connection of tube and plate) and the extension is placed between the two ends. Because the silicon tube slides through the encircling capsule very easily, the long proximal part of the tube can be advanced into the AC. Sometimes the conjunctiva/tenon has to be opened at the limbus to assist the (re)entrance of the tube into the AC.

In case the tube in the AC becomes too long, the diameter of the bulbus becoming smaller after lowering of the IOP, the AC can be filled with viscoelastics and the tube can be shortened intraocularly with fine vitreous scissors. The cut end is removed by vitreous forceps through the same paracentesis.

Studies of pediatric patients with glaucoma implants report motility disturbances in 0-16% after implantation. Similar findings (0-10%) were noted after implantation of an Ahmed or Molteno implant in pediatric patients. Motility problems are believed to be secondary to a mass effect from the equatorial filtering bleb, a Faden or posterior fixation effect induced by scarring under the rectus muscle, or fat adherence syndrome. In our study we found mild motility disturbances postoperatively in 7.3% of the patients. Strabismus surgery was necessary in only one patient, the motility disturbances in the other patients being transient after 4-6 months.

CONCLUSION

Glaucoma implants are effective and safe in the management of pediatric glaucoma, despite its propensity for tube related postoperative complications. One must be prepared to follow these patients a life time and deal with many possible complications, especially the tube related problems.

14

Shunt Surgery for Refractory Glaucoma

Jes Mortensen (Sweden)

In spite of the uncertainty surrounding the pathogenesis of the glaucoma the control of IOP retains a central position in glaucoma treatment: Damage to the optic nerve may occur mechanically or through interaction with the blood-flow to the papilla. The level at which the IOP poses a risk to the optic nerve is surely depended on individual factors such as genetic background.

What is known is that a very high pressure, over 40 mmHg, will accelerate the irreversible damage to the visual nerve.

REFRACTORY GLAUCOMA

The diagnosis of refractory glaucoma is given when the pressure reduction seen is not sufficient to protect the visual nerve of the eye, after all the various drugs, Pilocarpin, betablockers, adrenaline drugs, carbonic anhydrase inhibitors and prostaglandin analogues have been tested. The peroral carbonic anhydrase inhibitors are, due to the side effects, not an alternative to surgery in my opinion.

Refractory glaucoma is often seen in congenital glaucoma and secondary glaucoma. I have myself seen refractory glaucoma, in for example: Aniridia, congenital glaucoma with buphthalmia, Riegers syndrome, and glaucoma congenita tarda. Eyes with congenital cataract are also at the high risk of developing refractory glaucoma early or later in life. The largest group is secondary glaucoma: Post uveitis, after traumatic surgery for cataract or/and retinal detachment not to mention eyes which have silicone oil or have had silicone oil. A smaller group in our country is post-traumatic eyes. This group might differ from country to country. Penetrating keratoplasty is also a major risk factor, the risk increasing for every retransplant and episode of rejection. We are changing from penetrating keratoplasty to the lamellar keratoplasty technique, in eyes with a normal endothelium to minimize the risk of endure these complications.

In Sweden a vast majority of the population has the exfoliation syndrome. Glaucoma with exfoliation syndrome may quite commonly became refractory.

History of Glaucoma Surgery

Surgery for the management of glaucoma is much older than medication. Albecht von Graefe (1828 -1870) in Berlin operated on open-angle glaucoma back in the 19th century with iridectomy. All operations for glaucoma are meant to facilitate the outflow of the aqueous humor from the anterior chamber of the eye to the subconjunctival space. Many different operations have been tried, lately the

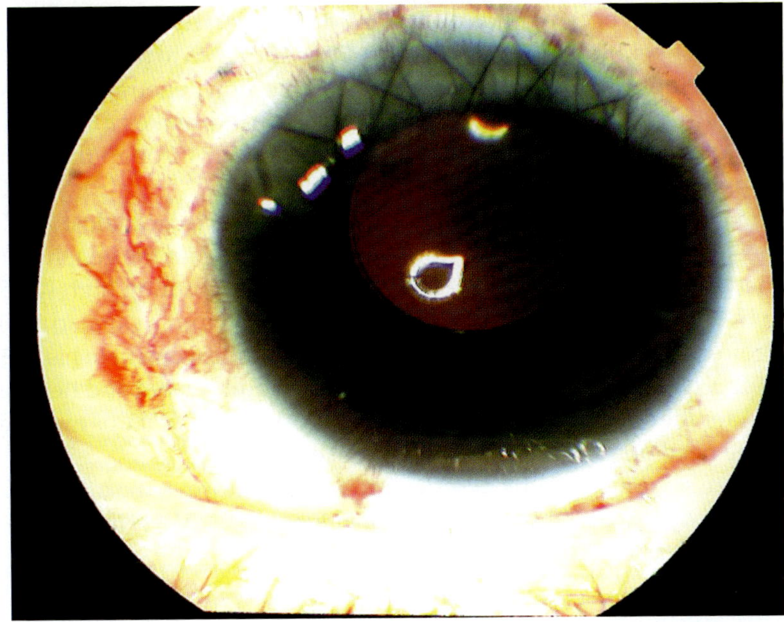

Fig. 1: Eye with aniridia, operated with and iris-prosthesis

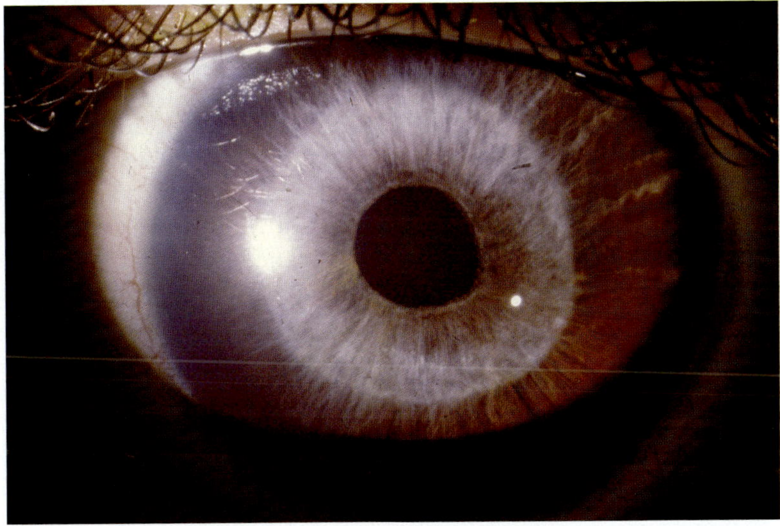

Fig. 2: Eye with Riegers syndrome

trabeculectomy has been regarded as the golden standard. The trabeculectomy is a well tested operation to lower the IOP. A new approach to trabecular surgery has been developed to minimize the complications, non penetrating trabecular surgery. Mermoud advocates a deep sclerectomy and makes a Descement´s window to facilitate percolation of the aqueous humor through this window from the anterior chamber.

Stegmann has another approach which he calls "viscocanalostomy". He uses a deep sclerectomy, deroofing of Schlemm´s canal and the generation of a Descement´s window. To facilitate the flow of aqueous humor, high -viscosity sodium hyaluronate (Healon GV) is injected into Schlemm´s canal to open the canal. Professor Stegmann has just published a new improvement to his method: he threads a 10:0 prolene suture through the Schlemm´s canal and ties it in the "lake" under the superior scleral flap. It is yet too early to say if this method will abolish the need of the glaucoma shunt devices.

There are several implants described to further improve the outflow of the aqueous humor, since 2001 we began at our clinic to use 1:0 PDS (polydioxanon) suture material as an implant.

When to Consider a Glaucoma Shunt Device

When the aforementioned surgical methods have been tested and even retested, the shunt operation is the next alternative. Some surgeons prefer to perform a cyclodestructive procedure before the shunt alternative, but in my opinion cyclodestruction is exactly what it says; destructive surgery which means that it is difficult to give the dose exactly. We have also tried the Express implant, first directly under the conjunctiva, then under a scleral flap. The results have not been promising. We still use the Express implant if we got a very old patient with refractory glaucoma, who can only tolerate a very short operation. We always add Mitomycin C 0.02%.

The basic design of the glaucoma shunt is a silicone tube that shunts aqueous humor from the anterior chamber of the eye to a plate which has been encapsulated by a fibrous capsule. The capsule serves as a reservoir. Six shunts are available today: Krupin-Denver valve implant, Molteno implant, Glaucoma pressure regulator, Baerveldt seton, Ahmed glaucoma implant and Schocket shunt. My own experience is limited to the Molteno, the Ahmed and to the Baerveldt implant. The Ahmed glaucoma implant has a pressure-sensitive membrane valve allowing aqueous humor flow to yield an IOP of at least 8 to 12 mm Hg.

Historical Aspects of the Shunt Procedure

Rollet and Moreau implanted a silk thread connecting the anterior chamber of the eye to the subconjonctival space back in 1906. In 1959 Epstein implanted a polythene tube and MacDonald and Pearce a silicone tube in 1965. All these operations failed due to scar formation stopping the flow or due to conjunctival erosion.

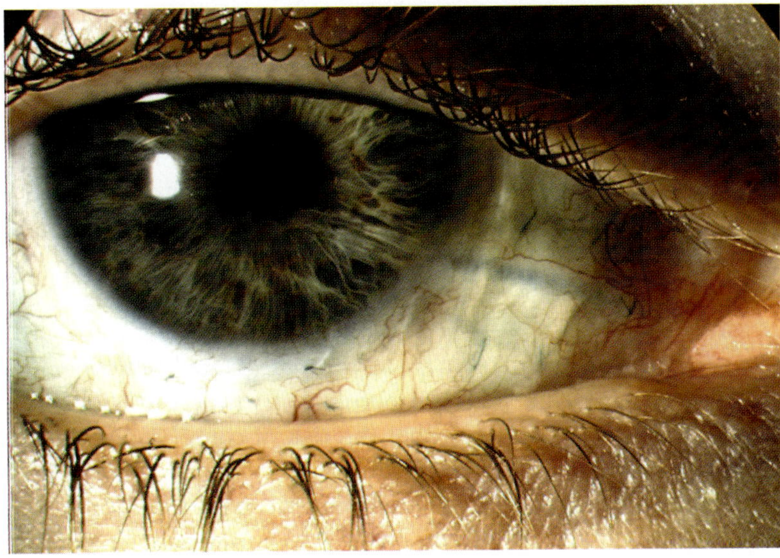

Fig 3: Eye with Baerveldt shunt controling the secondary glaucoma due to uveitis

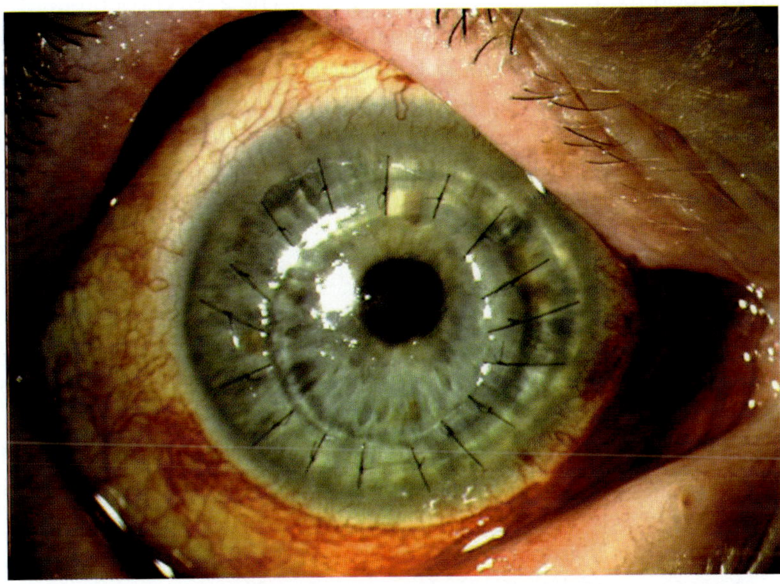

Fig. 4: Eye operated for keratoconus with a lamellar keratoplasty first postoperative day

In 1969 Molteno inserted an acrylic tube attached to a thin plate. Most of the early implants failed due to plate exposure or tube erosion and formation of fibrous encapsulation. In 1973 Molteno introduced the long silicone tube allowing the plate to be implanted 9-10 mm from the limbus. 1992 Molteno introduced the double plate implant with a surface area of 270 mm^2. In 1976 Theodore Krupin introduced an implant with a unidirectional valve. In 1993 Martenn Ahmed introduced the Ahmed implant with a unidirectional valve. 1992 George Baerveldt introduced a nonvalved silicone tube attached to a barium-impregnated silicone plate, available with three surface areas: 250 mm^2, 350 mm^2 and 500 mm^2.

The glaucoma drainage devices are as you can see not a new phenomenon; they are almost the same age as the trabeculectomy procedure, why has it not become more popular? I do think that the risk of complications during the operation and postoperation has made many surgeons reluctant to learn and perform the procedure. I shall now try to comment on the insertion of the shunt and the postoperative complications and how to minimize the risks.

Operating Technique

The first shunt I implanted was the Molteno, it was in the late 80-s, the tube was directly entered at the limbus no donor patch graft was used and no ligating suture was used around the tube to close the outflow in the postoperative period to hinder hypotony and choroidal detachment. The eyes chosen had more or less been given up: Eyes with neovascular glaucoma. The results mildly spoken were not good. In 1996, I heard a lecture about the Molteno shunt given by an ophthalmologist from Finland. He had good results using a Vicryl suture ligated around the tube and he even created a fenestration using a suture needle anterior to the ligature functioning as a primitive valve until the suture was resorbed after 6 to 8 weeks and the fibrous reservoir around the plate had developed.

Applying that technique was the start of much better results with the glaucoma shunt devices. I changed to the Ahmed shunt, but found that I got to much trouble with high pressure in the postoperative period. The Baerveldt shunt was marketed by the Pharmacia company, which at that time was a Swedish company, very successful in Ophthalmology. The Baerveldt shunt was pretty easy to place with its silicone plate and the two wings that were placed behind the rectus muscle. In the beginning a human patch graft was used to cover the tube. I found it easier to make a scleral flap 4 × 4 mm and insert the tube under the scleral flap. The silicone plate was sutured 10 to 11 mm from limbus. The anterior chamber was entered first by a 27-gauge needle parallel to the iris, to get the right direction before using the 23-gauge needle to make an insertion allowing the tube to enter the anterior chamber. The 27-gauge needle was put on a Healon© syringe to fill the anterior chamber, this method helps the silicon tube to place itself in a proper position.

Then a 7: 0 Vicryl suture is tight around the tube for ligation.

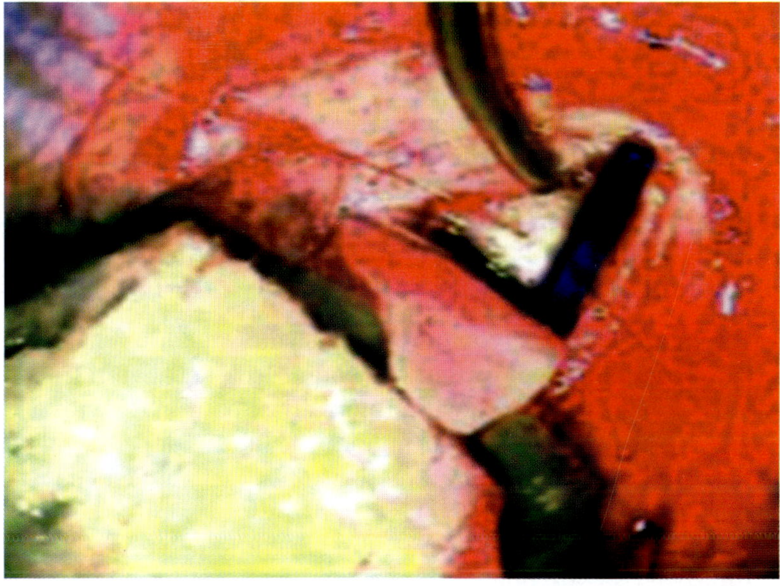

Fig. 5: Implant 1:0 PDS (polydioxanon) used by viscocanalostomy

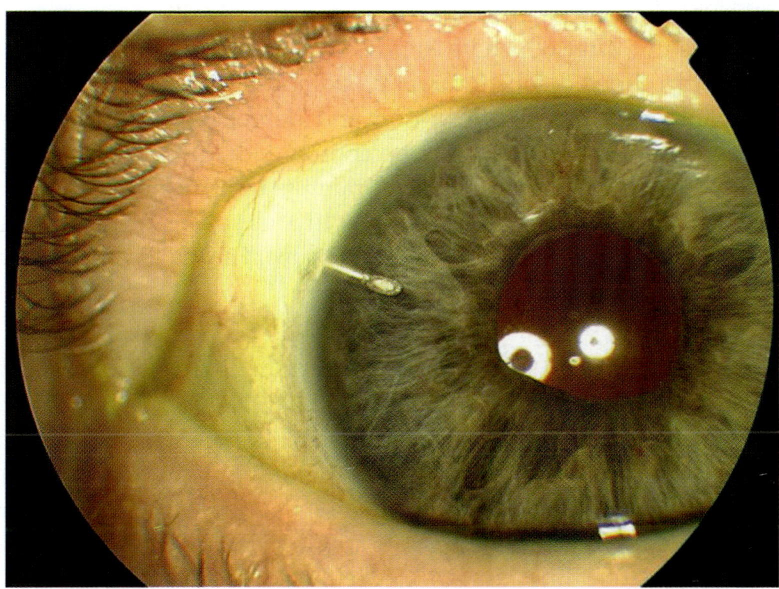

Fig. 6: Express implant

The major postoperative problem was hypotony until I began using biological glue, Tisseel. The glue is placed under the scleral flap and under the anterior part of the conjunctiva. You have to be careful that the glue does not flow backwards over the plate. The biological glue will secure that the closure of the conjunctiva to be watertight even with a scarified and thin conjunctiva after several earlier surgeries. With that technique you often see an eye with very little injection and a pressure of about 5 to 10 mmHg the day after operation.

Complications

Now to the complications. Hypotony with a shallow anterior chamber in the postoperative period. Often caused by wound leak and overfiltration. The incidence is as high as 20-30% with a nonvalved shunt, 9% with a valved shunt. With the ligating suture and "hiding" the tube under a scleral flap.

The risk is reduced and, in my experience, after using the biological glue (Tisseel©) is very seldom seen. If you get very low pressure in the immediate postoperative phase you must instruct the patient to be very careful not do heavy lifting even severe coughing can cause choroidal bleeding.

I operated on a man, who has been my patient for more than 20 years due to his glaucoma tarda. Left eye had light perception due to severe glaucoma damage. Right eye had good vision 20/20 with correction. The right eye earlier had surgery for glaucoma and cataract. The eye developed refractory glaucoma with an uncontrolled IOP of 35-40 mmHg. A Baerveldt shunt was placed and no problems was seen, the IOP was 5 mmHg . On the third day the patient coughed violently, after which he could see bleeding blinding the eye in few seconds. B-scan showed subchoroidal blood and even blood in the vitreous space. Visual acuity, light perception and defect location. Spontaneous resorption was allowed under thorough control with the B-scan ensuring that no retinal detachment occurred. After 6 months the subchoroidal blood has resorbed and even almost all blood in the vitreous space, the visual acuity is today 20/50 and will probably continue to improve. The IOP is stable 12 mmHg.

Hypertension Postoperatively

Is often seen in the valved glaucoma shunt group , but even after the nonvalved. As a matter of fact the most safe situation postoperatively is hypertony between 21 mm Hg and 30 mm Hg as rather mild antiglaucoma medication with eyedroppers can control the pressure until the strangulating suture round the tube is resorbed and the fibrous encapsulation develops around the plate.

If very high pressure is seen in the immediate postoperative phase an obstruction of the tube must be suspected, either from blood, fibrin, iris plug or vitreous. The ligature may also be too tight. You can try to wash the tube carefully leading a 27-gauge needle into the opening of the tube in the anterior chamber.

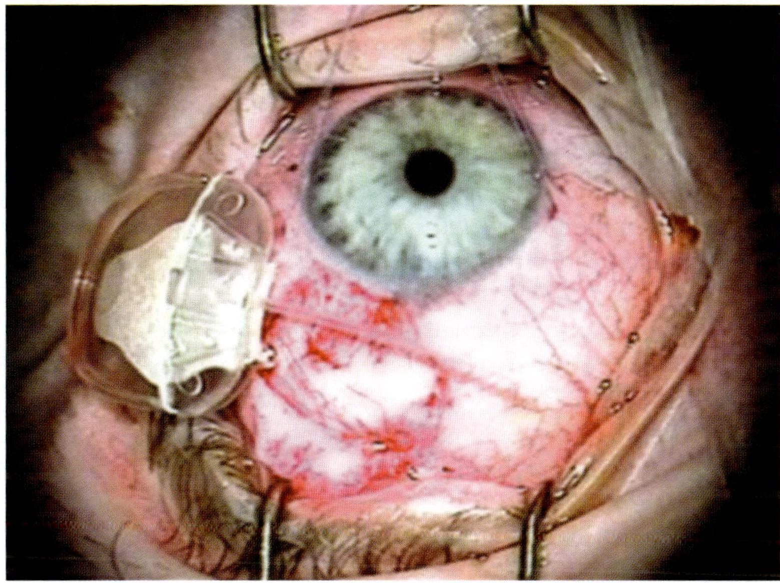

Fig. 7: Ahmed shunt

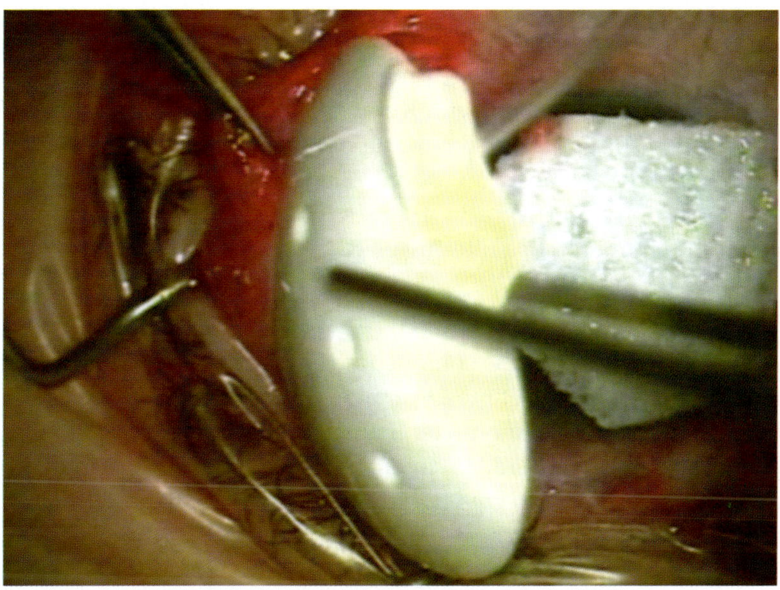

Fig. 8: Baerveldt shunt

We use Heparin in the washing water if we suspect coagulated blood in the tube and over the plate. If you suspect vitreous or an iris plug you can try to clean the opening of the tube with the Nd:YAG laser. A tight ligating suture can be cut with the argon laser.

If hypertension persists you should consider that the fibrous encapsulation bleb may be too small for appropriate resorption. Needling with the 27-gauge needle might solve the problem. If not I should try to open and remove the fibrous encapsulation and at the same time apply Mitomycin C 0.02% for three minutes.

If that does not solve the problem you have to consider a new shunt. I have one patient who underwent trabeculectomy at the age of 5 months due to congenital glaucoma. He is now 21 years of age, right eye blind from the very beginning, visual acuity of his left eye 20/60. He has three shunts, one Ahmed and 2 Baerveldt, the IOP has been controlled for the last 5 years, he is studying to become a teacher.

Corneal Decompensation

Corneal decompensation is not uncommon, the incidence following glaucoma drainage devices is as high as 10 to 20% and similar with both valved as non valved devices. The etiology is unknown. If the tube touches the cornea the tube shall be repositioned.

The risk of graft failure is also pretty high due to chronic inflammation and often multiple previous surgeries. I refer to an Article by professor Claes H. Dohlman. Combining surgery with Keratoprosthesis with an Ahmed shunt. From the Ahmed shunt plate a silicone tube was extended to the lachrymal sac or the ethmoid sinuses. The IOP was controlled and no infection was seen. That might be a solution to the intractable cases where scarring of the conjunctiva will hinder the formation of a filtering bleb.

Exposure of the Tube and the Plate of the Glaucoma Shunt

Erosion of the tube through the conjunctiva due to scarring and thinning from earlier surgeries is seen sometimes. We cover the exposed tube or plate with an amniotic patch or glue a human scleral patch or both.

If a large scleral flap is made to cover the tube 4 - 5 mm from limbus and the conjunctiva is carefully dissected avoiding perforations, you will seldom see that complication. In my experience using the biological glue will further minimize the risk of that complication.

The risk of getting an infection is extremely low. The lifetime risk of infection after glaucoma shunt operation is estimated to 0.1-0.5% as opposed to a lifetime risk of infection of 1-1.5% following trabeculectomy.

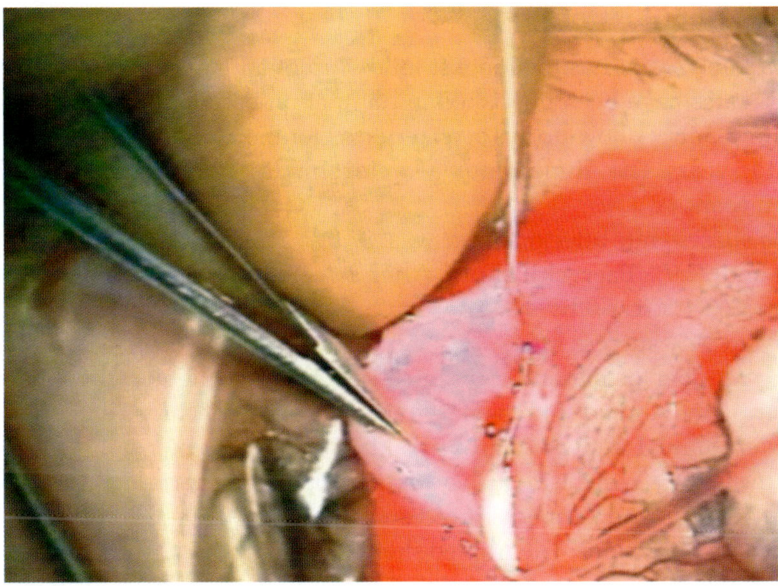

Fig. 9: Baerveldt shunt plate sutured to sclera 10 mm from limbus

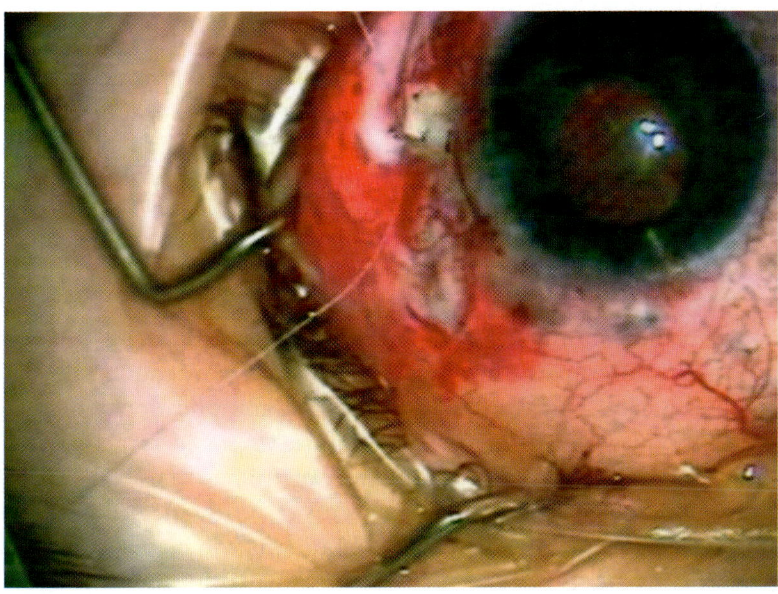

Fig. 10: The 7: 0 Vicryl suture is tight around the tube

Results from Literature

The Molteno shunt has the longest follow up of all glaucoma shunt devices. Success rates have been published in population-based studies on glaucoma shunt implants. Follow up has been reported for the Molteno shunt at 1, 2, 3 , 5, 10 and 15 years. The Ahmed and Baerveldt shunts have had follow-up time of 1 and 2 years.

The success rate after one year was: 87.0%, Molteno shunt. 82.7% Ahmed Shunt and 72.9% Baerveldt shunt. After 2 years the success rate was: 88.7%, 50% and 68.4% respectively. After ten and 15 years the Molteno shunt had 90.0% and 91% success rate.

The number of patients presented are often relatively few. One study comparing the Ahmed shunt versus trabeculectomy concludes that the success rates were similar in the two groups, although the trabeculectomy group had lower mean IOP, even the frequency of complications were comparable. Another study compares the Ahmed shunt versus the Baerveldt shunt for refractory glaucoma. Conclusions: The Ahmed shunt exhibited better control of the IOP in the early postoperative period (1 day, 1 week and 1 month) the Ahmed shunt had earlier encapsulation of the plate.

The surface area of the plate was thought to influence the success rate, the larger surface giving a better regulation; however a study comparing the 350 mm^2 versus the 500 mm^2 showed that the smaller implant is more successful than the larger.

The success rate for the Molteno shunt for each type of glaucoma has been investigated in different studies. The highest success rate was found in primary open angle glaucoma, 100% and the lowest in traumatic glaucoma 76%, even neovascular glaucoma had a very high success rate 87%. We do not however normally use glaucoma implants in neovascular glaucoma.

CONCLUSION

The first glaucoma shunt, The Molteno shunt was introduced almost at the same time as the trabeculectomy, in the late 60-s, but in my country never found the same popularity. This was surely due to the complications that was seen especially if the surgery was performed by unexperienced surgeons.

I do think that the glaucoma shunt technology has matured and that the many years experience from the numerous procedures performed all over the world indicates that the glaucoma shunt operations will increase. We still wait for the ideal glaucoma shunt device; easy to implant, lasting the patients lifetime, accessible for *in vivo* flow modulation and of a biocompatible material minimizing the scarring of the filtration bleb to give a better and longstanding reservoir.

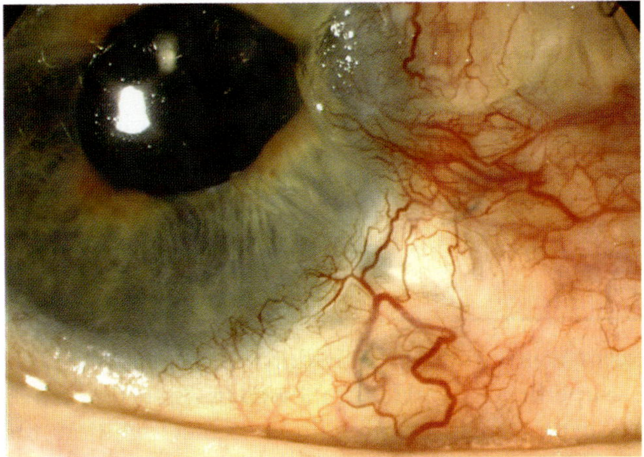

Fig. 11: The eye after 6 months. IOP 12, visual acuity 20/50

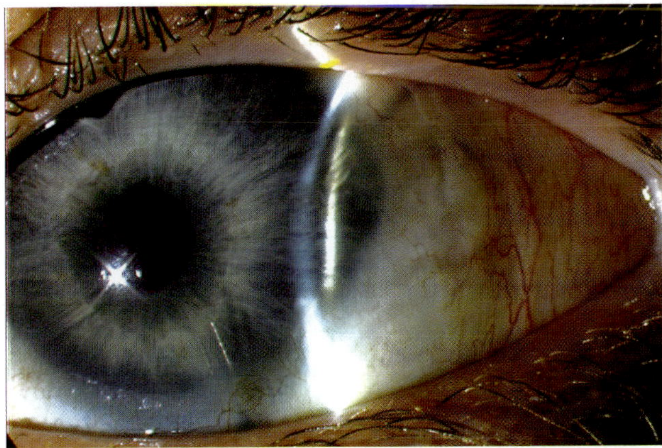

Fig. 12: The eye after 20 years. Two shunts are visible

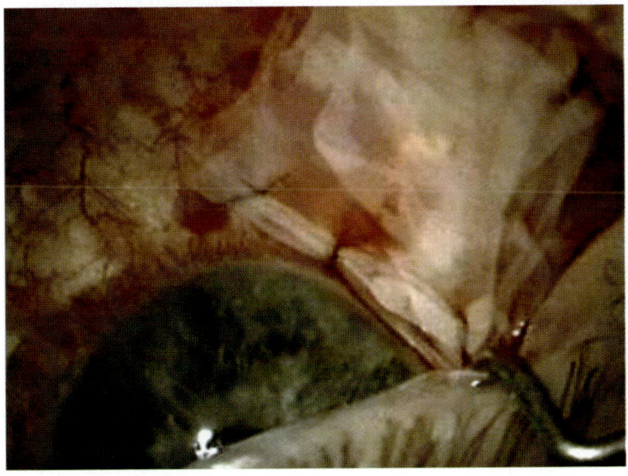

Fig. 13: Tube erosion covered with an amniotic patch

15

Trabeculotome-guided Deep Sclerectomy

Ahmed Mostafa Abdelrahman (Egypt)

INTRODUCTION

Deep sclerectomy was introduced by Fydorov in 1989. This procedure consists of dissecting a superficial scleral flap, followed by dissection of a deeper scleral flap that should expose an intact trabeculo-Descemet's window, through which the aqueous will percolate. In this way the major sites of aqueous outflow resistance in glaucoma, which are the inner wall of Schlemm's canal (SC) and juxtacanalicular meshwork, will be bypassed. The plane of dissection of the second flap *must* unroof the Schlemm's canal to expose the percolating Trabeculo-Descemet's membrane (TDM), and the roof of canal will be included in excised deep flap. Removal of the inner wall of the Schlemm's canal and juxtacanalicular trabecular meshwork will further increase aqueous percolation.

When compared to the standard trabeculectomy, deep sclerectomy is much safer (both short and long-term) because anterior chamber instability and bleb related infection occur less frequently. On the other hand, it is technically more difficult. The most difficult part of this procedure occurs during deep scleral flap dissection, especially for surgeons with recent conversion to the Non-Penetrating Glaucoma Surgery (NPGS); even experienced surgeons may miss the plane of Schlemm's canal.

The results from Dietlein et al showed that morphological signs of the removed parts of the outer wall of SC, along with the deep scleral flaps, were found in serial sections from 15 out of 29 patients, i.e. 52%. In 5 of these 15 patients, i.e. 17%, noticeable remnants of the juxtacanalicular trabecular meshwork were also found, although this was obvious in only one patient during surgery. In 14 out of 29 patients, i.e. 48%, there was no evidence of the deroofing of SC, although intraoperatively the dissection seemed to have been too superficial in only five patients. They concluded that deep sclerectomy, even when performed by experienced glaucoma surgeons, produces biopsy material of great morphological variability that does not always correspond to the intraoperative appearance of the operation site. Such variability may be of importance for the outcome of the surgery.

"Trabeculotome-guided unroofing of Schlemm's canal" is an alternative technique to the classic posterior approach, aiming to identify and unroof Schlemm's canal during NPGS. The technique is based on the identification of SC in the same way it is identified during trabeculotomy, one of the key surgeries in congenital glaucoma management.

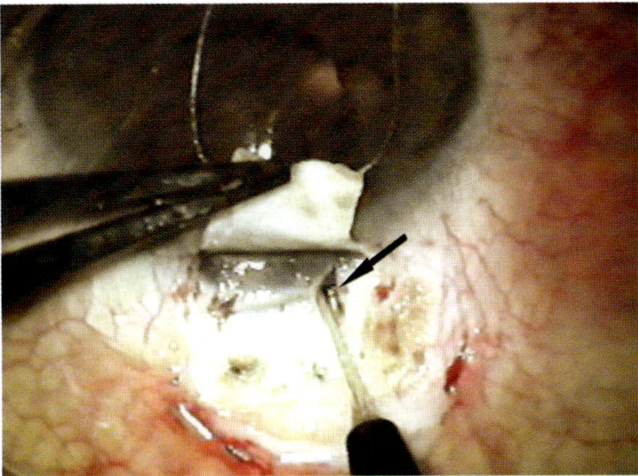

Fig. 1: Schlemm's canal identification. The initial vertical limbal incision to expose the canal. The arrow points to the opened canal

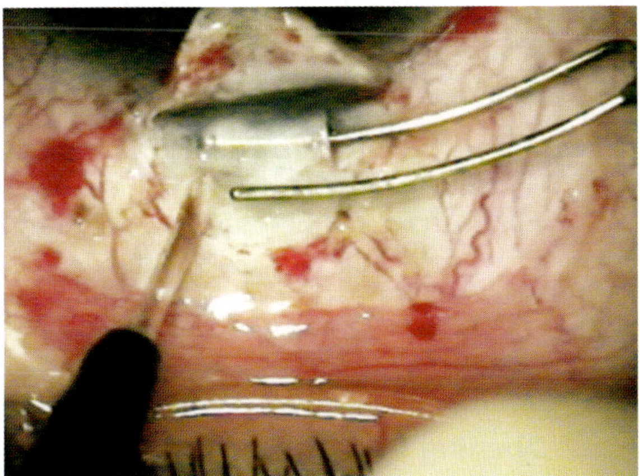

Fig. 2: Trabeculotome placement. The instrument is Introducing inside SC and pushed horizontally to the left while lifting the sclera up

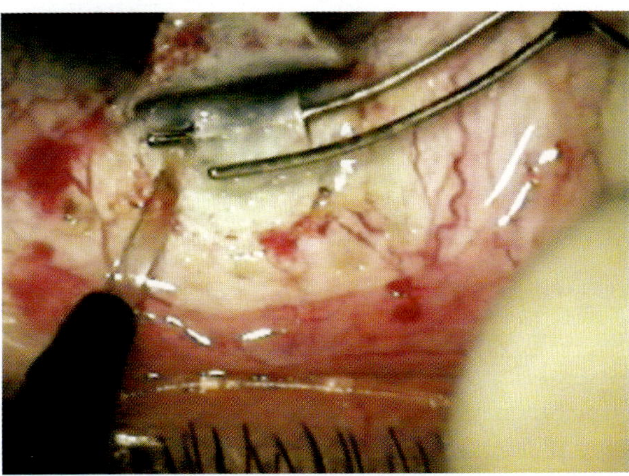

Fig. 3: Trabeculotome exist incision: Another vertical limbal incision is done directly over the instrument. Bottom right: The Trabeculotome exits through that second incision

SURGICAL TECHNIQUE

A Fornix – based conjunctival flap is prepared. Wet-field cautery is applied as little as possible to the bleeding vessels. A 5 × 5 superficial scleral flap is dissected. A Mitomycin-C ® soaked sponge (0.4 mg/Ml for 2 minutes) is placed deep and underneath the superficial scleral flap. The application area is abundantly washed with balanced salt saline solution (BSS).

Schlemm's Canal Identification

A vertical scratch incision is made at the sclero-limbal junction at one edge of the deep scleral flap. The scratch is gradually deepened under high magnification until SC is seen anterior to the circumferential fibers of the scleral spur (near the posterior aspect of the grey zone). Often, a small amount of blood or aqueous will reflux through the cut ends of the canal. To facilitate the identification of the canal, the assistant should keep the dissection area dry. The tissues can be pushed laterally with the cutting blade for a clearer vision of the SC.

Trabeculotome Placement

The Trabeculotome (Katena®) is introduced though this incision into the SC without resistance. It is then pushed horizontally in the canal while lifting the sclera up. This will avoid inadvertent trabeculotomy. At the other edge of the deep scleral flap, a direct vertical limbal incision is made over the trabeculotome, which will allow the instrument to exit. In this way, the trabeculotome will stabilize inside the SC in the area of the deep scleral flap. The handle of the trabeculotome is rotated towards the eye, and allowed to rest on its surface.

Schlemm's Canal Opening and Unroofing

The dissection of the deep flap is carried out as usual. As we approach the SC, the trabeculotome will start to show. A direct incision is made over the trabeculotome, opening the canal along its posterior border and unroofing it. Forward dissection of the deep scleral flap is continued to have adequate exposure of the trabeculo-Descemet's window. The deep flap is then excised, and the superficial flap is sutured with 2 10/0 Nylon sutures, one at each corner.

Combined Phacoemulsification and Deep Sclerectomy

The surgical steps will be as follows:

1. Fornix- based conjunctival flap.
2. Superficial scleral flap dissection and MMC application.
3. Separate corneal incision for phacoemulsification and IOL.
4. Trabeculotome placement inside SC and deep flap dissection. Percolation will not be evident at this step as the AC is filled with viscoelastic.
5. Irrigation/aspiration of the viscoelastic, and testing for percolation.

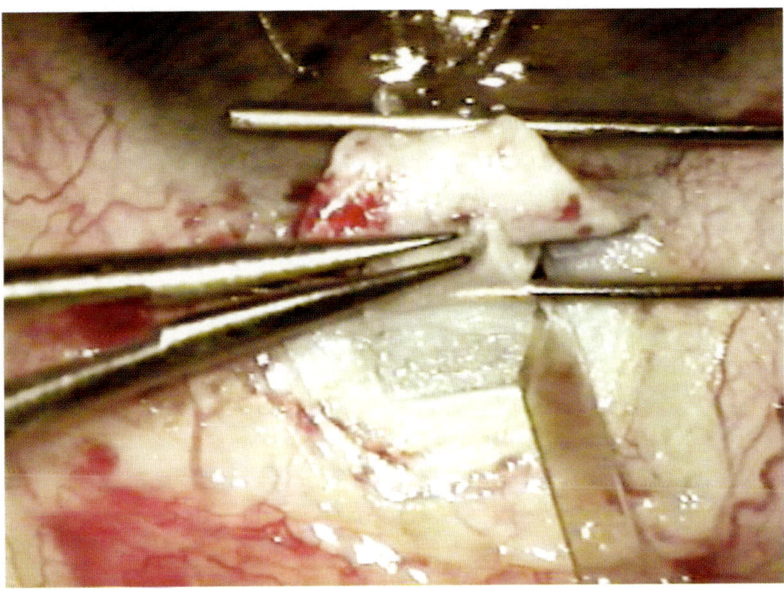

Fig. 4: Deep scleral flap dissection. The Trabeculotome starts to show as SC is approached

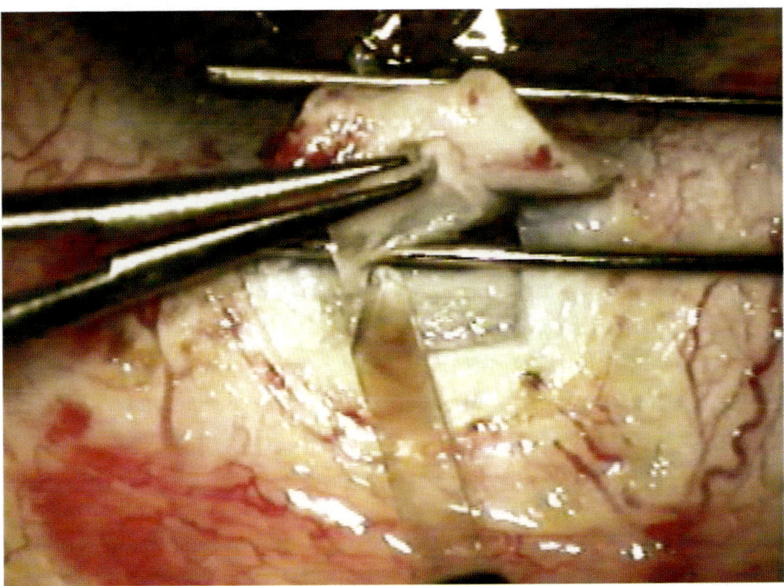

Fig. 5: SC unroofing. The posterior wall of the canal is incised directly over the trabeculotome

Advantages of the Technique

1. It facilitates identification and unroofing of SC, this might shorten the learning curve of NPGS (At least 200 cases are required to master deep sclerectomy using the standard posterior approach, *Dr. Elie Dahan, 5th international glaucoma symposium, Cape town, 2005*).
2. The second advantage is the ability to unroof SC without inducing severe thinning of the remaining scleral bed; classically the sclera has to be reduced to 10-5% of its thickness. Therefore the risk of scleral ectasia might be reduced.
3. Additional interesting finding is observing a reasonable trabeculo-Descemet's membrane exposure immediately after complete canal opening. This may be the result of tissue separation induced by the size of the trabeculotome.

Disadvantages

1. The relatively longer operative time compared to the standard deep sclerectomy; in fact deep sclerectomy beginners also consume longer operative time.
2. The SC has to be identified during the initial vertical limbal incision. Some practical points could help SC identification: a) Observing the horizontal-running scleral spur fibers, b) Detecting the transparency of the SC floor, c) Efflux of blood and aqueous.

CONCLUSIONS

Each surgical technique for deep sclerectomy has its Pros and Cons. The classic posterior approach is the standard technique for deep sclerectomy, yet it is still technically difficult with the possibility of missing the Schlemm's canal plane (up to 48%); in that situation dissection of a successful third flap is even much more difficult. The Trabeculotome- guided technique tries to minimize such an incidence, also it avoids severe surgical the induced thinning of the remaining scleral bed. On the other hand there are certain difficulties, namely the SC has to be identified initially, and longer operative time.

As **SC** identification and unroofing is a crucial step during NPGS, the Trabeculotome – guided technique increases the available surgical options to accomplish this step, *not aiming to replace the classic posterior approach,* a situation similar to nucleus management during phacoemulsification, where the surgeon is backed up by many techniques.

Although both techniques have technical difficulties, especially for beginners, Trabeculotome- guided technique could be of particular help to surgeons already performing trabeculotomy, as they share a common principle regarding SC identification and probing.

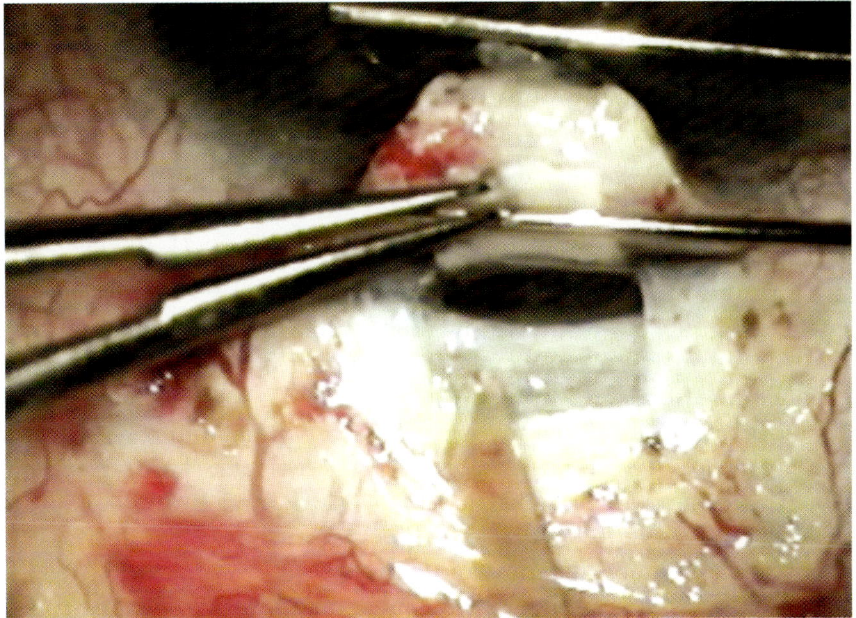

Fig. 6: Complete SC unroofing with release of the trabeculotome

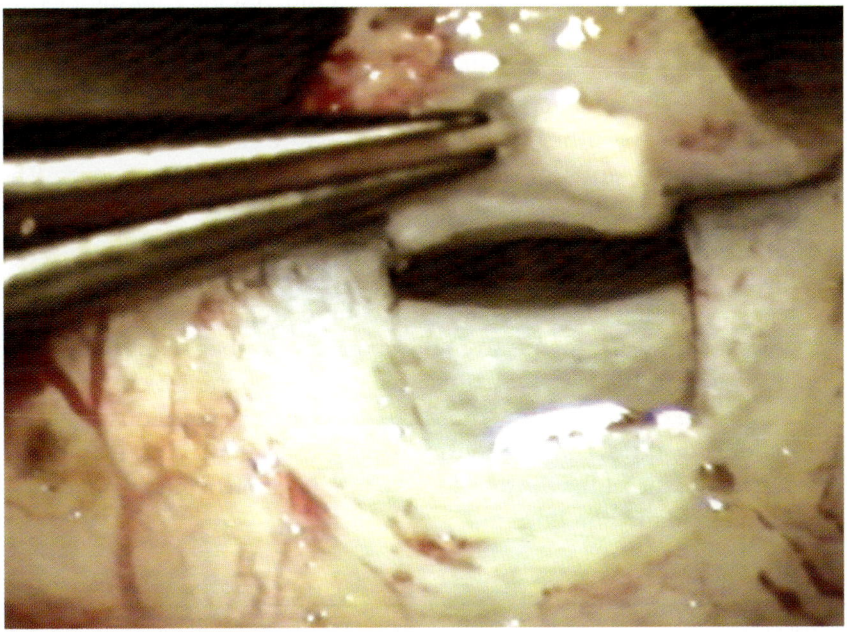

Fig. 7: The remaining scleral bed is of reasonable thickness

16

Glaucoma Drainage Implants

Mordechai Goldenfeld, Shlomo Melamed (Israel)

INTRODUCTION

The success of trabeculectomy, the most common glaucoma filtration surgery depends on two major factors, the patency of the sclerostomy site and the creation of a functioning filtering bleb.

In most cases trabeculectomy is a successful operation however, certain types of glaucoma have a considerable lower success rate. These types include Uveitic glaucoma, Neovascular glaucoma (NVG), and Juvenile glaucoma, glaucoma in eyes with previous intraocular surgery, like aphakia and pseudophakia, and repeated trabeculectomy.

In the minority of cases the cause of failure may be attributed the closure of the sclerostomy site. These cases include NVG, glaucoma in Iridocorneal endothelial syndrome, (ICE), endothelial down-growth and uveitic glaucoma, but in most cases, the cause of failure of the filtering operation is scaring of the conjunctiva. Different approaches have been made in order to improve the success of glaucoma surgery and to promote a functioning filtering bleb, and for that purpose the use of glaucoma drainage devices have been developed. These devices were commonly called Setons, but Setons are defined as solid devices, without a lumen that promote flow of aqueous along their outer surface. Historically Setons were the first attempt to bypass a closed angle and create a lasting flow from the anterior chamber into the subconjunctival space. These devices had only a limited success and are reviewed here only as a historical review. Later, tube shunts were introduced in order to improve the success of glaucoma surgery, by bypassing the closed angels, creating a permanent paten sclerostomy , avoiding the scarred anterior conjunctiva and creating a real shut that enables the flow of aqueous from the anterior chamber, using a tube, into a posterior subconjunctival reservoir, thus creating a functioning bleb. Tube shunts were also directed into the suprachoroidal space and the vitreous cavity. The idea of shunting fluid from the vitreous cavity in glaucoma was recently reintroduced by Baerveldt, who developed a modification of the original implant to the Pars plan glaucoma Implant.

HISTORICAL REVIEW

As early as 1906, horse-hair was used in order to promote flow from the anterior chamber and create a functioning filtering bleb, since then various materials have been tried in order to create flow from the anterior chamber into the

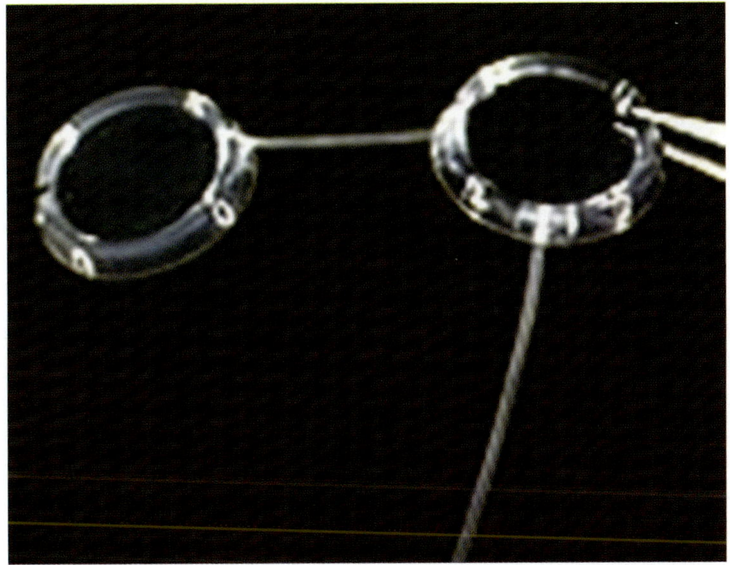

Fig. 1: Molteno glaucoma implants

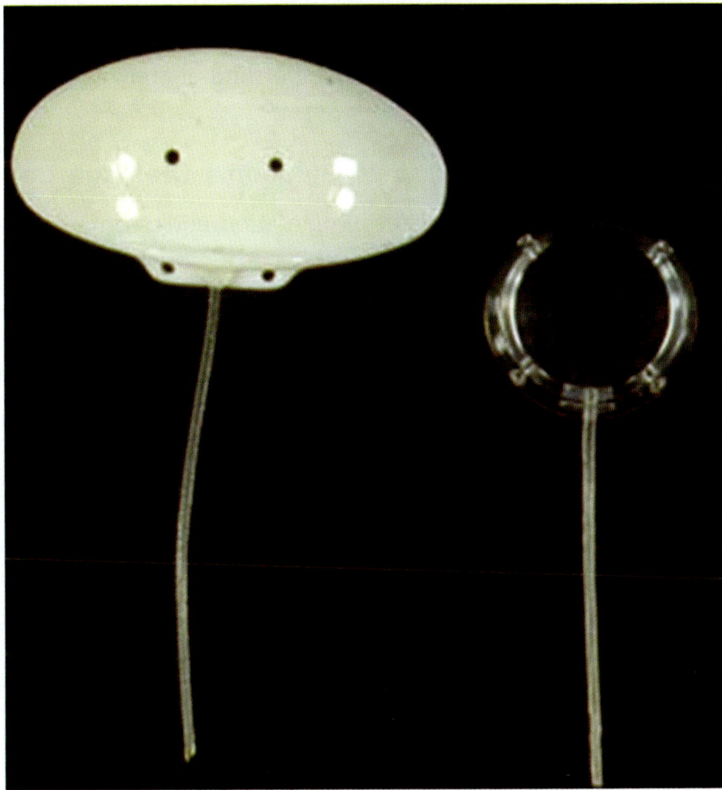

Fig. 2: Baerveldt and Molteno glaucoma shunt implants

subconjunctival space or from the vitreous cavity into the subconjunctival space, like platinum wire, Magnesium strip and other materials, however, in most cases the operation failed mostly due to local inflammation and scarring, mostly due to biocompatibility problems. Others tried to create a shunt into the lacrimal sac, vortex veins, or to the conjunctival-tear surface,. All were abandoned eventually due to very limited success. Attempts were made to create a shunt from the anterior chamber, using a trans-limbal approach, to the sub-conjunctival space, placing the explant drainage site close to the limbal are, but in most cases success was limited mainly due to excess scaring of the bleb, but also due to local complications like corneal complications and patient intolerance due to foreign body sensation. Later observations revealed the when encircling buckles used in retinal detachment operations, had to removed from the eye, they were usually removed easily with little scar tissue around them , and the result was that shunt tubes were developed in order to shift the flow not just out of the anterior chamber to the perilimbal area , but mainly to create a shunt from the anterior chamber into the posterior conjunctiva and sub-Tenon's space, thus by-passing the closed angle with scarred Trabecular meshwork ,avoiding the excess scaring of the perilimbal area and creating a functioning posterior bleb. The first to publish data that employs the principle of posterior shunting was Molteno, that originally used an explant placed in the immediate perilimbal area and later moved the explant from the perilimbal area, posteriorly, thus creating a large posterior bleb.

Principles for the Implantation of Glaucoma Drainage Device

Several key points are in the basis of the implantation, and essentially all modern glaucoma shunts follow the same principles:

1. The creation of a shunt from the anterior chamber into the posterior conjunctival and sub-Tenon's space.
2. Direct communication between the anterior chamber and the bleb at the posterior sub-conjunctival and sub-Tenon's space.
3. Placement of the collecting device in the posterior sub-conjunctival and sub-Tenon's space that enables the creation of a large bleb, thus enabling a greater reduction of intraocular pressure.
4. Placement of the collecting device posteriorly, allows better protection of the implant, reducing the risk of exposure.

These key points have been confirmed in histological studies that demonstrated the tissue surrounding the posterior fibrovascular bleb is capable of passive aqueous flow through its walls.

Types of Glaucoma Tube Shunts

The first tube shunt was described by Molteno, who was the first to introduce the principal of directing the flow of aqueous from the anterior chamber towards

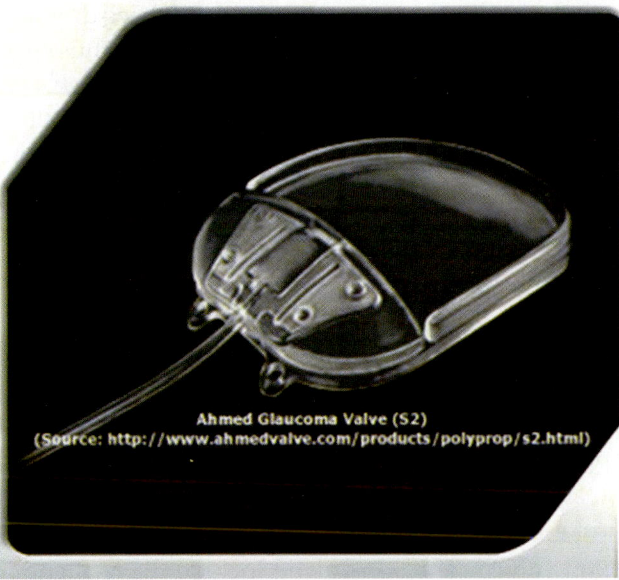

Fig. 3: Ahmed glaucoma valves

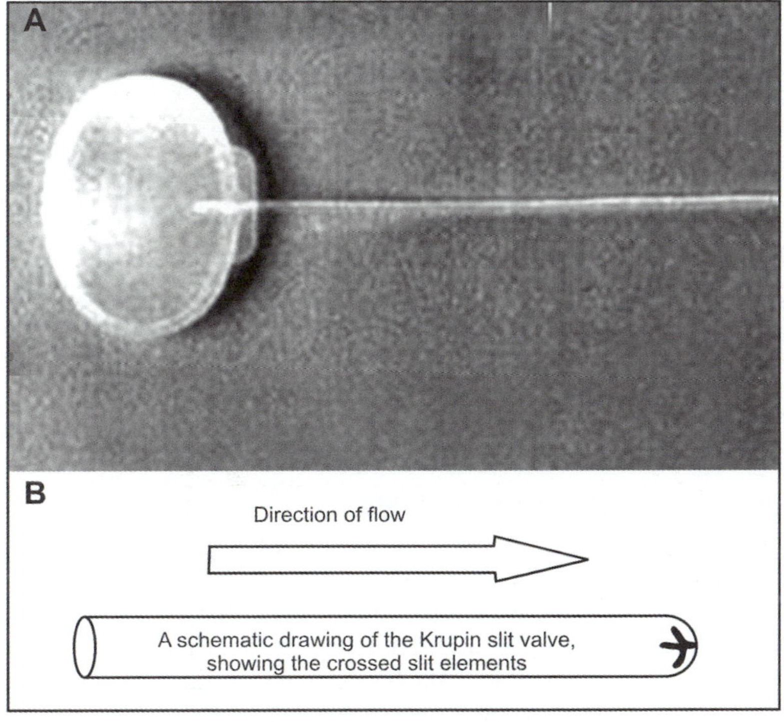

Fig. 4: Krupin valve with disk

the posterior sub-conjunctival/sub-Tenon's space. Molteno directed the posterior opening of the tube onto the plate explant upper surface, thus ensuring that the flow is directed superiorly, promoting separation of the bleb's walls from the opening of the tube on the plate, minimizing the risk of tube closure with scar tissue at its posterior orifice. Experimental perfusion studies demonstrated the there is a linear relationship between the drainage capacity of the filtering bleb around the explant and it's surface area, and that the resistance of the capsule to perfusion is related to the thickness of the bleb walls. These findings, reassured that the initiative for new versions of tube shuts with larger explants and multiple explants were rational, and that use of anti fibrotic materials in order to create a relatively thin-walled bleb was justified. Currently used shunt implants follow the principle introduced by Molteno, using a long tube that drains posteriorly to an episcleral plate that acts as a bleb-spreading device. Recently, a new device the ExPress Shunt was developed. This implant uses a different concept, promoting flow to the perilimbal area, and will be discusses separately.

The Posterior tube-shunt implants can be divided essentially into two groups, Valved and Non-valved. The non-valved include the Molteno implants, the Baerveldt implant, and the Schocket shunt to an encircling tube. Valved implants include the Krupin valve with disk, the Ahmed valve, the Joseph implant, Optimed implant, and the White pump-shunt. Interestingly, all use the same internal tube diameter of 0.3 mm. The outer diameter varies between 0.58 mm (Krupin and Joseph) and 0.64 mm (Schocket, Baerveldt, Joseph, Optimed, White Ahmed); The Molteno is the only one with outer diameter of 0.63 mm

Table 1: Characteristics of commonly used posterior tube shunt implants

Shunt	*Restrictive*	*Surface area(mm^2)*	*Shape*	*Height*
Optimed	Yes	18	Rectangular	1.40 mm
Krupin valve with disk	Yes, Valved	180	Oval	1.75 mm
White pump	Yes	280	Round	
Joseph valve	Yes	765	Rectangular band	
Ahmed valve	Yes, Valved	184	Pear	1.90 mm
Baerveldt valve	No	250, 350, 425	Curved semilunar	1.00 mm
Schocket	No	300	Rectangular band	
Molteno	No	134	Round	1.5 mm

Non-restrictive Glaucoma Implants

The Molteno Implant. (IOP, Inc., Costa Mesa, Calif).

The Molteno is a non-restrictive implant, allowing bidirectional flow of aqueous.

It consists of a circular, 13 mm diameter, convex, rigid explant made of polypropylene. A silicone tube is attached to the plate, passes through the rim and opens onto the convex upper surface of the plate. The proximal end of the tube is placed into the anterior chamber through a limbal paracentesis wound

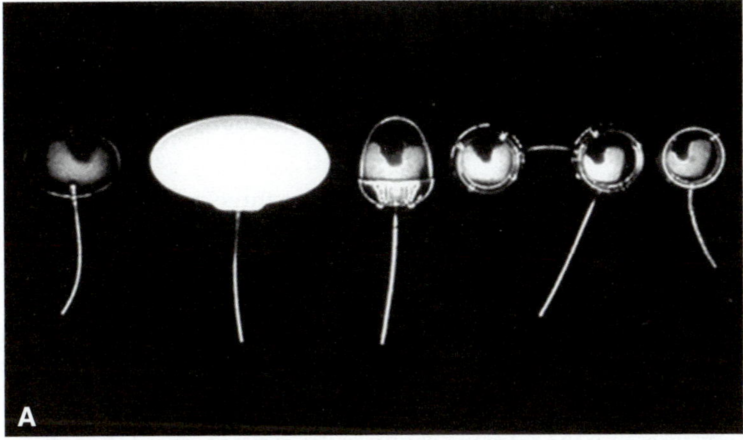

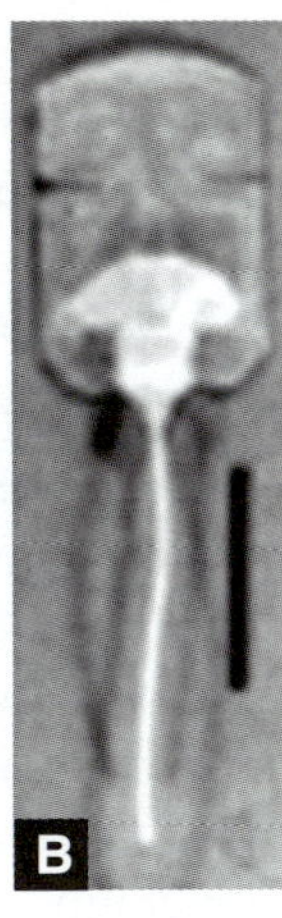

Fig. 5A Glaucoma drainage devices are shown. From left to right, Krupin drainage device, Baerveldt drainage implant (350 mm^2), Ahmed implant, double plate Molteno device, and single plate Molteno device

Fig. 5B: Optimed pressure regulator

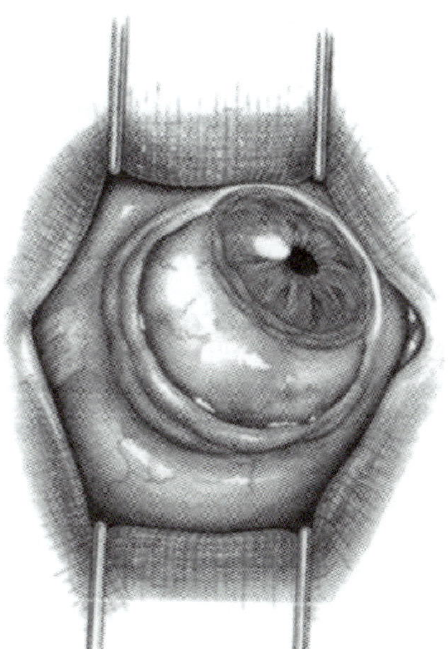

Fig. 6: Fornix base conjunctival incision

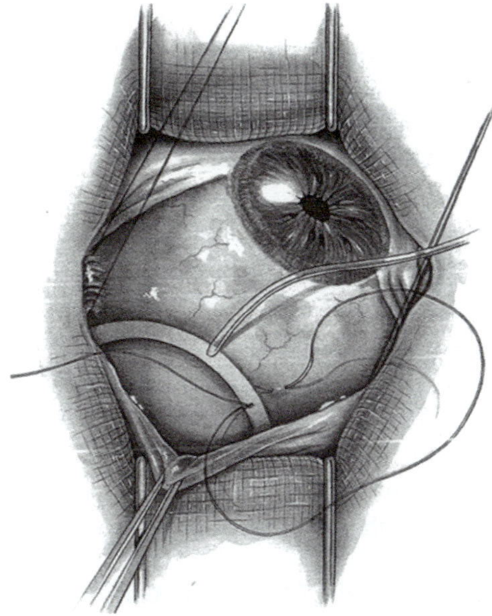

Fig. 7: Insertion of the posterior plate explant

that may be passed directly using a full thickness tract, or underneath a partial thickness scleral flap. Aside from the single plate Molteno implant, dual and even quadruple plate Molteno valves are available. And also a pediatric size.

The Baerveldt Implant (Iovision, Irvine, Calif)

The Baerveldt implant is a silicone implant available in three sizes .The explant is placed with the silicone plate underneath two adjacent recti muscles in the nasal or temporal ocular quadrant. The Baerveldt episcleral plate includes fenestration holes that allow growth of fibrous tissue through the plate and to the other side of the bleb wall, thereby reducing the volume of the bleb. Recently a new version of the Baerveldt implant The Pars Plana Glaucoma Implant was introduced, and is designed for placement during or following a pars plana vitrectomy, communicating the vitreous cavity to the explant.

The White Pump Shunt (Tamcenan Corp, Sioux Falls, SO)

The White pump shunt consists of a tube made of silicone that is inserted into the anterior chamber, while it's end is connected to a 16-18 mm balloon which has an outlet into the retrobulbar space. The distal end of the tube contains two unidirectional valves. The valves open at a pressure between 5 and 15 mmHg thus minimizing hypotony. And preventing reflux of aqueous into the anterior chamber from the reservoir. Digital massage or blinking activity, pumps aqueous into and out of the balloon, maintaining continuous flow from the anterior chamber.

Schocket Band Implant

The Schocket anterior chamber tube shunt to an encircling band is based on the diversion of aqueous to a reservoir of an encircling band from which fluid is postulated to diffuse into the orbit. It consists of a Silastic tube sutured into the grooved portion of a silicone band; Originally Schocket used a 30 mm long tube with a 0.3 mm inner and a 0.64 mm outer diameter. A 360° #20 or #220 Silicone band is used as the external scleral explant, creating a drainage surface area of approximately 300 mm^2. Being a non-valves shunt, early hypotony with shallow anterior chamber limited its use.

Ex-PRESS™ Miniature Glaucoma Implant (Boston Scientific, Inc, MA)

This shunt is not a substitute for posterior shunt procedures indicated for refractory glaucoma, but is reviewed here because it is, by definition a glaucoma shunt device enabling flow from the anterior chamber to the anterior perilimbal area. Essentially it is designed to be implanted all instances in which the surgeon would normally first elect to perform a trabeculectomy. The miniature Ex-PRESS™ is constructed of implantable, biocompatible stainless steel approved

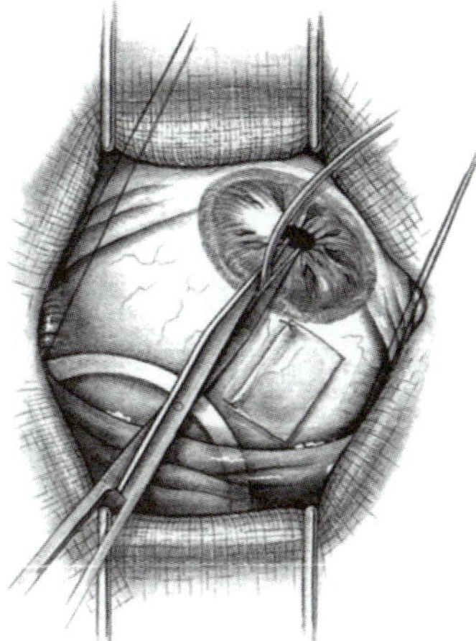

Fig. 8: Tube trimming

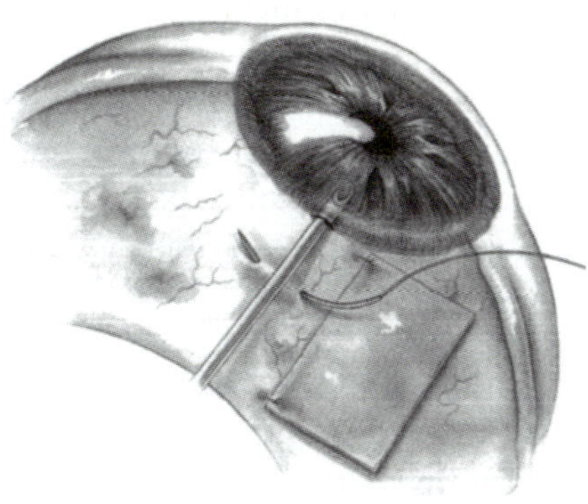

Fig. 9: Tube suturing and fixation to the epi-sclera

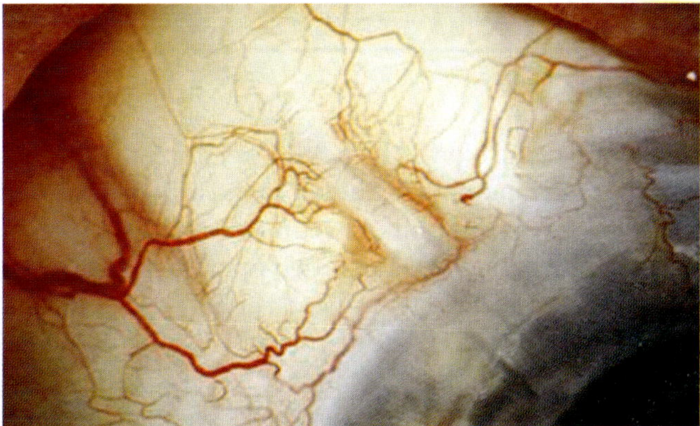

Fig. 10: Tube erosion through the overlying conjunctiva

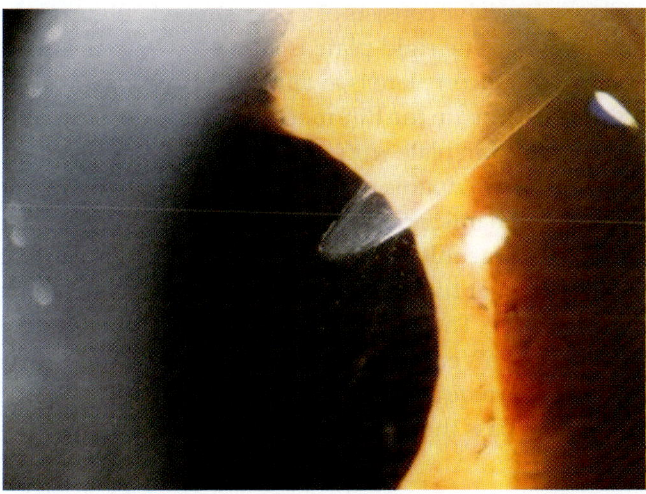

Fig. 11: Vitreous plugging the tube

for human use. It is 2.96 mm long and has an outer diameter of 400 μm. The lumen size of the product (R-50) is 50 μm. The shunt's penetrating tip is blunt and needle-shaped in order to minimize tissue damage and facilitate insertion. While the distal end has a flat, angled flange to prevent intrusion and blend with the limbal anatomy, the proximal end has a beveled spur to prevent extrusion, and the distance between the spur and the shunt's distal flange equals the scleral thickness. The angles of the disk and spur are designed to follow the normal anatomy of the limbal area. The shunt's proximal end also features three additional transverse orifices to prevent plugging by the iris, blood, or inflammatory membranes. The device comes loaded on a disposable inserter. The concept of the Ex-PRESS mini-glaucoma shunt is similar to that of trabeculectomy; both divert aqueous humor from the anterior chamber to the perilimbal subconjunctival space. Thus , promoting the flow to the anterior perilimbal area. The flow-restricting unit inside the shunt's lumen provides a fixed resistance to flow.

RESTRICTIVE GLAUCOMA IMPLANTS

The Joseph Valve

This is a modification of the Non-valved Schocket implant designed in order to prevent postoperative hypotony attributed to the lack of a restricting valve. It consists of a curved tube with a slit valve in the upper surface of the silicone tube that functions as a valve with a reported opening pressure between 4 and 20 mmHg.The tube is connected to a silicon rubber strap which is attached to 180° of the scleral circumference . The silicon rubber strap allows accumulation of aqueous using a surface area of 765 mm^2

The Ahmed Valve (New World Medical, Inc, Rancho Cucamonga, Calif)

The Ahmed Glaucoma Valve consists of a pear-shaped polypropylene or silicon explant. The polypropylene rigid plate is 13 mm × 16 mm, and has a surface area of, 184 mm^2. The silicon plate is available in two sizes, a 9.6 mm × 10 mm with a surface of 96.00 mm^2 in the PF8 model used in pediatrics or small globes, and a 13.00 mm × 16.00 mm plate with a surface of 184 mm^2 in the PF7 model for regular use. There is also a double plate model, the F×1. The Ahmed valve uses the Bernoulli's hydrodynamic principle, by which the velocity of a fluid increases as it travels from the large inlet to the smaller outlet port. The aqueous passes from the anterior chamber tube between two layers of a thin membrane on the upper surface of the plate. The membrane is enclosed within the anterior portion of the implant, creating a Venturi effect on aqueous flow through the device. A force of 8 to 12 mmHg is required to separate the layers of the silicone membrane and allow aqueous to pass through the valve, into the reservoir.

The Optimed Implant (OGPR;Optimed, Inc., Int., Santa Barbara, Calif)

The Optimed Glaucoma Pressure Regulator (OGPR) employs the principle of capillary flow. It consists of a polymethyl methacrylate (PMMA) matrix of conductive resistors that establish the egress of aqueous flow from the eye. The Optimed implant's "flow-restricting" unit is made up of multiple microtubules providing a pressure gradient, governed by Poiseuille's formula. The tubules connect to an anterior chamber silicone tube that connects to an explant 18 mm^2 surface. There are three models that vary according to the length (not number) of capillary passageways, the longer the length of the tubules the flow is reduced. The Optimed regulator enables aqueous outflow when pressure within the eye exceeds 10 mmHg.

Krupin Valve With Disk (Hood Laboratories, Pembroke, Mass)

The Krupin valve consists of a Silastic tube connected to a Silastic disk the distal end of the tube is sealed and contains horizontal and vertical slits that function as a unidirectional and pressure-sensitive valve. The valve requires a force of approximately 9 mm Hg to 11 mm Hg for aqueous flow through the device

Two types of external scleral explants have been used with the long glaucoma valve implant: The episcleral plate shaped to fit the curvature of the globe .The anterior edge of the explant differs from other explants by having a platform for the fixation of the explant to the sclera and not permanent holes. This design enables the surgeon to fixate the explant more easily, not having to fixate the plate at predetermined areas.

Alternatively, the tube can be connected to a #220 Silastic band as with a Schocket procedure.

Glaucoma Implants—Indication for Use

Although originally the use of glaucoma implants was limited only to refractory glaucoma in eyes with little visual potential, in recent years the introduction of newly designed and valved devices, and the use of excellent inert biocompatible material have greatly improved the results and favored the surgical outcome of implant surgery. As a rule glaucoma implants are used in refractory glaucoma, but primary use has been reported in pediatric glaucoma and in pseudophakic glaucoma and active neovascular glaucoma (NVG) ICE syndrome.

There are no universally accepted guideline regarding the implantation of glaucoma implants, however we recommend their primary use in pediatric glaucoma, NVG, ICE syndrome, and as a second line in cases where previous trabeculectomy with the use of anti-metabolites have failed. (Aphakic and pseudophakic glaucoma, uveitic glaucoma, glaucoma following penetrating keratoplasty, glaucoma in cases of extensive conjunctival scaring such as following retinal surgery). If however the visual acuity is less than 20/200 we believe that a cyclodestructive procedure is more appropriate.

Technique

Basically, most of the procedure is extraocular, the only intraocular step is the introduction of the tube into the anterior chamber, and the procedure is very similar in all types of shunt surgery. Valved shunts can be implanted I a one stage operation. Non-valved shunts require either a two-stage insertion or a legation of the tube in order to prevent early postoperative hypotony and flat anterior chamber and choroidal detachment or hemorrhage.

The One Stage Insertion

Consists of the following steps:

1. A fornix-based conjunctival flap superiorly
2. Tenon's capsule is undermined to expose the sclera
3. The appropriate recti muscles are exposed.
4. The explant is inserted under the conjunctiva and Tenon's capsule and sutured to the episclera
5. A clear cornea paracentesis is made away from the surgical site.
6. We recommend the use of an anterior chamber maintainer (ACM) connected to a balanced salt solution (BSS) infusion; alternatively viscoelastic material can be injected into the chamber through the paracentesis we prefer to use the ACM because the viscous material may clog the orifice of the tube in the anterior chamber or may adversely affect the function of Valved implants. Also the use of viscoelastics may artificially deepen the chamber and can contribute to inaccurate tube placement.
7. The anterior chamber is entered. The entry track is made at an oblique angle, parallel to the plane of the iris. This can be made either under a partial thickness scleral flap or full-thickness track. We prefer the full-thickness track, using a 23 gauge needle, and to cover the tube with a sutured partial thickness preserved donor scleral flap, alternatively preserved pericardium or preserved dura have been used. Dissection of a scleral flap improves visualization of the limbal anatomy and allows more accurate tube placement into the anterior chamber, however the use of a partial thickness lamellar scleral flap may lead to oozing of aqueous around the tube and create hypotony and flat anterior chamber. (In cases of aphakia or pseudophakia, after careful vitrectomy the tube can be inserted through the parsplana.)
8. The tube is trimmed bevel-up to extend 2 to 3 mm into the anterior chamber. The length of the tube is estimated by laying the tube across the cornea
9. The tube is inserted through the entry track into the anterior chamber with smooth forceps.
10. A single 10-0 nylon episcleral suture is tied around the tube midway along its course to reduce tube movement and to maintain tube contact with the

sclera. The suture knot is rotated and buried into the sclera to prevent external erosion.

11. The tube is covered with a partial thickness preserved donor sclera. Alternatively preserved pericardium or preserved dura have been used.
12. The conjunctiva is draped down towards the limbal area and is sutured tightly to the limbus, ensuring that the closure is water-tight. A drop of fluorescein is used to ensure a negative Seidel test. In cases where conjunctival closure is difficult, due to conjunctival scars, it is most important to ensure that the explant is completely contained in a water-tight conjunctival bleb. The remaining conjunctiva can be sutured down to episcleral, and eventually will cover the bare episclera anteriorly. In some cases, a conjunctival autograph can be used from the inferior fornix or a preserved, partial thickness donor scleral flap may be used to cover the exposed areas.

Two-Stage Insertion

After the explant is sutured to the episclera, the open end of the tube is placed under the plate or beneath a rectus muscle. The tube is than sutured to the episcleral. The use of black silk suture is recommended in order to facilitate locating the tube at the second surgical stage. If the IOP is very high and the danger to damage of the optic nerve is imminent, than a trabeculectomy may be performed in order to provide a temporary reduction of the IOP. This is the end of the first stage and tenon's capsule and conjunctiva are sutured and closed.

At the second operative stage, 2 to 6 weeks later, the insertion of the tube into the anterior chamber, is performed. The conjunctiva is opened and the tube is recovered and inserted into the anterior chamber as previously described. The two-stage procedure is recommended in all high risk patients. (High myopia Aphakia/pseudophakia, Shallow anterior chamber). In the two-stage operation the reduction of the IOP is not immediate, since the aqueous flow is limited due to the initial small size of the filtering bleb, or the formations of a Tenon's cyst, this may results an initially high IOP, necessitating the aggressive use of anti glaucoma medication and topical steroids. The use of the double plate Molteno tube shunt has been advocated in order to reduce this hypertensive phase.

Another approach to prevent early postoperative hypotony is the temporary occlusion of the tube, which prevents aqueous flow from the anterior chamber until the episcleral plate becomes encapsulated. The tube can be legated with an absorbable suture, alternatively a releasable suture can be tied around the tube with it's end exposed through the conjunctiva and pulled at the appropriate time. A black suture can be visualized through the conjunctiva and opened with the use of laser. Insertion of an absorbable suture into the lumen of the tube, passing it through the explant orifice and through the conjunctiva has been describes, the suture is occluding the lumen of the tube until it dissolves or it may be pulled out.

Success

The overall success rate of the most popular glaucoma drainage implants is between 72-79% . Table 2 contains only the results of the Molteno, Ahmed, Krupin and Baerveldt implant; this is because the Schocket, the Optimed, the White shunt pump and the Joseph implants, all lack substantial peer-reviewed literature. Success is usually defined as IOP between 5-22 mmHg with or without the use of anti-glaucoma medication. The Double plate Molteno has the highest reported success rate.The higher rate of success may be due to the larger surface area of the explant, however, this conclusion is challenged by another study that compared the 350 mm^2 vs. 500 mm^2 Baerveldt implant, and did not find a statistical significant difference in the overall surgical success rate or IOP control. In another study that compared the double plate Molteno (270 mm^2) to the 350 mm^2 Baerveldt implant there was no advantage to the greater size of the Baerveldt im-plant. Chain-Huey Hong et al conclude that the optimal size may be the 270 mm^2 size of the Double plate Molteno and that a larger surface area has no benefit. Stratifying the successes rate according to glaucoma type revels that the lowest rate of success is reported in epithelial down-growth. Favorable results are reported for use in glaucoma following keratoplasty, in Neovascular glaucoma (NVG) treated with the Krupin valve, 35.7 -67 %, and up to 95% in cases of NVG treated with the Schocket implant, however in the later the rate of prolonged flat anterior chamber was 74%. In another series of refractory glaucoma treated with the Ahmed valve, the mean success rate at 3 years was 73%, the most frequent indications for use of the drainage device were: neovascular glaucoma (45.7%), no response to other glaucoma surgery (20%), Aphakic glaucoma (10%) and traumatic glaucoma (8.5%).A report published on the successes rate of the Joseph implant had a 94% success , but follow-up was only 6 months. A similar success rate of 89% was reported by White using the White glaucoma pump shunt, this high rate of success was contrasted by another report who had a success rate of only 31%.

Use of Antifibrotics (Mitomicin-C and 5-FU)

Antifibrotic agents are commonly used in glaucoma surgery. They enhance bleb survival and increase the success rate of trabeculectomy. The role of these agents in glaucoma drainage surgery is not clear. On one hand they may promote the creation of a thinner walled bleb and increase flow across the bleb walls, but on the other hand may create a greater risk of outer plate erosion though the overlying conjunctiva . Reports from the literature are mixed, and show a higher complication rate in the anti-fibrotic treated group, while the final IOP in the anti fibrotic treated patients was similar to the control group. Currently we do not know why the use of anti-fibrotic agents in glaucoma drainage surgery, does not have the same advantages as in trabeculectomy.

Table 2: Results of glaucoma shunts implantation					
Data	*Molteno shunt without modification*	*Molteno with modification*	*Baerveldt implant*	*Ahmed glaucoma valve*	*Krupin valve*
Number of published studies	6	27	9	8	2
Total no. of patients (all studies)	234	1297	550	526	75
Mean follow-up (months)	23.1±10.8	27.1±14.2	18.6± 7.8	16.0± 7.5	21.3±11.2
% change in IOP	59±3	51±6	54±8	51±8	62±5
Surgical success, %	75±12	77±13	75±10	79±8	72±11

Modified from: Glaucoma drainage device. A systemic Literature review and current Controversies. Chain-Huey Hong et al. survey ophthalmol Vol 50 number 1 January-February 2005

Complications

Aside from complications that may occur in any ocular surgery, (Infection, hemorrhage, ect), Tube shunt have unique complication, that can be divided into early postoperative and late postoperative. Table 3 summarizes these complications

Table 3: Complications of glaucoma drainage implants	
Early Postoperative	*Late Postoperative*
Hypotony	Tub/explant erosion
Shallow/flat anterior chamber	Diplopia
Tube blockage	Corneal decompansation
Tube-corneal/Iris touch	Explant encapsulation

Early Postoperative Complications

Hypotony :In case that a Non-valved shunt is used , excessive flow of aqueous humor before encapsulation around the posterior explant has occurred may result in a flat anterior chamber, hypotony, and choroidal detachment. This can be avoided by a two-stage approach, or by using various techniques of flow restriction that were previously discussed. Aqueous may also leak around the tube entrance into the anterior chamber; this is usually self limited and can be treated with a pressure patch.

Flat anterior chamber: can be reformed with viscoelastics that can create a temporary tamponade of the tube and reform the anterior chamber.

Tube Blockage: inflammatory debris, vitreous strands or red blood cells blocking the orifice of the tube may be fragmented by Nd: YAG laser, another method may be flushing of the tube, using the corneal paracentesis.

Tube-corneal/iris touch: If there is corneal touch, the tube is too long, in this case the tube needs to be extracted, trimmed and reintroduced into the anterior chamber. If there is iris touch, it may be sufficient to resuture the tube to the episclera. Applying a tight ligature to the tube, usually lifts it's end upwards, towards the cornea, away from the iris.

Late Postoperative Complications

Tube/Explant Erosion of the tube through the overlying conjunctiva may be due to the donor scleral/pericard graft melting over the tube, sometimes, the cause is a protruding suture, not properly buried under the tube. This may start an inflammatory reaction, and the graft, lacking blood supply is subjected to melting. Melting is treated by resuturing a new grat over the exposed tube and covering it with conjunctiva. Explant exposure is a more serous issue, necessitating removal of the device in many cases.

Diplopia

Diplopia is complication that is best prevented by careful placing the implant in the superotemporal quadrant, avoiding the extraocular muscles .it is usually caused by improper placement of the explant, resulting in pressure over the recti muscles; a large encapsulation of the explant may also cause diplopia due to a mass effect, limiting globe movement. The highest rate of diplopia is reported with the Baerveldt implant and is probably related to the insertion of the wings plate underneath the recti muscles. Later studies reported a much lower rate of diplopia, between 6% and 18%. Diplopia may be related to the height of the bleb or due to the adhesions to the recti muscles as the Baerveldt end-plate is inserted under the muscle belly. Diplopia from the other implants appears to be related to the height of the bleb and is significantly less than the Baerveldt implant.

Corneal Decompensation

Corneal decomposition is one of the most serious complications following glaucoma drainage device surgery. Any complication of glaucoma drainage device surgery, (inflammation, shal-low anterior chamber with tubecorneal endothelial touch, tube-iris touch), could contribute to corneal edema or corneal graft failure. The reported rate of corneal decompensation is as high as 51%. The highest rate (up to 51%), of decompensation is reported in postkeratoplasty patients implanted with glaucoma drainage devices. These eyes probably have initial lower endothelial cell count due to previous intraocular surgeries, and previous episodes of inflammation coupled with intermittent elevations of IOP, that adversely affect the endothelial cell with subsequent corneal decompensation.

SUMMARY

Aqueous humor drainage implants are an essential tool for the treatment of refractory glaucoma. In recent years the success rate has improved, and complications have been reduced. Larger explants provide lower IOP, and valved tube technologies reduced the rate of hypotony, and hypotony related complications. In the future Bleb-less technology may reduce postoperative complications such as bleb fibrosis and erosion. Such developments are shunts between the anterior chamber and the supraciliary space.

17

Managing Aphakic Glaucoma in Children with AGV Valves

Keiki R Mehta, Cyres K Mehta (India)

INTRODUCTION

Aphakic glaucoma in children, has always been a difficult problem to manage. Trabeculectomy, customarily has a high failure rate with or without the adjunctive use of antimetabolites. Medical therapy would need to be continued as a routine despite surgery, which in children can lead to problems. Often the surgeon has to resort to ciliary body ablative procedures such cyclodiode laser, which has only short-term benefits and may occasionally result in a late hemorrhage.

Valved and non valved tubes have been available for many years. Over the past few decades the non-valved implants such as the Molteno, Baerveldt, and Shocket tube have been in use but they had the problem of excessive drainage leading to flat chambers. The advent of the valved implants such as Krupin, Ahmed and Optimed have made have made a great deal of difference. The safety and efficacy of surgery using these implants compared to trabeculectomy, as a primary procedure or primary open-angle glaucoma has been well authenticated. In various studies, the success rates have ranged from 45 to 90%. Coleman mentioned the success rate of 70% and 61% over one and two year period.

In all these valves, the aqueous flow drains out onto the plate over the sclera, and thence onwards by capillaries and lymphatics into venous outflow.

SURGICAL PROCEDURE

The Ahmed valve we have utilized routinely is model S2 from New World medical. The Ahmed glaucoma valve implant (New World Medical, Rancho Cucamonga, CA, USA) was introduced to the market in 1993. It is composed of a silicon drainage tube (0.635 mm outer diameter, 0.317 mm inner diameter) and a 184 mm^2 polypropylene body (16 mm long × 13 mm wide × 1.9 mm thick). The body consists of a specially tapered chamber, with a large inlet to a small outlet, to create a venturi-flow effect and to provide resistance to aqueous flow. We used this valve as routine for many years. This analysis recounts our success in utilizing it in children. Indications for insertion were intraocular pressure not controlled by medical therapy or cases, which had previous trabeculectomy or cycloablation, both unsatisfactory.

Diagnosis of glaucoma was mainly based on changes in the optic disks and intraocular pressure. Indications for valve insertion included intraocular

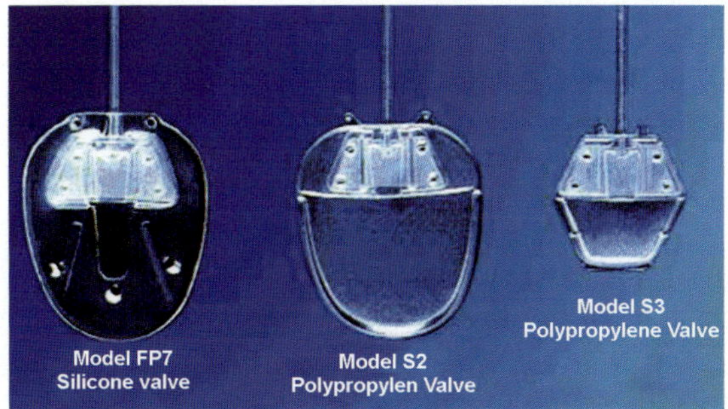

Fig. 1: Different AGV valves. The Ver S2 is ideal for children

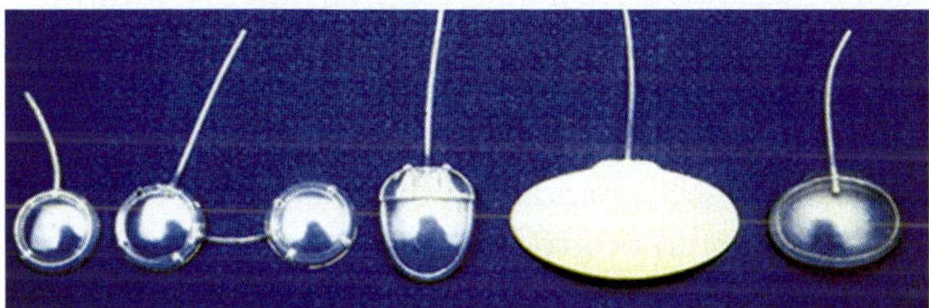

Fig. 2: Molteno-single and double, Ahmed valve-single , Baerveldt valve, Krupin valve

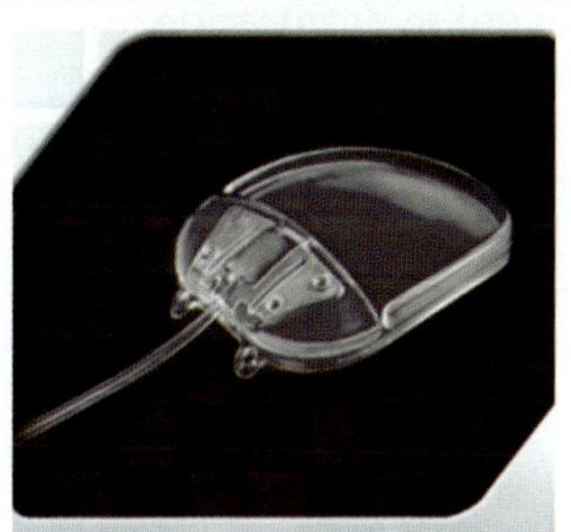

- Valved plate body: Medical grade polypropylene
- Drainage tube: Medical grade silicone
- Valve: medical grade silicone, elastomer membrane
- Thickness: 1.9 mm
- Width: 13.00 mm
- Length: 16.00 mm
- Surface area: 184.00 mm^2
- Tube length: 25.00 mm
- Tube inner diameter: 0.305 mm
- Tube outer diameter: 0.635 mm

Courtesy: New World Medical, Inc.

Fig. 3: Ahmed glaucoma valve parameters

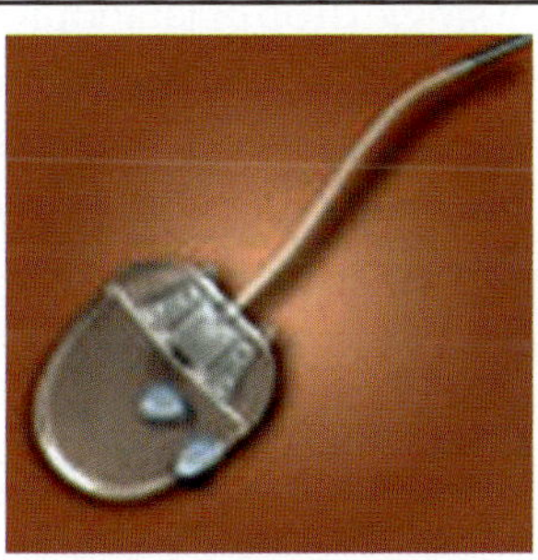

- The implant should be examined and primed prior to implantation. Priming is accomplished by injecting 1cc balanced salt solution or sterile water though the drainage tube and valve, using a blunt **26 gauge cannula**

Courtesy : New World Medical, Inc

Fig. 4: Priming the implant

pressure not controlled by medical therapy or other forms of surgery—namely, cycloablation and or trabeculectomy.

The Surgical Technique Involved

A fornix based conjunctival flap is made in the superonasal or superotemporal quadrant. Mitomycin-C in a oncentraion of 0.05 mg/ml is applied to the sclera and subconjunctiva for a period of two minutes. The tube was primed using BSS until the liquid spurted freely under the valved. A pocket was made utilising a blunt spatula and dis-secting backwards over the recti. The plate was slipped into position and sutured with 6.0. prolene sutures. Using a graded micrometer blade horizontally 6 incisions were made , each 4.0 mm in width, and 0.3 mm in depth. This therefore gave us 3 scleral bands under which the tube can be pushed following a blunt dis-sension with an iris repositor. The most proximal band was 5 mm from the cornea, and the most distal 5 mm from the plate. The tube is allowed to go under the bands and then permitted to lie on the cornea and trimmed so that it would protrude, 2 mm into the anterior chamber. The anterior chamber was entered using a 1 mm diamond knife. The tube is then introduced into the chamber. No further sutures are required, but a single suture is tied snugly onto the tube, in between the first and second band, with 8.0 Polyglactin(Vicryl) This suture is basically to prevent over filtration and does not need to be opened as it will dissolve in 8 to 10 days time .

Results

37 eyes of 28 children were operated over 2 years.

Of ages spanning from 2years to 18 years , followed up for 48 months, (mean 32 months)

14 eyes had previous surgical procedures such as cycloablation or trabeculectomy. Mitomycin-C was used at surgery in all patients .

Average IOP decreased from 32.8 ± 6.2 before surgery to 14.6 ± 5.0 postoperatively ($P < .0001$).

Pressure control maintained: 29eyes (78.3%) achieved intraocular pressure control of 15 mmHg or less with a valve alone or with a single drop of latanoprost-nghtly , followed up to a 8 months period, 24 eyes, (64.8%) maintained their control up to 16 months. Upto 32 months, the 21 eyes managed to maintain their control (56%) . These included the 9 eyes had valve needling with Healon GV between 6 to 19 months following surgery after surgery.

Bottom of Form

The average number of medications used decreased from 2.5 ± 1.97 to 1 ± 2.0 ($P < .0001$).

Some complications occurred in 16 eyes (43.2%) .Although most resolved or were treated successfully, 2 patients had severe visual loss during the follow-up).

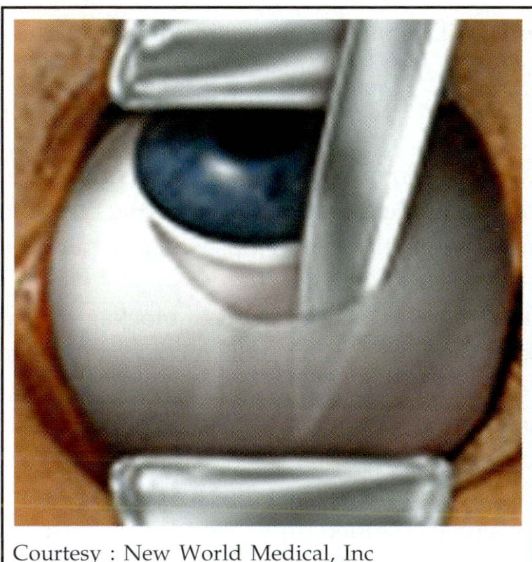
Courtesy : New World Medical, Inc

Fig. 5: The fornix-based incision is made through the conjunctiva and Tenon's capsule. A pocket is formed at the superior quadrant between the medial or lateral rectus muscles by blunt dissection of Tenon's capsule from the episclera

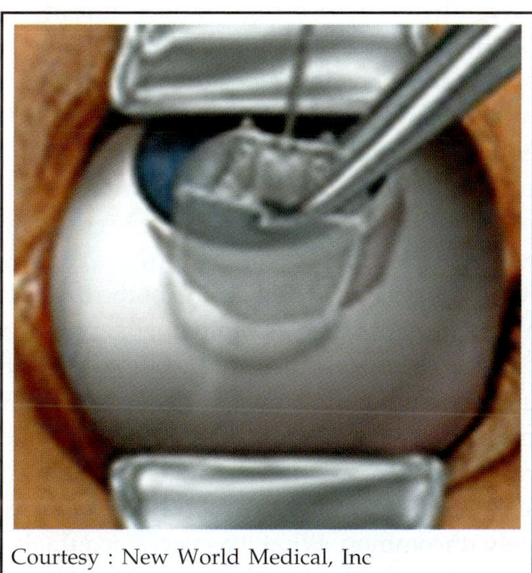
Courtesy : New World Medical, Inc

Fig. 6: The valve body is inserted into the pocket between the rectus muscles and sutured to the episclera. The leading edge of the device should be at least **8-10 mm from the limbus**

They included:

1. Excessive drainage. Despite the vicryl suture around the tube—4 cases
2. Tube retraction may occur if the silicone tube has been cut too short. Its needed to bring the body of the implant a bit forward which solved the problem—in 5 cases
3. Erosion through the conjunctiva. Making the strap system prevents it as does the use of donor scleral flap placed over the tube in the last 6 mm. We saw only one case where the scleral lops were too thin . Solved using donor sclera.
4. Drainage failure may occur as a result of blockage of the end of the tube from debris, thrombosis or iris tissue. Seven cases needed to be flushed. Four maintained patency.
5. Double vision can occur if the plate passes under a muscle—No case.
6. Inflammatory response over plate. Seemed to be quite common in the first two months perhaps due to the fact that we used Mitomycin-C in all cases, but it was transient and settled down rapidly.
7. Encapsulation and scarring of plate sometimes if the drainage is insufficient, the capsule over the implant needed to be needled in 9 eyes.
8. Aqueous misdirection to the vitreous has been reported but we did not see any.

DISCUSSION

Trabeculectomy has always had a high failure rate in Aphakic children irrespective as to whether antimetabolites are used. Tube shunts have been there for a number of years but had never been considered very seriously till the presnt where a new alternative would now need to be looked into. The alternative following any regular trabeculectomy was to continue the use of medical support. However in children medical support is often to maintain as the child is completely dependent on the care giver to place his drops at the appropriate time. Often the result has been that the disease process continues despite all the efforts as simply total irregularity in the timing of the drops takes place.

Many , nonvalved implants such as Molteno, Baerveldt, and Schocket and valved implants such as Krupin, Ahmed, and Opti-Med,have been used in children. The Ahmed valve was first used in 1993. We chose the Ahmed valve because it was simple to use, can be done in a single stage and most important of all, functioned well. We were worried about the possibility of its shifting with rubbing the eyes (children are inveterate eye rubbers) but were pleasantly surprised that it was extremely uncommon. What was very encouraging was the limited tendency for a flat chamber developing. Certainly the use of glaucoma drainage implant devices has improved the outcome in neovascular glaucoma and in glaucoma following post-penetrating keratoplasty,uveitis and aphakia.

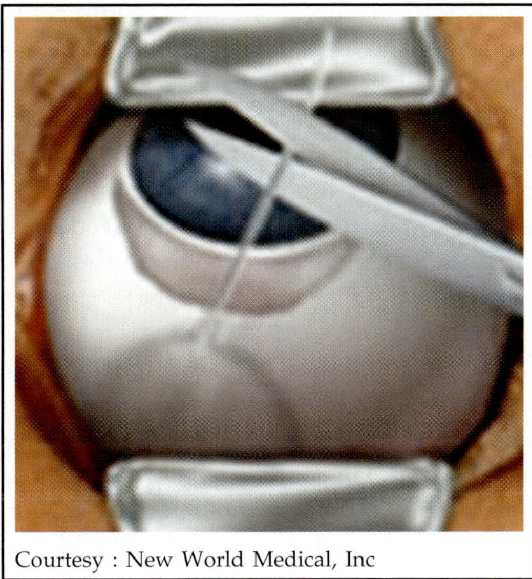

Courtesy : New World Medical, Inc

Fig. 7: The drainage tube **is trimmed to permit a 2-3 mm** insertion of the tube into the anterior chamber (AC). The tube should be bevel cut to an anterior angle of 30° to facilitate insertion

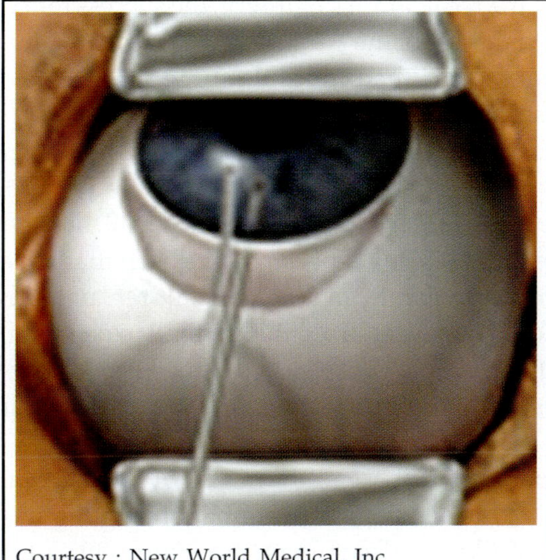

Courtesy : New World Medical, Inc

Fig. 8: A paracentesis is performed, and the AC is entered at the limbus with a sharp **23 gauge needle**, parallel to the iris. **Caution:** Care must be taken to insure that the drainage tube does not contact the iris or corneal endothelium after insertion

In an effort to analyze the results, if one takes an intraocular pressure below 21 mmHg, as a criteria of success in the procedure , then the success in the literature ranges from about 45 to 90%.

Coleman et al reported an overall success rate of 78% and 61% while Englert reported a success rate of 91%and 58% during a 1 year and 2 year follow up.

Morad et al commented on a diminished success rate of 71% and 46% after 36 and 48 months after surgery. Donahue et al showed a greater success rate with drainage implants for aphakic glaucoma in those who had only one previous surgery.

The other surgical techniques such as trabeculectomy with mitomycin are 59% and 67% at 12 and 24 months and cycloablation 66% and 44% at 6 months and 57 months.In Mitomycin augmented Trabeculectomy, Beck and Freidman for children under 2 years of age,aqueous shunt devices offered a better chance of successful glaucoma control in the first 2 years of life.

Looking through the literature as enumerated above, our results compare rather favorably. Interestingly we have managed to achieve a lower IOP than the usual, but perhaps it is because the valve is dipped into dilute (1 in 10 solution of 2 mg concentration) Mitomycin-C prior being inserted, kept in position for 2 minutes and them washed off with BSS. In many of the cases the reduction was exceptional and a follow up of up to 6 years has now shown that the pressures are remaining stable.

Again it was initially thought that in cases with multiple failure where the glaucoma has become recalcitrant to surgery, the success rate would be severely compromized with the use of the Ahmed valve. We were pleasantly surprised. Analyzing our cases which had multiple surgeries, such as cycloablation or trabeculectomy, as illustrated in 14 of our patients.

In cases where the pressure has risen after a few months, needle revision of failed and failing trabeculectomy blebs with adjunctive 5-fluorouracil has proven useful. Literature regarding the same Broadway et all. has shown similar good results with the technique. Our experience has been that if it is going to encyst it tends to occur more frequently in younger children and often commences by the 6 months period. We have utilized this method to needling of the valve with 23 gauge needle. The conjunctiva is elevated using Healon GV. A useful indicator of successful response is the finding of a drop in intraocular pressure immediately

The initial hypertensive phase was reported by Ayyala et al and Kooris et al. who commented on the histological examination, highlighting the emergence of a dense layer of fibrous tissue over the plate with a consequent rise in intraocular pressure. The hypertensive phase may be transient in some patients. Shiu-Chen Wu, 2003 commented that its presence early in the postoperative period may be associated with an unfavorable outcome and most of these eyes may need continuing medical therapy.

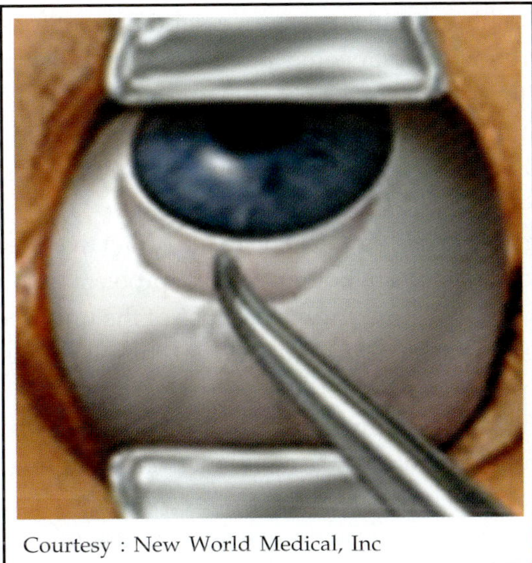

Courtesy : New World Medical, Inc

Fig. 9: The drainage tube is inserted into the AC approximately **2-3 mm**, through the needle track and parallel to the iris. The leading edge of the device should be **8-10 mm from the limbus**

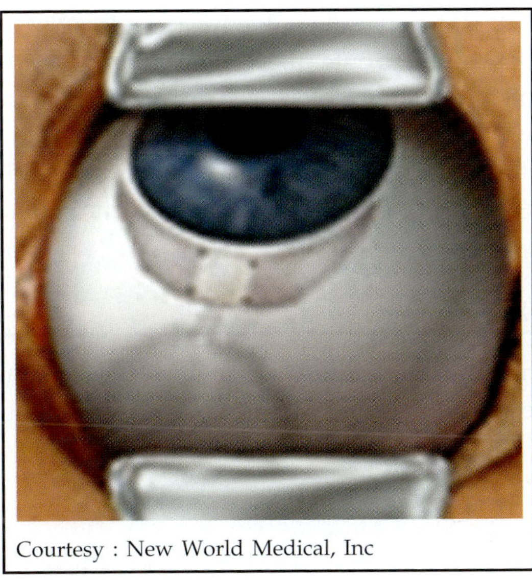

Courtesy : New World Medical, Inc

Fig. 10: The exposed drainage tube is covered with a small piece of preserved donor sclera or pericardium, which is sutured into place, and the conjunctiva is closed

Mitomycin-C is now established as an essential agent for trabeculectomies in most forms of refractory glaucoma and in other high risk patients. It carries potential side effects both long and short-term, such as bleb leakage and infection. Our rationale and that of Shiu-Chen Wu, 2003 in using it in some patients is to reduce Tenon cyst formation and bleb encapsulation over the valve.

We have so far, found no complication in the adjunctive use of Mitomycin- C.

Fortunately postoperative hypotony , a major problem with all valve implants is less common with the Ahmed valve because of the unidirectional flow. The special valve mechanism is designed to prevent complications of overfiltration in the immediate postoperative period.

Shiu-Chen Wu, 2003 commneted on the use of SF6 gas as an technique to manage postoperetive hypotony. He mentioned encountering hypotony in two eyes with choroidal detachment and one required anterior chamber reformation. He used SF6 gas which remains in the eye for 72 hours, giving enough time for aqueous production and the increase of intraocular pressure to a level sufficient to prevent hypotony.

Looking at complications, corneal touch with the tip of the tube is avoidable and usually simply needs to be revised. Tube exposure however needs to be urgently handled. Our technique of using the banded sclera approach seems to have obviated to a large extent the problem. Encystment of the valve can be simply managed by needling. In three of our cases the valve had got blocked with pigment but flushing out the valve by a needle (27 G) inserted via the limbus at 6 o'clock position to enter the lumen of the valve and flushing seems to immediately open up. Often a blob of pigment is visualized just next to the valve exit on the body of the implant.

Considering the good results we have achieved, it would be reasonable to mention that the AGV procedure was an excellent technique and can be cited as a primary choice especially in children.

CONCLUSION

Ahmed valve implantation surgery alone or in combination with medical therapy is successful and safe in the management of pediatric aphakic glaucoma.

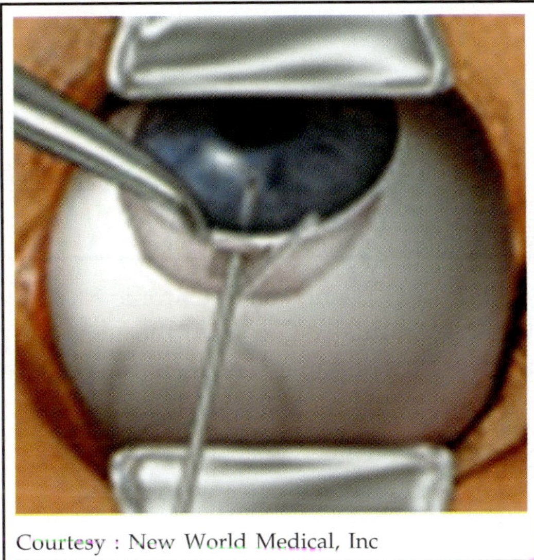

Courtesy : New World Medical, Inc

Fig. 11: **As an alternative to Step 7**, a 2/3 thickness limbal-based scleral flap may be made. The tube is inserted into the AC through a **23 gauge needle** puncture made under the flap and the flap is sutured closed

18A

Absolute Glaucoma

Ranjit S Dhaliwal (India)

INTRODUCTION

Chronic Primary Open Angle Glaucoma or Chronic Narrow or Closed Angle Glaucoma, if untreated, gradually goes into the terminal phase called the Absolute Glaucoma. This final stage may or may not be preceded by intermittent subacute attacks.

Clinical Features

The eye is:

- Painful,
- Irritable and
- Totally blind (no perception of light).

On examination:

- Anterior ciliary veins are dilated, causing circumcorneal ciliary congestion,
- Prominent and enlarged vessels may be seen in long standing cases (caput medusae),
- Cornea is clear , but sensitivity is reduced in early cases,
- Later on cornea becomes hazy, and bullous keratopathy or filamentary keratitis may set in,
- Anterior chamber becomes shallow,
- Iris is atrophic,
- Pupil is dilated and fixed, and may exhibit a green hue,
- Total glaucomatous optic atrophy is seen, and
- Intraocular pressure is very high and the eyeball is stony hard.

Complications

Prolonged high intraocular pressure causes in

- Corneal ulceration (due to reduced corneal sensitivity and epithelial edema), which may even perforate,
- Ciliary or even equatorial staphyloma (due to scleral thinning because of high intraocular pressure), and finally
- Atrophic bulbi (due to degeneration of the ciliary body).

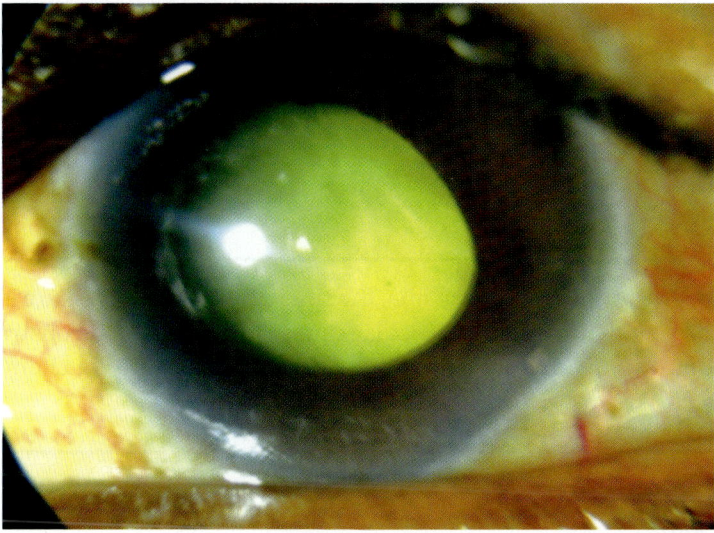

Fig. 1: Absolute glaucoma—Fixed dilated pupil with a green hue

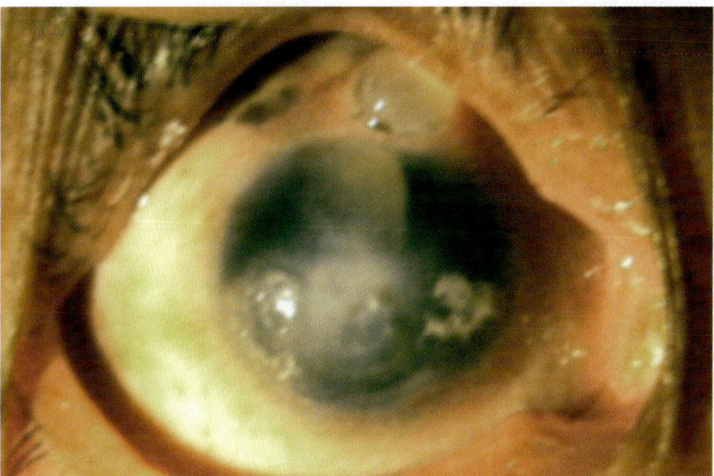

Fig. 2: Absolute glaucoma—Corneal degeneration and ciliary staphyloma

Treatment

- Retrobulbar injection of 1ml of absolute alcohol, under local anesthesia, to reduce the pain by destroying the ciliary ganglion.
- Cyclodestruction by cryo, diathermy or photocoagulation to destroy the secretory ciliary epithelium.
- Enucleation of the eyeball in recalcitrant cases not amenable to conservative treatment. Enucleation is also justified by the high frequency of presence of malignant growths in painful blind eyes.

18B

Primary Narrow Angle Glaucoma

Ranjit S Dhaliwal (India)

INTRODUCTION

In Primary Narrow Angle Glaucoma, the rise in Intraocular pressure is usually bereft of any evident systemic or ocular cause, and is due to the obstruction to the aqueous outflow due to a narrow or closed angle of anterior chamber.

ETIOLOGY

Predisposing Factors

Anatomical

- Hypermetropic eyes having a shallow anterior chamber,
- Eyes having anteriorly placed iris lens diaphragm,
- Eyes having a narrow angle of anterior chamber, due to
  - Small eyeball,
  - Large lens,
  - Micro-cornea and
  - Large ciliary body, and
  - Plateau Iris.

General

More common in:
- The 5th decade of life,
- Females (M : F :: 1 : 4),
- Nervous people,
- The rainy season,
- Individuals having positive family history.

Precipitating Factors

- Dim illumination,
- Emotional stress and
- Use of mydriatic drugs.

Mechanism of rise of IOP

Anatomically predisposed eye →
Effect of precipitating factors →

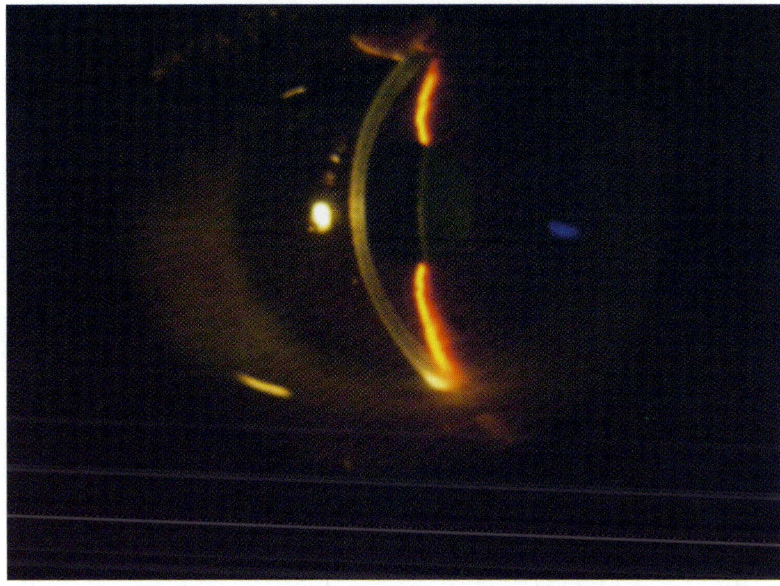

Fig. 1: Narrow angle of the anterior chamber

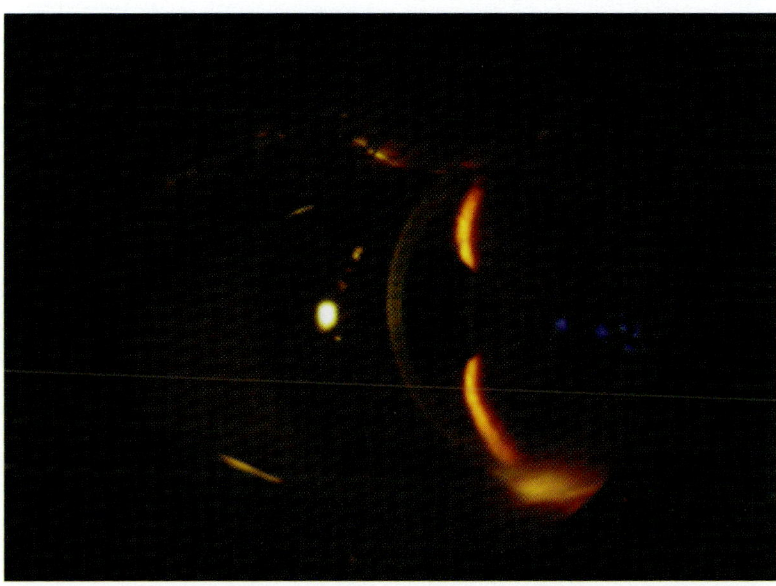

Fig. 2: Narrow angle of the anterior chamber and iris bombe

Mid dilatation of pupil →
Apposition between the lens and pupillary margin increases →
Relative papillary block →
More aqueous collects in the PC →
Iris bombe (flaccid iris pushed forward) →
Irido – corneal contact →
Appositional closure of the angle of AC →
Rise in IOP →
Synechial angle closure (due to peripheral anterior synechiae) →
Attack of raised IOP.

Clinical Features

Stages of Narrow Angle Glaucoma

- Prodromal glaucoma
- Intermittent or subacute glaucoma
- Acute congestive glaucoma
- Chronic closed angle glaucoma
- Absolute glaucoma

Symptoms

- Transient blurring to impairment of vision,
- Colored haloes around light sources,
- Mild to severe frontal headache,
- Mild eye ache to severe pain in the eye,
- May be associated with nausea, vomiting and prostrations,
- Photophobia, and
- Lacrimation.

Signs

Depend on the stage of the disease—

- During prodromal stage and in between attacks {revealed by oblique illumination (Van Herrick's classification) and gonioscopy}—Only narrowing of angle of AC.
- During attacks
  - Eyelids—oedematous,
  - Conjunctiva—chemosed and congested,
  - Cornea—edematous and sensitivity is decreased,
  - Anterior chamber—shallow, aqueous flare and cells maybe seen,
  - Angle of AC—completely closed (gonioscopically),
  - Iris—discoloured,
  - Pupil—semi dilated, vertically oval and fixed (no reaction to both, light and accommodation),

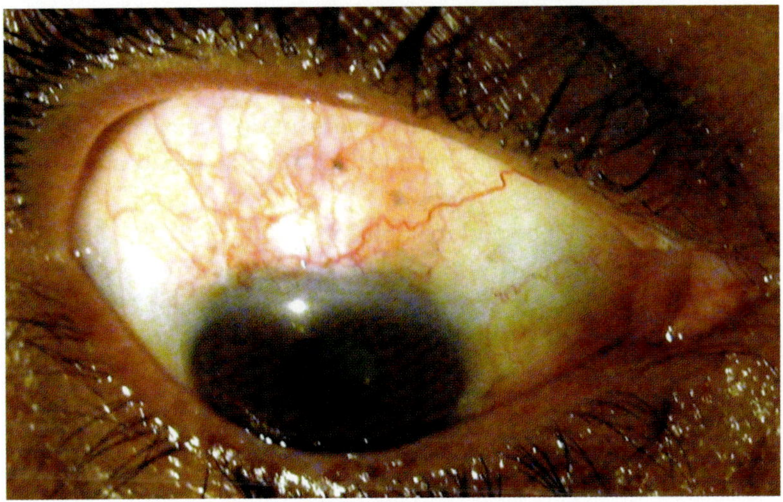

Fig. 3: Trabeculectomy bleb—Functioning

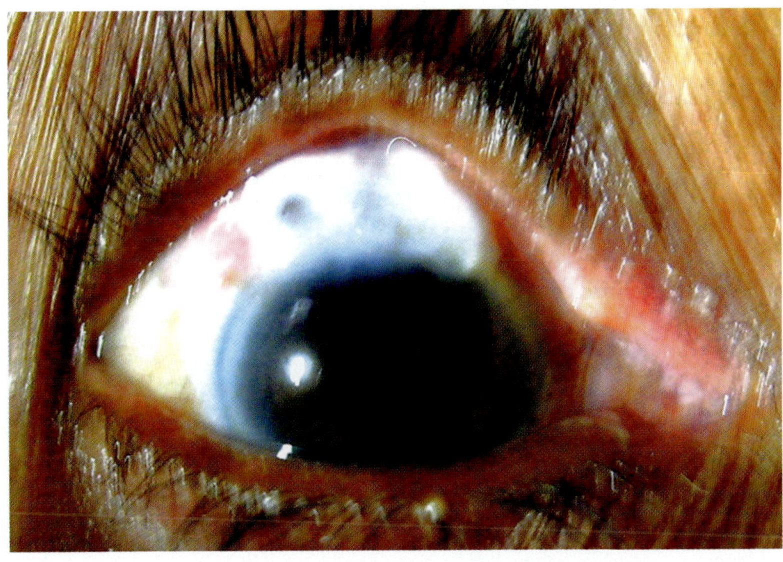

Fig. 4: Cystic Trabeculectomy bleb—Non-functioning

- Intraocular pressure—elevated (40 – 70 mmHg),
- Optic disk—hyperaemic and edematous, and
- In the other eye—shallow AC and narrow angle.

- Chronic narrow or closed angle glaucoma is due to extensive and progressive peripheral anterior synechiae after an attack of acute narrow angle glaucoma. The eye in this stage is—
  - Constantly congested and irritable, or
  - Painless and white as in Primary Open Angle Glaucoma (when due to gradually progressive peripheral anterior synechiae),
  - Visual field defects as in Primary Open Angle Glaucoma,
  - Glaucomatous cupping of optic disk,
  - Visual acuity is diminished, and
  - Angle of anterior chamber closed.

Diagnosis

- History of colored haloes (along with other symptoms),
- Presence of narrow or closed angle of anterior chamber, on gonioscopy,
- Provocative tests
  - Prone—darkroom test,
  - Mydriatic test.

Differential Diagnosis

- Acute conjunctivitis,
- Acute iridocyclitis,
- Phacomorphic glaucoma,
- Acute neovascular glaucoma, and
- Glaucomatocyclitic crisis.

Treatment:

Medical management:

- Parenteral analgesic, immediately,
- Systemic hyperosmotics
  - I/V Mannitol (1 gm/kg body weight),
  - Urea,
  - Glycerol orally (1.5 gm/kg body weight),
  - Acetazolamide orally.
- Pilocarpine eye drops
- Beta-blocker eye drops, e.g. Timolol, Betaxolol.
- Steroid eye drops.

Surgical Management

- Peripheral iridectomy,
- Laser iridotomy,
- Filtration surgery (Trabeculectomy).

Prophylactic Management (of the other asymptomatic eye)

- Laser iridotomy,
- Peripheral iridectomy.

Prognosis

Good, if managed in time.

18C

Sturge-Weber Syndrome

Ranjit S Dhaliwal (India)

INTRODUCTION

This syndrome is named after William Allen Sturge and Frederick Parkes Weber.

Sturge-Weber syndrome is one of the phakomatoses, and is also known as **encephalotrigeminal angiomatosis.** It does not have a hereditary tendency and occurs sporadically, unlike other neurocutaneous disorders (phakomatoses).

It is an embryonal developmental anomaly, resulting from errors in mesodermal and ectodermal development. It is caused by an arteriovenous malformation that occurs in the cerebrum of the brain on the same side as the physical signs described above.

Normally, only one side of the head is affected, but interestingly, the case shown here has involvement of both sides of the face.

Clinical Features

It is a rare congenital neurological and skin disorder, and is often associated with—

- **Seizures** at birth and in infancy and may worsen with age. **Convulsions** usually happen on the side of the body opposite the birthmark, and may vary in severity.
- **Developmental delays** may occur later in life. While some children will have **mental retardation**, but most will have glaucoma.
- **Large port-wine stain** on the forehead and upper eyelid, one side of the face. The birthmark varies in color from light pink to deep purple, and is due to an abundance of capillaries around the ophthalmic branch of the trigeminal nerve, just beneath the surface of the face.
- **Ipsilateral leptomeningeal angioma**—there is malformation of blood vessels in the pia-mater overlying the brain, on the same side of the head as the birthmark. This causes calcification of tissue and loss of nerve cells in the cerebral cortex. There may be muscular weakness on the same side.
- **Glaucoma** (increased intraocular pressure) can be present at birth or develop later. Increased pressure within the eye can cause the eyeball to enlarge and bulge out of its socket (buphthalmos).

Sturge-Weber syndrome rarely affects other body organs.

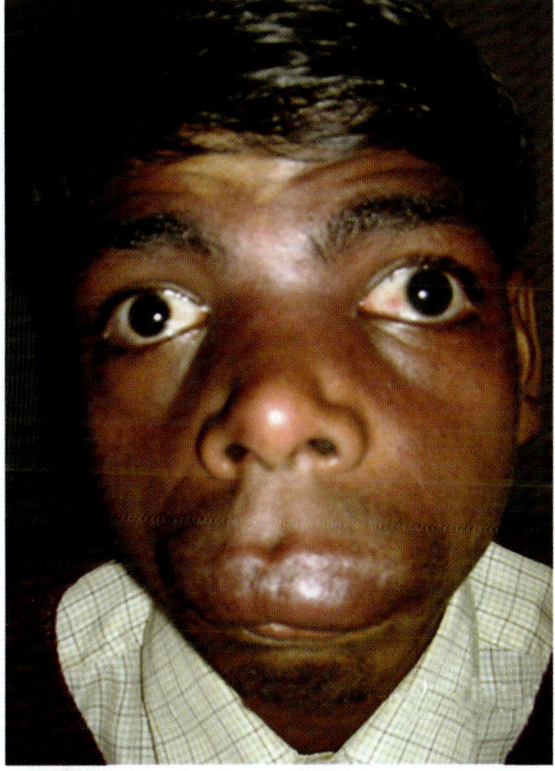

Fig. 1: Sturge-Weber syndrome—Front profile

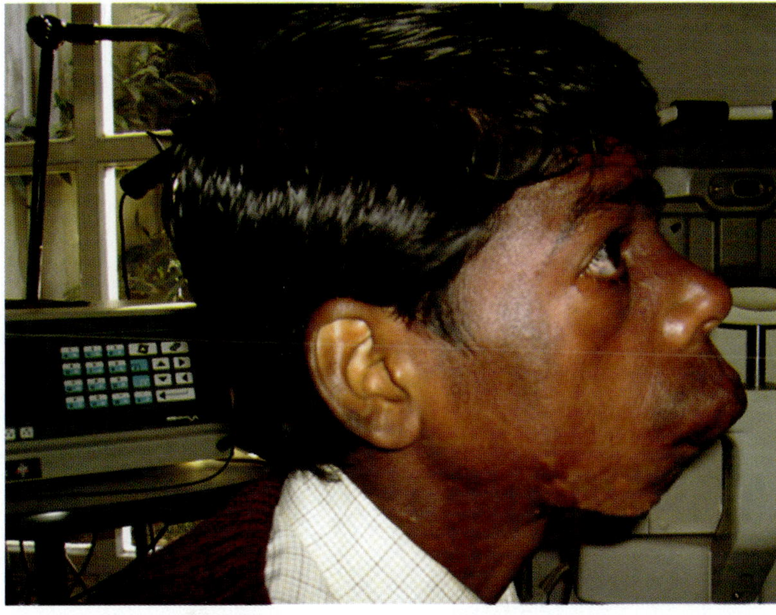

Fig. 2: Sturge-Weber syndrome—Right profile

Treatment

Treatment for Sturge-Weber syndrome is symptomatic.

- **Anticonvulsant** medications may be used to control seizures.
- **Laser** treatment may be used to reduce or remove the birthmark.
- **Monitor for glaucoma**, and surgery may be needed in serious cases.
- **Physiotherapy** should be considered for infants and children with muscle weakness.
- **Educational therapy** is often prescribed for those with mental retardation or developmental delays, but there is no complete treatment for the delays.
- **Neurosurgery** involving removal of the portion of the brain that is affected by the disorder can be considered. This is successful in controlling the seizures.

Prognosis

- While it is possible for the birthmark and atrophy in the cerebral cortex to be present without symptoms, most infants will develop convulsive seizures during their first year of life.
- Possibility of intellectual impairment, when seizures start before the age of 2, and are resistant to treatment.

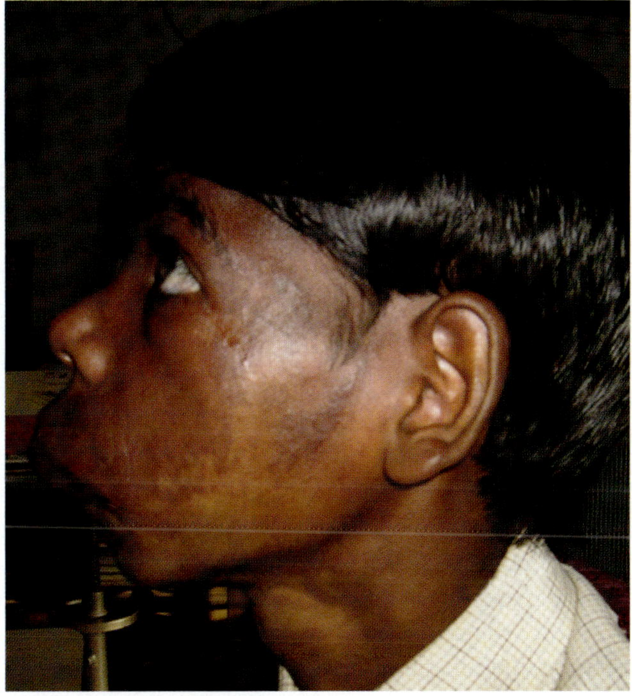

Fig. 3: Sturge-Weber syndrome—Left profile

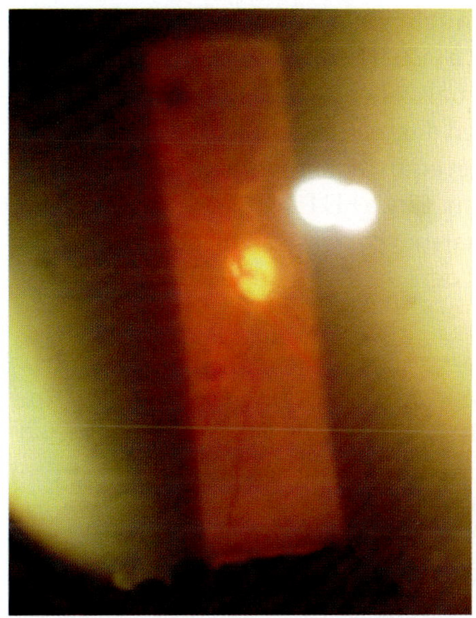

Fig. 4: Sturge-Weber syndrome—Partial glaucomatous optic atrophy OD

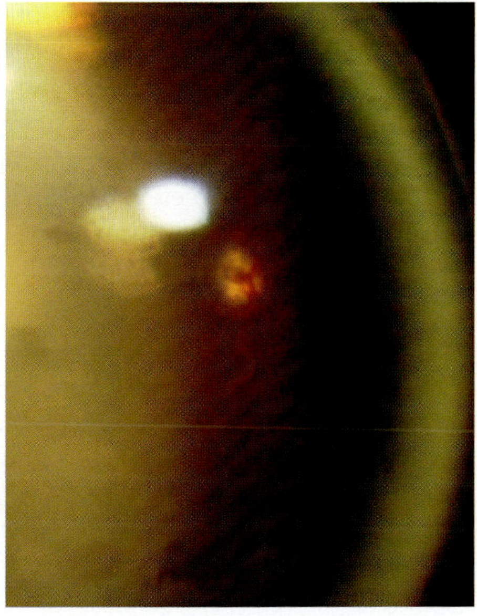

Fig. 5: Sturge-Weber syndrome—Total glaucomatous optic atrophy OS

19

New Investigations in Glaucoma

Tanuj Dada, Shibal Bhartiya, Shweta Jindal (India)

FREQUENCY DOUBLING PERIMETRY

Introduction

Frequency Doubling Technology (FDT) perimeter (Welch Allyn and Humphrey Instruments, Inc) uses a large low spatial frequency sinusoidal grating (<1 cycle/degree) that consists of black and white bars undergoes a rapid counter phase flicker (>15 Hz) leading to a frequency doubling illusion in which, at a certain level of contrast, the number of visible lines appears to double.

- It incorporates a moveable binocular cowling piece which shields ambient room light. A viewfinder slides from side to side to allow monocular viewing without the need of patching. A video display unit presents 10 degree square target and a central 5 degree radius target.
- Used for screening, diagnosing and monitoring glaucoma.

Principle

- It is assumed that the large-diameter optic nerve fibers (M) are preferentially damaged in the early stages of glaucoma. Also, as per the Reduced Redundancy Theory, it is assumed that a visual field test will be more sensitive to early loss if only a subset of the visual system is tested.
- The standard FDT target is a square ten degrees in diameter, which is much larger than the size III Goldmann target equivalent that shines a spot of light 0.43 degrees in diameter on to the retina. Since FDT tests larger areas, it may detect certain subtle diffuse changes that maybe missed with other perimetric tests ,but may miss shallow localized defects.

Method

- The patient is asked to fixate a small central spot on video monitor and fixation is monitored and responses to the stimulus presented are recorded.
- Stimulus consists of a monochrome sine-wave sinusoidal pattern of vertical gray stripes of spatial frequency 0.25 cycles per degree and temporal frequency of 25 Hz.

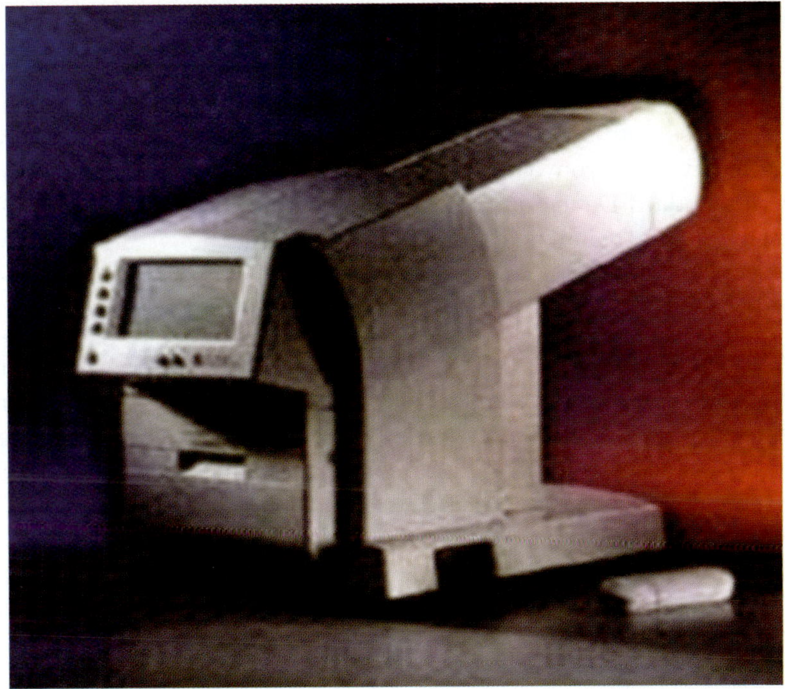

Fig. 1: FDT perimeter

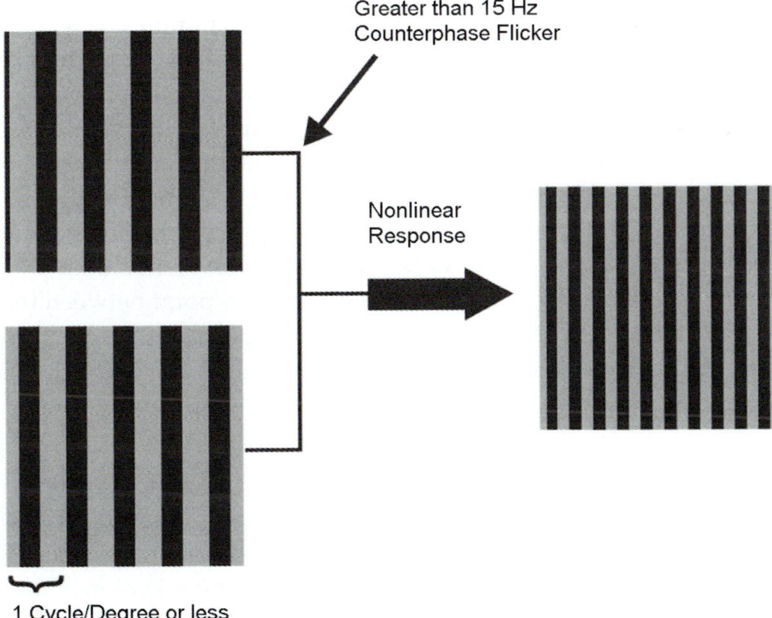

Fig. 2: FDT principle

Evaluating FDT Printouts

Number of points depressed , location of involved points, pattern of involved points, depth of depression, comparison between the two eyes, correlation of any field loss with ocular examination ,Reliability indices ,Mean Deviation (average deviation from a normal visual field based on age-related norm) and Pattern Standard Deviation Indices (a measure of how locations differ from each other in the overall field) for the threshold tests.

Testing Modes

Suprathreshold Strategy

Test options include a screening field (Screening C-20-1) in which gratings with three contrast levels are shown at 17 locations in the central 20 degree field and it takes about 45 seconds. Other is suprathreshold screening C-30 program. FDT screening mode perimetry is considered abnormal if there is:

- Any defect in the central five locations
- Two mild or moderate defects in the outer 12 squares
- One severe defect in the outer 12 squares
- Screening test time greater than 90 seconds per eye.

Full Threshold Strategy

Two variants: In C-20, central 20 degree is examined at 17 locations whereas in N-30 additional 2 nasal points (total 19 locations) are also examined. C-20 takes about 3 1/2 minutes while N-30 takes about 6 minutes.

Threshold sensitivity is measured using either method of adjustment (MOA) or by modified binary search (MOBS). In method of adjustment, three contrast threshold adjustments are made for each stimulus pattern and the geometric mean of the three trials is used as the final contrast threshold value. Modified binary search (MOBS) procedure is a staircase test strategy which continues until a criterion number of response reversal have occurred and the difference between the upper and lower stack values is equal or less than a specified interval. Final threshold is then defined as the mid point between the upper and lower limits when both of these criteria have been met.

Two other newer strategies are rapid efficiency binary search technique (REBS) and zippy estimation of sequential testing (ZEST).

Custom 24-2 FDT Perimetry

Custom designed FDT perimetry (Quadravision) uses 54 stimuli with 4° target using 24-2 stimulus presentation pattern with modestly higher sensitivity for detection of early glaucomatous loss and better characterization of the pattern of visual field loss, but the takes approximately twice as long.

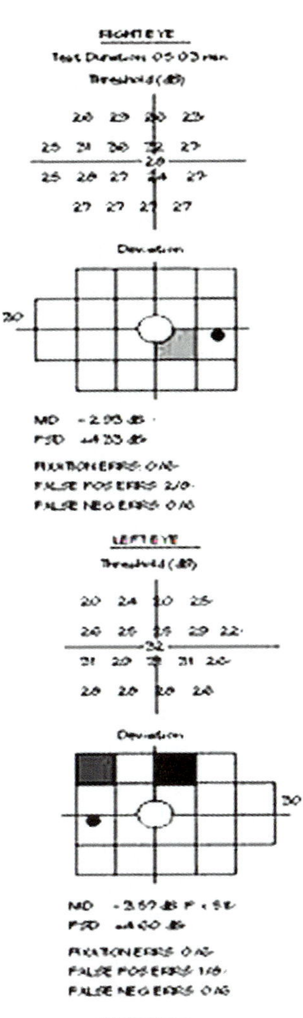

Fig. 3: FDT full threshold field of a patient (HFA 30-2 was normal). FDT shows one point abnormal with $p < 2\%$ and another point abnormal with $p < 5\%$ in right eye. In left eye one point is abnormal with $p < 0.5\%$, another point is abnormal with $p < 1\%$ and four points abnormal with $p < 2\%$

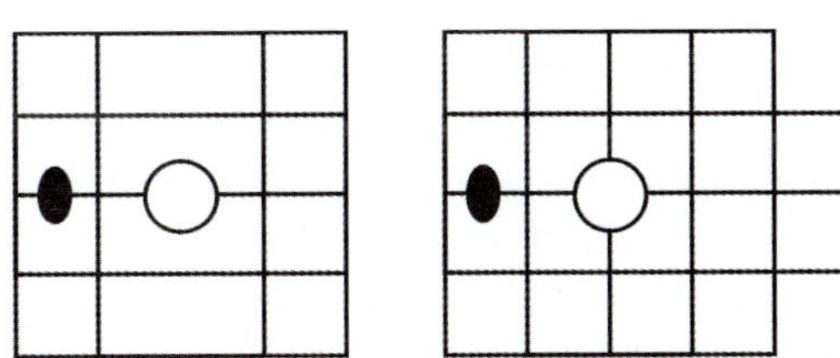

Fig. 4: C-20 and N-30 for FDT perimetry

Matrix FDT Perimetry

The Humphrey matrix (FDT2) is a second generation instrument using similar small FDT stimuli has recently became available for clinical use. It provides up to 69 stimuli, 5° × 5° each, to fully characterize visual field defects and can also be used to perform a serial analysis to determine progression. Here, except foveal stimulus, the stimuli are 5 degree square windows of a vertical grating with spatial frequency of 0.5 cyc/deg, counterphase flickered at 18 Hz. It uses a Bayesian strategy specifically ZEST (Zippy estimation of sequential testing), with a fixed number of presentation at each test location and a flat previous probability density function (PDF). By this strategy the test time for full threshold perimetry is reduced to half without affecting the accuracy or reliability of the measurements. Threshold testing using the FDT Matrix and SAP is comparable when the 24-2 test pattern is used and the global visual field indices mean deviation (MD) and pattern standard deviation (PSD) of FDT and SAP correlate highly and the test –retest variability of FDT2 is uniform over the measurement range of the instrument.

Screening Tests

The Humphrey Matrix offers two suprathreshold tests (Table 19.1) for rapid screening that take less than 2 minutes per eye, similar to the ones available on the original FDT perimeter. The difference with using the matrix is that moving fixation to examine the 2 nasal points is not required.

The 24-2-5(-1) is the additional screening test found in Matrix. Each test location is assigned one of two probability levels (1% or 5%) similar to the N-30 screening, depending on the test selected. What changes in this test is that 55 smaller targets (5°) are used in a testing pattern based on the 24-2 HFA test, to analyze the central 24°. This screening method may be slightly longer than the N-30 test, but greater spatial information about possible localized defects is given, due to the use of a greater number of smaller targets.

Threshold Tests

The Humphrey Matrix offers 5 threshold testing methods (Table 1) that provide quantitative measurements of the VF function at each location. Results are then compared to a normative database based on over 270 individuals (18 to 85 years of age). The Matrix threshold tests all use a test algorithm known as Zippy Estimation of Sequential Thresholds (ZEST), and differ in eccentricity tested, pattern, and target characteristic (size and spatial frequency).

The N-30-F test is essentially the same 19 point threshold test found on the original FDT. The only minor differences are that Matrix uses a two-reversal MOBS strategy (instead of four reversals) for determining threshold, which tends to be a more efficient and time saving algorithm, and moving fixation is not required.

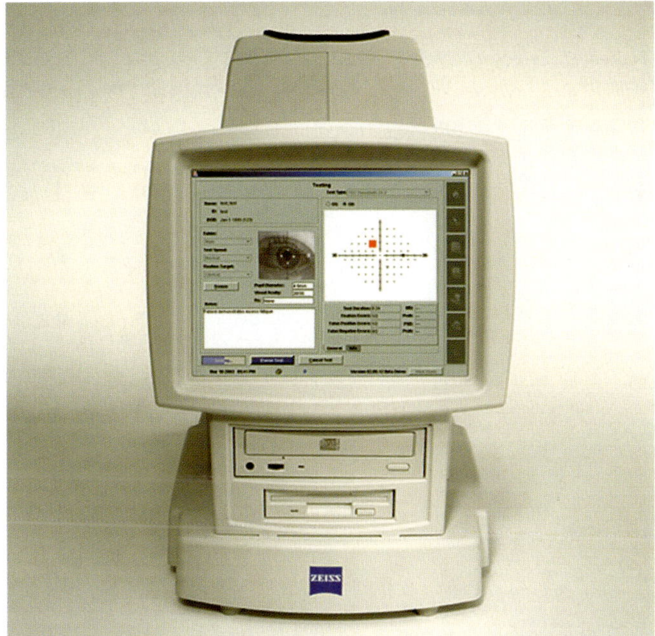

Fig. 5: Humphrey-matrix

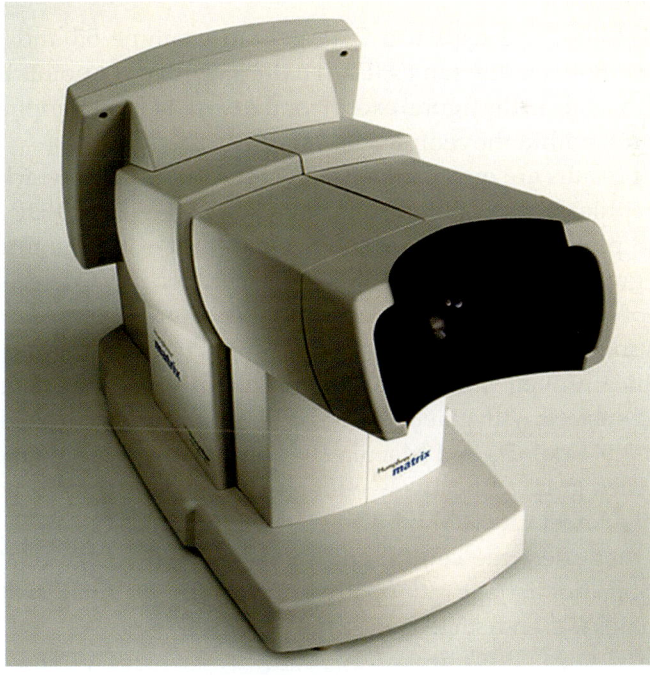

Fig. 6: Humphrey-matrix

Table 1: Humphrey matrix test characteristics

	N-30-5(−1) screening	*24-2-5(-1) screening*	*N-30-F threshold*	*24-2 threshold*	*30-2 threshold*	*10-2 threshold*	*Macula threshold*
# of VF locations	19	55	19	55	69	44	16
Eccentricity (degrees)	30	24	30	24	30	10	4
Stimulus (St) size (°)	10	5	10	5	5	2	2
St spat. freq. (c/deg)	0.25	0.5	0.25	0.5	0.5	0.5	0.5
St temp. freq. (Hz)	25	18	25	18	18	12	12
#Fixation catch trials	3	10	6	10	10	10	6
#False + trials	3	10	6	10	10	10	3
#False – trials	0	0	3	6	6	6	0
Test strategy	Supra-threshold	Supra-threshold	MOBS	ZEST	ZEST	ZEST	ZEST
Test time 1 eye (min)	< 1	< 2	< 3	< 5.5	< 6.5	< 4.5	< 2

The 24-2 and 30-2 tests use 5° targets to examine 55 and 69 locations respectively. Both use the same HFA II pattern, with most points being similar (indicated in white in the figure) except for the extra 14 most peripheral locations (shaded gray) within the central 30° tested with the 30-2 test.

The test results are quite similar to the HFA II printout, which include the various graphical representation of results (gray scale, TDP, PDP and both TD and PD dB plots), VF indices (MD, PSD and GHT), and the three reliability indices. A greater spatial and detailed representation of VF defects is provided by the use of smaller sized and a greater number of targets compared to the prior FDT. This may be advantageous in detecting VF defects earlier , which are topographically well defined, and consequently used in diagnosing and monitoring subjects with glaucoma and other ocular and neurologic disorders.

The 10-2 (44 points) and Macula (16 points) tests examine the central 10° and 5° (shaded gray) respectively with targets 2° in size that are counterphase flickered at a lower rate (12 Hz). These testing methods are more beneficial in disorders that affect the central and macular VF (like age-related macular degeneration and diabetic retinopathy) or when only a small central island of vision remains (i.e. end-stage glaucoma).

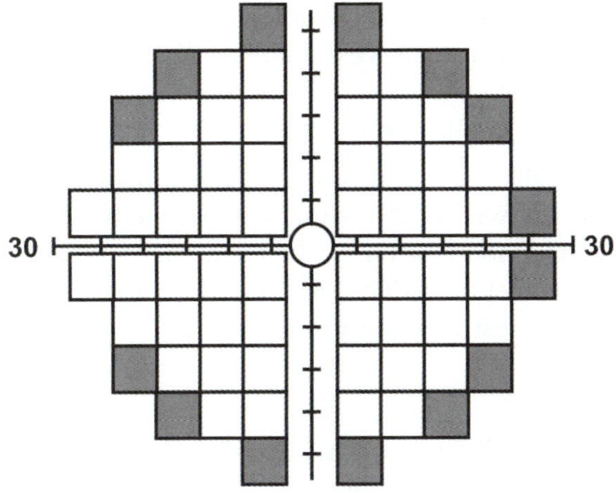

Fig. 7: FDT matrix 30-2

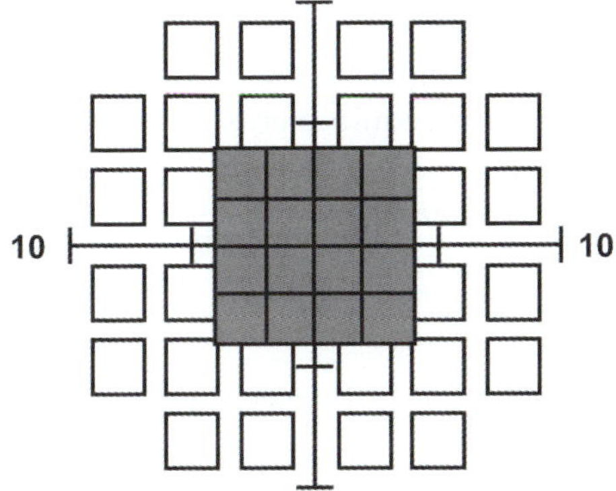

Fig. 8: 10-2 FDT matrix

The smaller stimulus size and lower flicker rate preclude the appearance of frequency doubling, so the test is essentially a flicker sensitivity procedure.

Threshold Strategy Algorithm

The Humphrey Matrix uses a threshold determination procedure based on Bayesian statistics known as ZEST, similar to the Swedish Interactive Threshold Algorithm (SITA) found in the HFA. The advantages offered by this algorithm over other strategies include reduced test time (by about 50%), greater efficiency, lower intra and inter test variability, and similar levels of accuracy.

Advantages of FDP

- Short test duration(4-5 min for full threshold)
- Very tolerant to defocus and blur (± 6 dioptres sphere)
- Patients can wear spectacles with bifocals
- Not affected by pupil size
- Useful for glaucoma screening
- Test – retest reliability is good
- Can follow glaucoma progression with MD and PSD values
- Less stringent dark room requirements
- Portable and cheaper
- Easily learned by patient and examiner
- Feasible in children
- Disadvantages
- May miss focal defects
- Central 20 degree field may miss nasal steps
- Lack of longitudinal data
- Difficult to follow up early progression.

ANTERIOR SEGMENT OPTICAL COHERENCE TOMOGRAPHY

Introduction

- Optical coherence tomography (OCT) is a cross-sectional, three-dimensional, high-resolution imaging modality that uses low coherence interferometry to achieve a high axial resolution ranging from 10-20 μm, "optical biopsy".
- Anterior segment imaging using OCT was first demonstrated in 1994 by Izatt using light with a wavelength of 830 μm, with 1.3 μm wavelength ASOCT by Radhakrishnan.

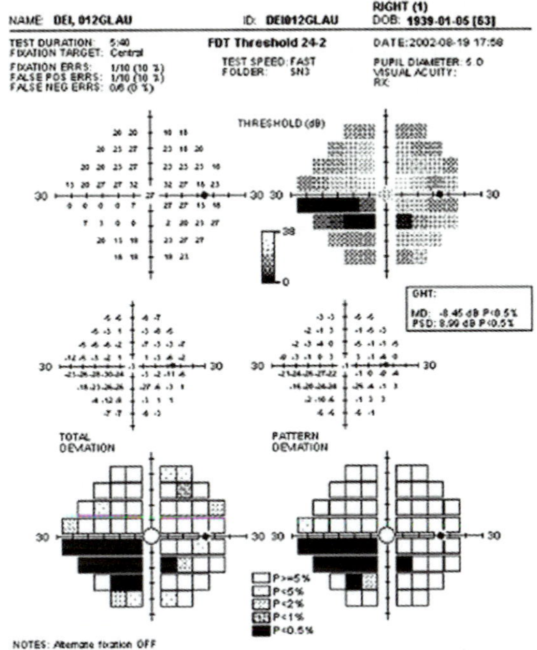

Fig. 9: Humphrey matrix FDT 24-2 printout

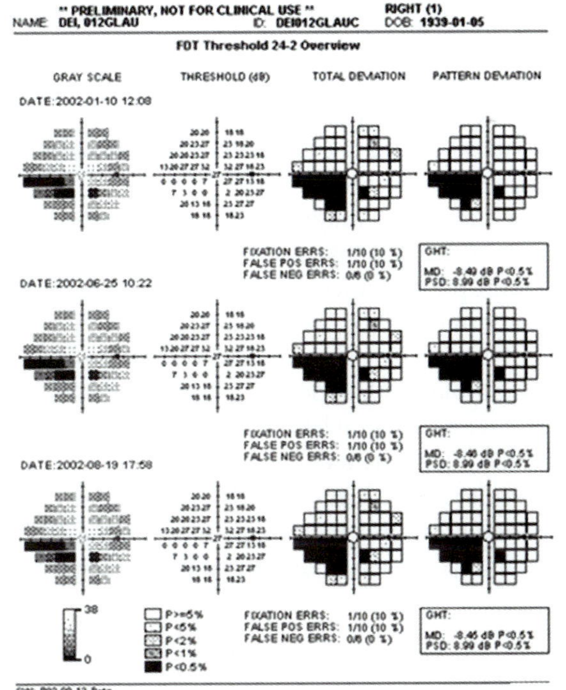

Fig. 10: Humphrey matrix FDT 24-2, serial field analysis for progression

Optical Principle

- Light (wavelength range of 800–1550 nm) from a broadband, near-infrared source is split into two one leading to a reference mirror and the second focused into the tissue.
- An optical detector detects the interference between the reference and tissue signals.
- Reference-arm mirror is scanned at a constant velocity, allowing depth scans (analogous to ultrasound A-scans), and the beam scanned laterally constitutes an optical B-scan of the anterior chamber.
- Lateral resolution is 60 μm and the axial resolution is 18 μm compared to 50 μm and 25 μm respectively by UBM.

Uses

1. Digital gonioscopy: allows objective anterior chamber angle assessment which is non-contact, accurate, quantitative and rapid and can be performed without slit-lamp illumination and artifactual widening of the angle.
2. Cornea: Pachymetry for the entire cornea or any lamellar segment, flap and stromal bed, anterior and posterior curvature of cornea, total corneal power measurement and its change after refractive surgeries.
3. Anterior segment biometry: Including AC depth, AC diameter, pupil diameter, assessment of posterior chamber phakic IOL and accommodating IOL.
4. Corneal pathologies: Ectatic disorders, keratoplasty assessment and planning of post PKP glaucoma management.
5. Iris imaging: ASOCT imaging can help in diagnosing and follow-up of cystic diseases of and atrophic areas.
6. Assessment of tumors of anterior segment depth of penetration and extrascleral extension, also invasion of angle.
7. Study of dynamic physiological changes of anterior segment in response to light and accommodation, dark room and the prone provocative tests.
8. Mechanism of secondary angle closure glaucomas specially post-penetrating keratoplasty glaucoma.
9. Evaluation of laser peripheral iridotomy, iridoplasty, glaucoma drainage devices and trabeculectomy blebs.
10. Bleb revision under ASOCT guidance for failing blebs
11. Evaluation of ocular trauma including angle recession, hyphema
12. Evaluation of dry eye by tear meniscus height measurement.

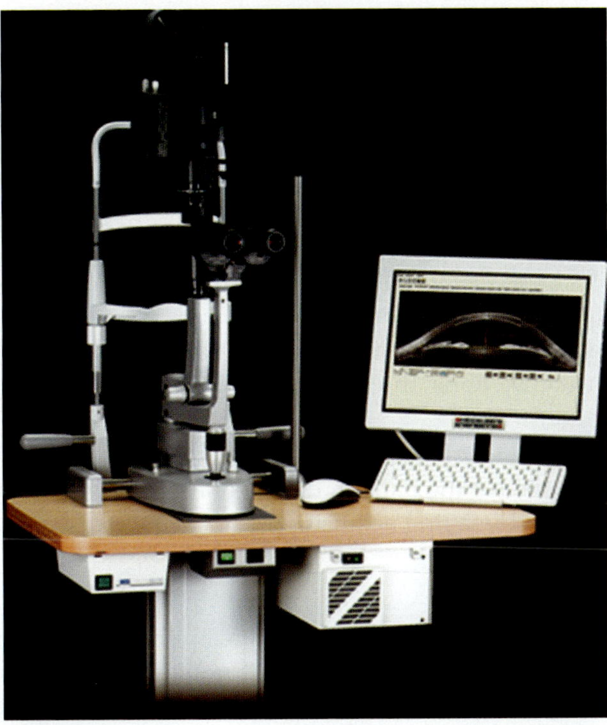

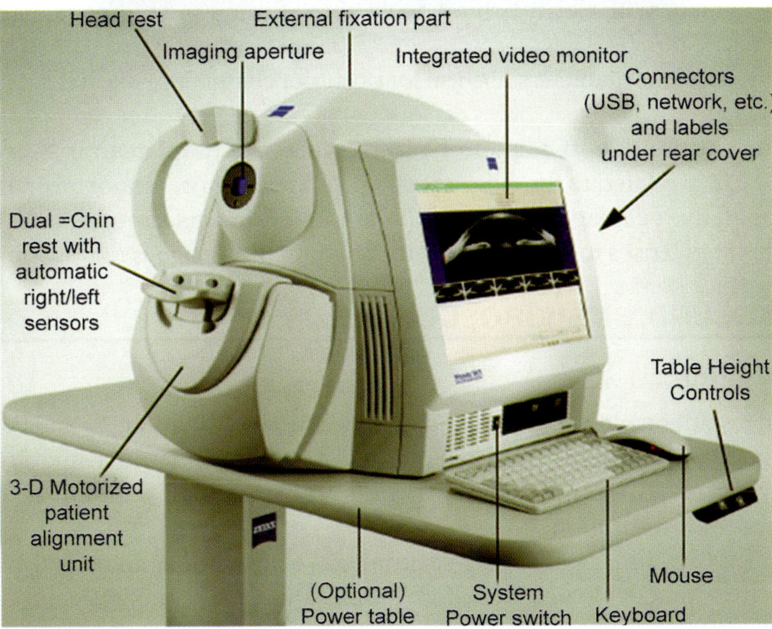

Figs 11 and 12: The Visante AS-OCT (*Carl Zeiss*) and SL-OCT (*Heidelberg Engineering*)

Advantages of ASOCT

- Non-contact method therefore no indentation of the angle by placement of the scleral cup on the eye.
- No risk of corneal abrasion or punctuate epithelial erosions.
- It is a more physiological examination as patient is imaged sitting upright.
- Shorter imaging time ,rapid image acquisition. (Eight frames captured per second, allowing operator to choose best image).
- Requires less expertise to perform , less inter-operator variability, small learning curve for the operator.
- Incorporated Optometer provides accommodation stimulus to measure changes in ACD, Lens thickness, iris thickness and angle during accommodation.
- Very useful inbuilt LASIK flap tool and pachymetry map.
- More comfortable for the patient, due to non-contact technique, upright. position and rapid imaging acquisition.

Limitations of ASOCT

- Since the posterior layer of the iris (pigment epithelium) is not transparent for infrared light, the posterior chamber is not visualized in most cases.
- entire thickness of the sclera is not visible.
- cannot image with clarity behind dense corneal scars and pigmented limbal lesions.
- Sulcus to sulcus diameters , critical for posterior chamber phakc IOLs, cannot be measured.
- Angle closure due to a anterior placed ciliary body (plateau iris) or any other cause related to the ciliary body (swelling, tumor) cannot be imaged.
- Preoperative evaluation in eyes with traumatic cataracts, pseudoexfoliation, subluxated lenses to identify amount of zonular damage is not possible.

ULTRASOUND BIOMICROSCOPY

Introduction

- High resolution ultrasound technique developed by Pavlin, Sherar and Foster.
- High-frequency ultrasound technology that allows noninvasive *in-vivo* imaging of structural details of the anterior ocular segment at near microscopic resolution.
- Detailed two-dimensional gray-scale images of the various anterior segment structures and evaluates them both quantitatively and qualitatively.

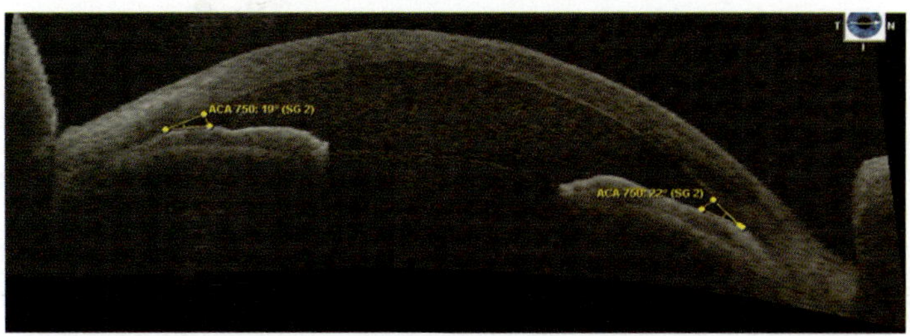

Fig. 13: Digital gonioscopy, SL-OCT image showing narrow angles

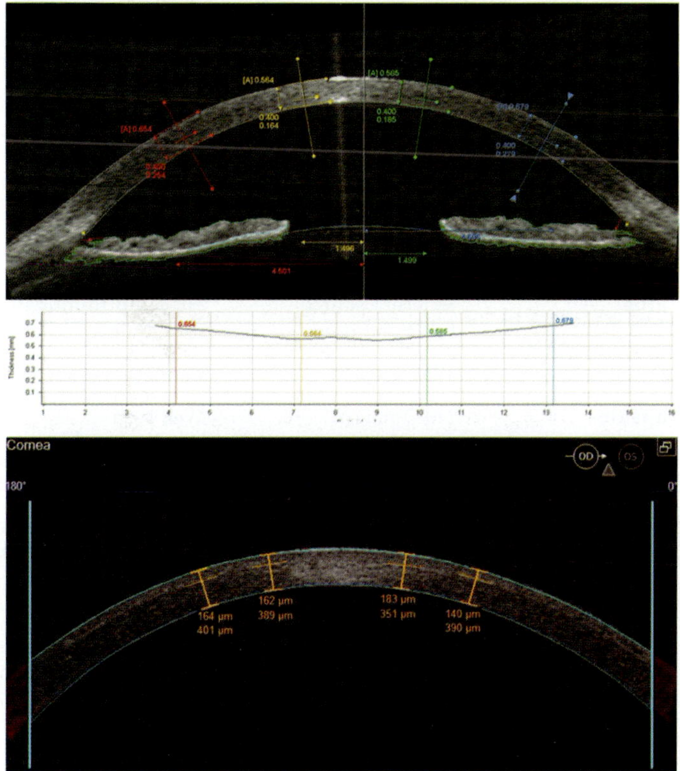

Figs 14 and 15: Pachymetry report and flap thickness and RSB (residual bed thickness) using the LASIK flap tool (Visante)

Comparison of UBM versus ASOCT

	UBM	*ASOCT*
Method of examination	Contact	Non contact
Technique	Skilled operator	Easy to perform
Topical anesthesia	Required	Not required
Patient positioning	Supine	Sitting
Patient discomfort	Yes	No
Source	Ultrasound 50 MHz frequency	1310 nm diode laser
Imaging time	Longer	Shorter
Coupling medium	Required	Not required
Field of view	5 mm across	16 mm across
Image quality	Grainy	Clearer
Axial resolution	50 microns	18 microns
LASIK flap tool	Not available	Available
Stimulus for accommodation	External source	Inbuilt in the hardware
Light stimulus	External source has to be used	Slit-lamp illumination (SLOCT)
Ciliary body, zonules	Well imaged	Cannot image behind iris
Posterior capsule	Not imaged	Well seen
Optical axis marker	Not present	Present can check centration
Number of scans	One axis at one time	Quad scan
Eyelids	No obstruction	Obstruct imaging along vertical meridian
Contraindication	Open globe injury	Can be performed
Early postoperative period	Risk of ocular injury and contamination	No risk involved

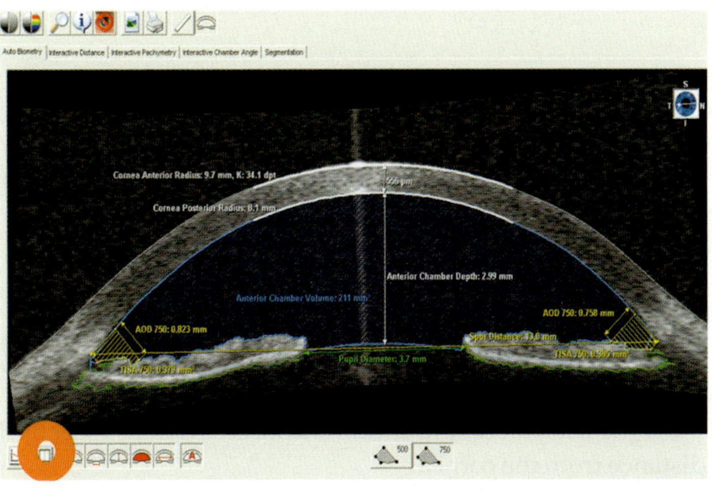

Biometry Results

Parameter	Value
Cornea Anterior Radius	9.7 mm, K: 34.1 dpt
Cornea Posterior Radius	8.1 mm
Central Cornea Thickness	560 µm (Min.: 552 µm)
Anterior Chamber Depth	2.99 mm
Anterior Chamber Volume	211 mm³
Spur Distance	12.9 mm
Pupil Diameter	3.7 mm

Left Chamber Angle

Parameter	Value
AOD 500	0.629 mm
TISA 500	0.183 mm²
AOD 750	0.874 mm
TISA 750	0.392 mm²

Right Chamber Angle

Parameter	Value
AOD 500	0.573 mm
TISA 500	0.241 mm²
AOD 750	0.776 mm
TISA 750	0.407 mm²

Figs 16 and 17: Biometry from SL OCT with the printout

Principle

- The transducer frequency of the UBM instrument is 50 MHz
- Provides much higher image resolution (approximately 25 µm of axial and 50 µm of lateral resolution).
- Reduced depth of penetration of the ultrasonic beam (limited to approximately 5 mm for a 50 MHz UBM instrument).
- Smaller angular field.

Examination Technique

- After informed consent from the patient instill topic anesthesia (0.5% proparacaine) prior to insertion of an appropriate sized eye cup.
- insert the cup, fill it with coupling fluid and insert the transducer tip, keeping a safe distance from the cornea.
- Ask the patient to look up at a target on the ceiling to minimize accommodation, do not apply undue pressure on the eye cup and standardize illumination.
- Start scanning from 12 o′ clock and move in a clock wise direction to scan each quadrant , keeping probe perpendicular to the limbus or area of interest. When you save an image, mention the axis or cock hour being scanned.
- Do both an axial and transverse scan over a pathological area and also use overlay of a scan to see reflectivity of the lesion. Adjust the echogenecity of the signal to an optimal level and reduce noise.
- Use calipers and angle software to make measurements and write the report. Use a lower frequency probe (35 MHz) instead of the 50 MHz one if a large field of view is to be captured.
- Gently take off the eye cup, clean the coupling fluid and ask the patient to wash his eyes, after which a drop of antibiotic may be instilled.
- Analyze the images and transfer to a computer or data storage device.

The following parameters are used for doing an objective analysis of the anterior chamber angle structures, with the scleral spur taken as the reference point.

1. The trabecular iris angle (TIA) or anterior chamber angle (ACA, θ_1) is measured with its apex at the iris recess and the arms of the angle passing through a point on the trabecular meshwork at 500 µm from the scleral spur and the point on the iris perpendicularly opposite.
2. The angle opening distance 250/500 (AOD 250 and AOD 500) is the distance between the posterior corneal surface and the anterior iris surface measured on a line perpendicular to the trabecular meshwork, 250 or 500 µm anterior to the scleral spur.

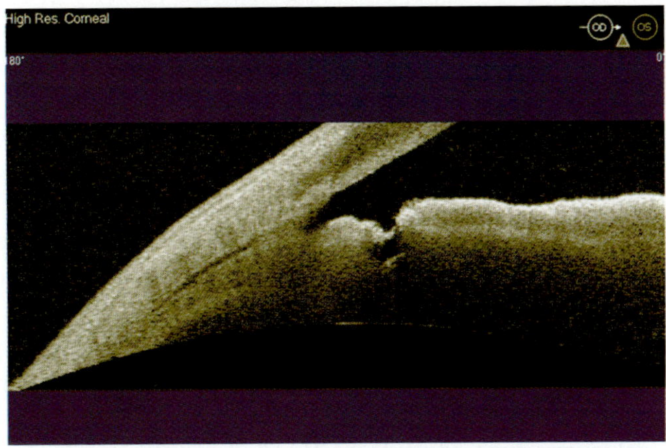

Fig. 18: ASOCT (Visante) image showing an eye with primary angle closure post laser iridotomy

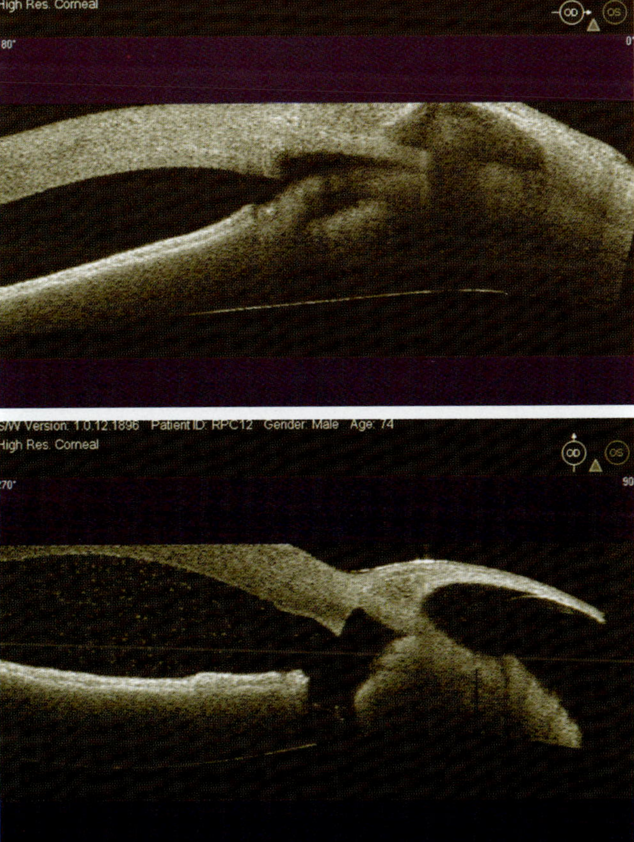

Figs 19 and 20: ASOCT image of a bleb showing the intrascleral course of the aqueous and a patent iridotomy

3. The trabecular-ciliary process distance (TCPD), is measured on a line extending from the corneal endothelium at 500 µm from the scleral spur perpendicularly through the iris, to the ciliary processes.
4. The iris thickness 1 (ID-1), is the iris thickness measured along the same line as the TCPD. ID-2 is the iris thickness at 2 mm from iris root and ID-3 is maximum iris thickness near pupillary margin
5. The iris-ciliary process distance (ICPD), is the distance measured from the posterior iris surface (iris pigmented epithelium to the ciliary process along the same line as the TCPD).
6. The iris-lens contact distance (ILCD), is measured along the iris pigmented epithelium from the pupillary border to the point where the anterior lens surface leaves the iris.
7. The scleral ciliary process angle (SCPA) between the tangent to the scleral surface and the axis of the ciliary process.
8. Iris zonule distance (IZD)—it is a part of TCPD at a point just clearing the ciliary process.
9. Angle recess area (ARA)—triangular area bordered by the anterior iris surface, corneal endothelium, and a line perpendicular to the corneal endothelium drawn to the iris surface from a point 750 µm anterior to the scleral spur.
10. Iris convexity or concavity—a line is first created from the most peripheral point to the most central point of iris pigment epithelium. A perpendicular is extended from this line to the iris pigment epithelium at the point of greatest concavity or convexity. This parameter is useful in determining the dynamic iris configuration changes.
11. UBM-anterior chamber depth (UACD)—from the corneal endothelium to the anterior lens surface.
12. Central corneal thickness (CCT)—from the corneal endothelium to the corneal epithelium when the probe is well centered and the pupil is well visualized.
13. Iris lens angle (ILA, θ_2)—the angle at which the iris leaves the lens surface.

Contraindications

- Fresh postoperative cases
- Open globe injury
- External ocular infection.

Uses

UBM is used for the evaluation of the following:

1. Examination of the anterior chamber angle details including PAS, iris bombe, etc. occludability of the angle, mechanisms of congenital glaucoma, etc.

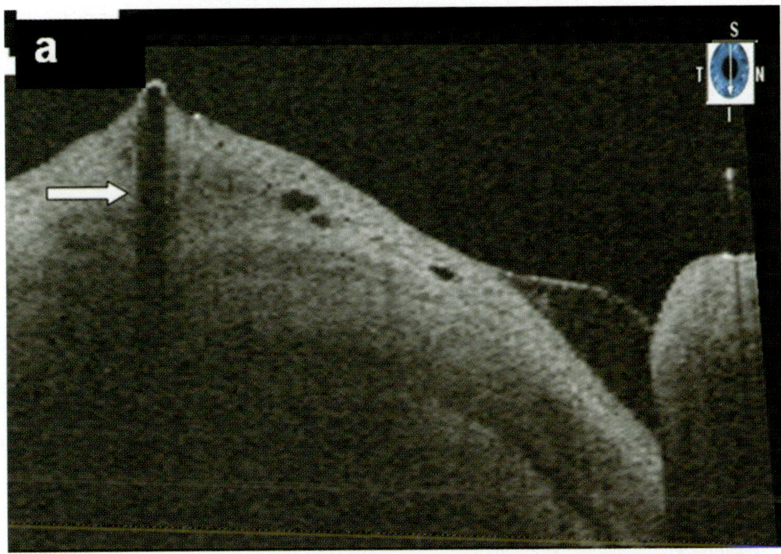

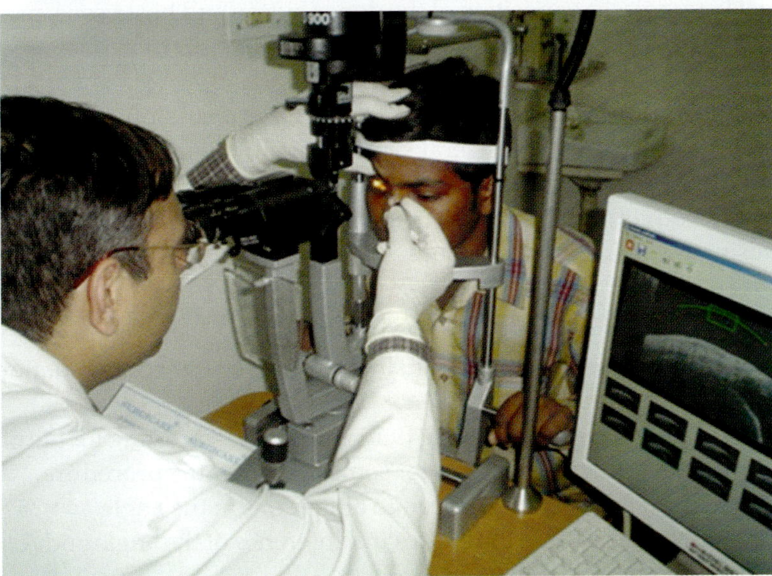

Figs 21 and 22: SLOCT guided needling of a failing bleb (needle track – arrow)

2. Biometry of the anterior segment—the corneal thickness, anterior chamber depth, posterior chamber depth, IOL thickness, iris thickness, ciliary body thickness, scleral thickness, etc.
3. Determining the mechanism of glaucoma: post-traumatic , pseudophakic and lens induced glaucoma, malignant glaucoma.
4. Evaluation of cysts and tumors causing angle closure.
5. Determining patency and effect of laser iridotomy, functional status of a filtering surgery, non-penetrating deep sclerectomy, goniopuncture, aqueous drainage devices.
6. Evaluation of the bleb function and postoperative complications after trabeculectomy.
7. Congenital malformations of the anterior segment associated with a cloudy or opaque cornea, adherent leucomas, anterior staphyloma, corneal dystrophy, ICE syndrome.
8. Descemet detachment in non-resolving corneal edema, bullous keratopathy, band shaped keratopathy.
9. Post keratoplasty apposition of the donor button and host tissue, presence or absence of vitreous or iris incarceration in the incision, interface following lamellar keratoplasty, etiology of opaque grafts.
10. Evaluation of trauma: iridodialysis , angle recession, cyclodialysis, hyphema, foreign body, scleral laceration, vitreous in anterior chamber, partially absorbed or subluxated crystalline lens.
11. Ciliary body tumors, anterior uveal melanomas invading the angle and causing secondary angle closure.

Limitations

- It is a contact investigation with risk of causing ocular contamination and injury (corneal abrasion).
- Use of the eyecup with a coupling fluid is very discomforting for the patient and can cause blurring of vision for some time after the procedure.
- Pressure from the eye cup can lead to alterations in the angle.
- Takes a long time to scan the entire circumference of the angle and requires a skilled operator.
- Need for the patient to lie supine during the procedure instead of being sitting as in most other investigations. Supine position leads to backward shift of the iris-lens diaphragm due to gravity.
- It cannot be used in the immediate postoperative period due to risk of injury and transmission of infection.
- Contraindicated in suspected open globe injuries as it can aggravate the damage.

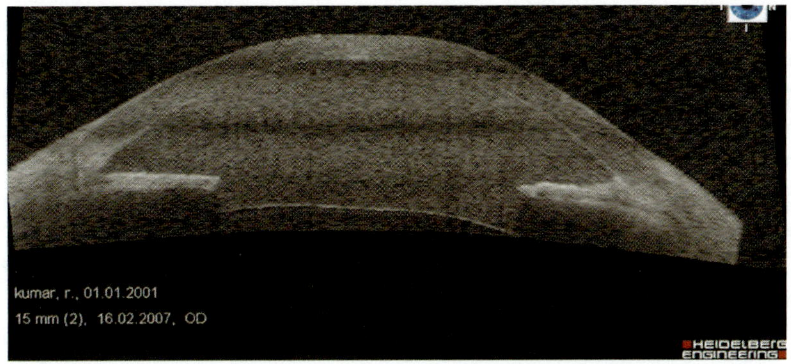

Fig. 23: SL-OCT image of a post-traumatic case showing total hyphaema

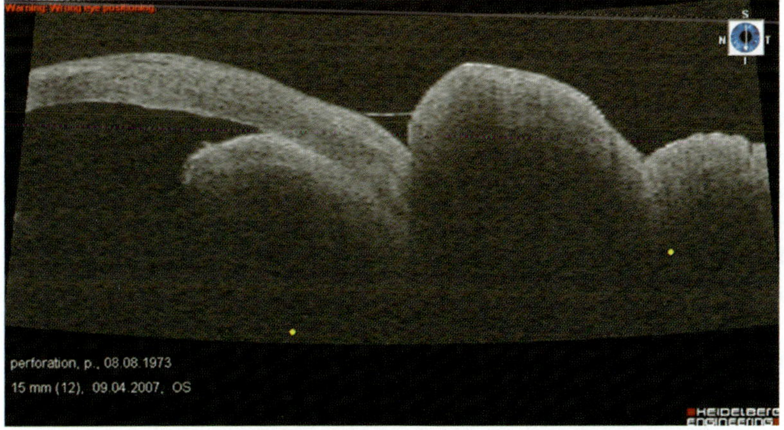

Fig. 24: Tear meniscus

- The invasive nature of the modality may preclude its use in younger children and uncooperative adults and may necessitate the use of sedation or even general anesthesia to accomplish the same.
- Inability to capture the posterior lens capsule due to limited penetration precludes its use in the preoperative assessment of traumatic cataracts or posterior polar cataracts to preoperatively analyze whether a pre existing posterior capsular defect is present or not.
- Only one part of the angle can be imaged at one time and it is difficult to pin-point the exact clock hour of imaging.
- There is no optical axis marker and exact centration while imaging is difficult to achieve.

RETINAL NERVE FIBER LAYER ANALYSIS USING SCANNING LASER POLARIMETRY

Introduction

- RNFL defects are the earliest sign of have found occur prior to visual field loss and optic nerve head (ONH) changes.
- Scanning laser polarimetry is a method of measuring RNFL using a scanning laser ophthalmoscope with polarization modulation, a cornea polarization compensation, and a polarization detection unit utilizing the birefringent properties of the RNFL.
- A scanning laser polarimeter is basically a confocal scanning laser ophthalmoscope with an integrated ellipsometer to measure retardation.

Principle of Scanning Laser Polarimetry

The retinal nerve fiber layer (RNFL) is made of highly ordered parallel axon bundles which are the source of RNFL birefringence. Birefringence is the splitting of a light wave by a polar material into two components which travel at different velocities creating a relative phase shift termed retardation proportional to the thickness of the RNFL.

Retinal scanning laser polarimetry (SLP) determines the RNFL thickness, point by point in the peripapillary region, by measuring the total retardation in the light reflected from the retina.

Anterior Segment Birefringence and Variable Corneal Compensation (VCC)

The axis and magnitude values from the anterior segment can be computed by analyzing the non-uniform retardation profile around the macula due to the birefringence from the anterior segment. The axis of the anterior segment

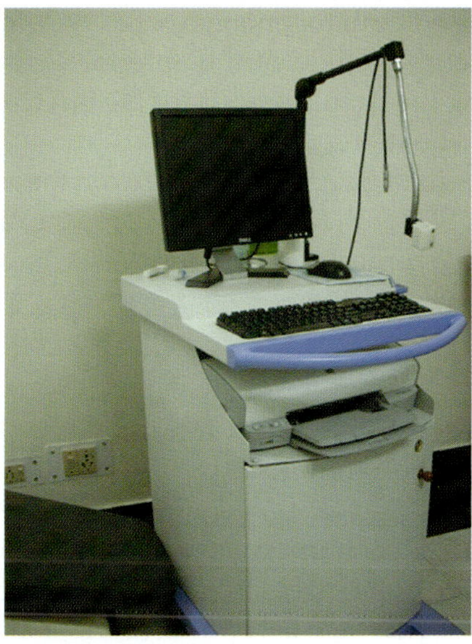

Fig. 25A: UBM machine (Appasamy Associates, India)

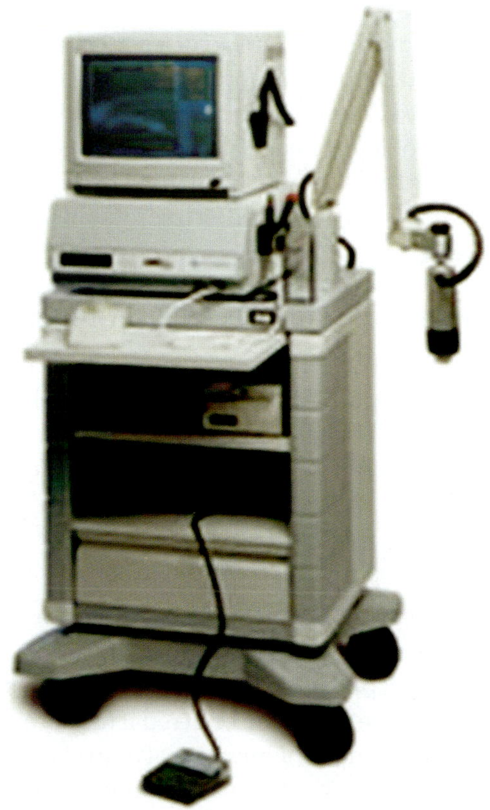

Fig. 25B: P 40 UBM machine from Paradigm (Salt Lake City, Utah, USA)

birefringence is determined by the orientation of the 'bow-tie' birefringent pattern in the macula and the magnitude of the anterior segment birefringence is calculated by analyzing the circular profile of the birefringence in the macula according to standard equations.

If the corneal values for a given eye deviate from the assumed values of the fixed compensator, the SLP with fixed corneal compensation FCC image is less comparable. The variable corneal compensation (VCC) scan therefore results in a more accurate RNFL measurement.

RNFL Measurements

The raster scan using a beam of a near-infrared laser (780 nm) captures an image with a field 40° horizontally by 20°vertically, including both the peripapillary and the macular region generating two images: a reflectance image and a retardation image . Each image is made up of 256 (horizontal) × 128 (vertical) pixels, or 32,768 total pixels. For an emmetropic eye, 1 pixel is .0465 mm in size, and the total scan field is 11.9 mm (horizontal) × 5.9 mm (vertical).

Measurement Technique

It is performed with an undilated pupil of at least 2 mm diameter and total time for the examination and output is less than 3 minutes for both eyes.

The test is totally objective and the reproducibility of images is 5-8 micron per measured pixel. Looking at image allows one to see if the ellipse was placed properly and the ellipse can be manually aligned to conform to the disk margin. The diameter of the ellipse is displayed in microns and gives an idea about the actual disk diameter.

Clinical Interpretation of the GDx VCC Printout

For each GDx VCC scan, an age-matched comparison is made to the normative database and any significant deviations from normal limits are flagged as abnormal with a p value.

Quantitative RNFL evaluation is provided through four key elements of the printout.

The Thickness Map

The Thickness map shows the RNFL thickness in a color-coded format (blue to red) up to 120 microns. Each quadrant is analyzed and actual deviation from normal, in microns, is displayed. Deviations from normal are highlighted in yellow if they are borderline ($p < 0.10$), or in red if they are outside normal limits ($p < 0.05$). The normal pattern is a symmetrical hourglass shape of bright colors superior and inferior and dark colors nasal and temporal.

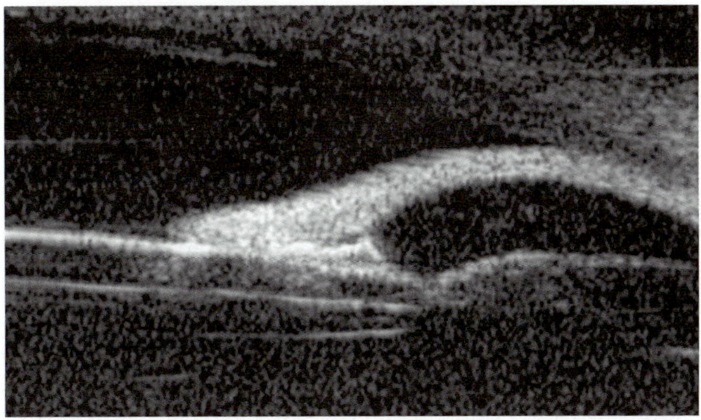

Fig. 26: Iris bombe

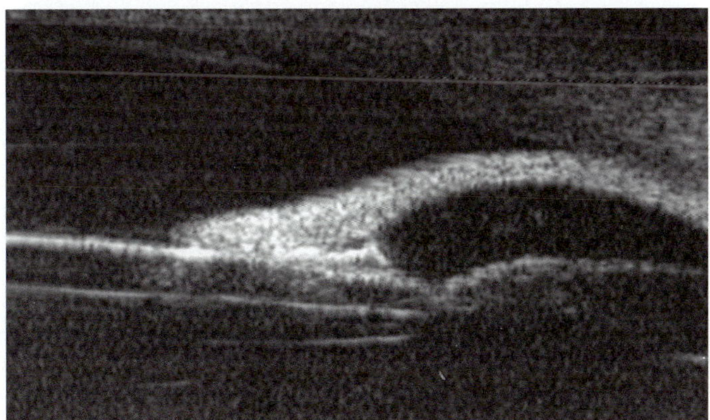

Fig. 27: Peripheral anterior synechiae

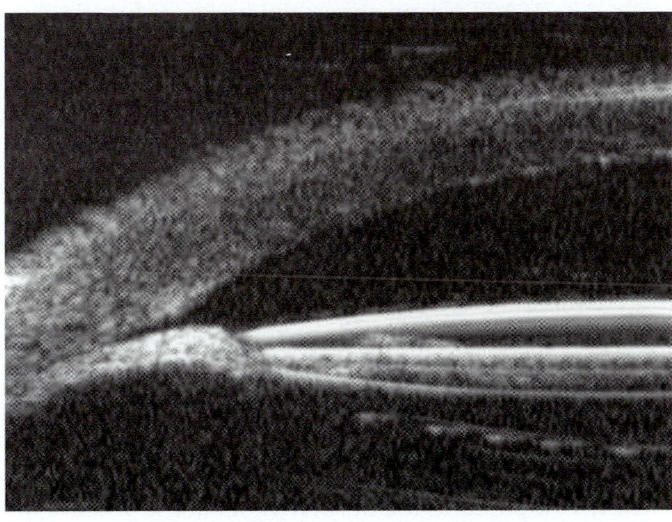

Fig. 28: ACIOL and secondary angle closure

An Abnormal pattern may include any/all of the following:
1. Diffuse loss of RNFL.
2. Focal defects are seen as concentrated dark areas (visible on fundus image as well).
3. Asymmetry between superior and inferior quadrants.
4. Asymmetry between the two eyes.
5. Higher than normal nasal and temporal thickness.

The Deviation Map

The Deviation map reveals the location and magnitude of RNFL defects over the entire thickness map. The Deviation Map analyzes a 128 × 128 pixel region (20° × 20°) centered on the optic disk. Dark blue squares represent areas where the RNFL thickness is below the 5th percentile of the normative database. This means that there is only a 5% probability that the RNFL thickness in this area is within the normal range, determined by an age-matched comparison to the normative database. Light blue squares represent deviation below the 2% level, yellow represents deviation below 1%, and red represents deviation below 0.5%. The deviation map uses a grayscale fundus image of the eye as a background, and displays abnormal grid values as colored squares over this image.

The TSNIT Map

The TSNIT stands for Temporal Superior Nasal-Inferior—Temporal and displays the RNFL thickness values along the calculation circle starting temporally and moving superiorly, nasally, inferiorly, and ending temporally. In a normal eye the TSNIT plot follows the typical *'double hump'* pattern, with thick RNFL measures superiorly and inferiorly and thin RNFL values nasally and temporally. The TSNIT Graph shows the curve (or function) of the actual values for that eye along with a shaded area which represents the 95% normal range for that age. When there is RNFL loss, the TSNIT curve will fall below shaded area, especially in the superior and inferior regions. In the center of the printout at the bottom, the TSNIT graphs for both eyes are displayed together. In a healthy eye there is good symmetry between the TSNIT graphs of the two eyes and the two curves will overlap.

The Parameter

Parameters are displayed in a table in the center of the printout. The TSNIT parameters are summary measures based on RNFL thickness values within the calculation circle. The calculation circle is a fixed circle (a fixed size band) centered on the Optic Nerve Head (ONH). The band is 0.4 mm wide, and has an outer diameter of 3.2 mm and an inner diameter of 2.4 mm. These parameters are automatically compared to the normative database and are quantified in

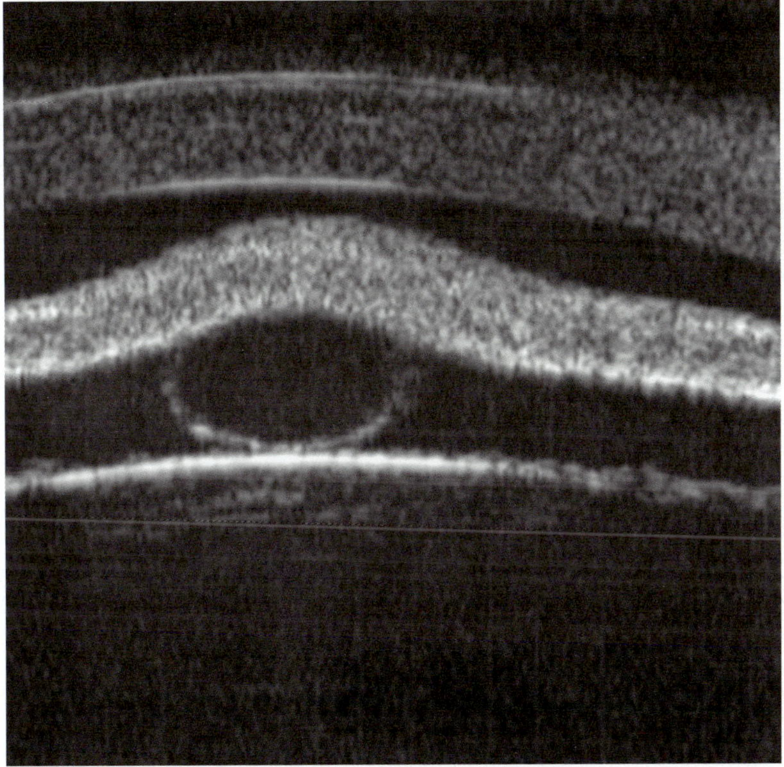

Fig. 29: Iris pigment epithelial cyst

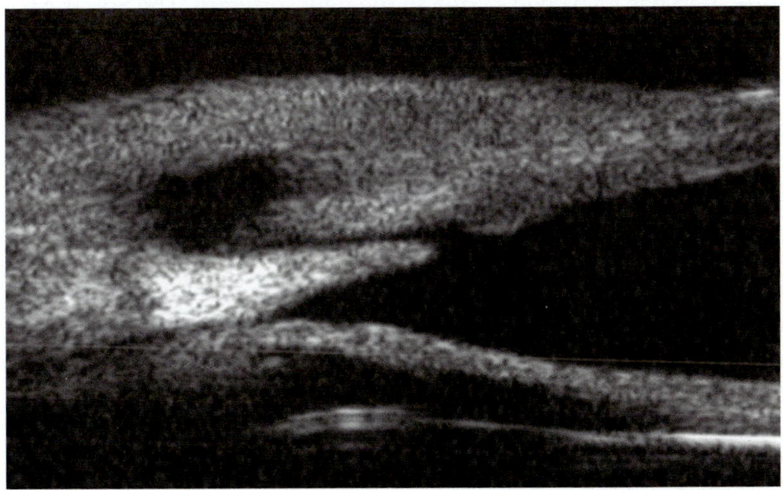

Fig. 30: Trabeculectomy

terms of probability of normality. Normal parameter values are displayed in white, abnormal values are color-coded based on their probability of normality same as the Deviation Map

The five TSNIT parameters are: TSNIT Average, Superior Average, Inferior Average, TSNIT Standard Deviation (TSNIT SD), and Inter-eye symmetry.

The nerve fiber indicator (NFI) : The NFI is a global measure based on the entire RNFL thickness map. It utilizes information from the entire RNFL thickness map to optimize the discrimination between healthy and glaucomatous eyes. The output of the NFI is a single value that ranges from 1 to 100 and indicates the overall integrity of the RNFL. Output values range from 1 to 100, with classification based on the ranges: 1 to 30 as normal, 31 to 50 as borderline, 51+ abnormal.

Abnormal Scan

TSNIT average, superior average, inferior average, TSNIT standard deviation, Intereye symmetry or NFI is Abnormal at $p < 1\%$ level .They are considered Borderline at $p < 5\%$ level .NFI is > 47 at the $p < 1\%$ level or >30 at $p < 5\%$ level, the scan is abnormal).

Detecting Progression of RNFL loss: Serial Analysis

The serial analysis printout has five key elements that should be considered when assessing RNFL change over time: Thickness Maps, Deviation Maps, Deviation from Reference Maps, Parameters Tables and TSNIT Graph. A change probability map has also been added in the new software. The Serial Analysis can compare up to four exams.

Thus progression of the RNFL over a period provides key data regarding:

1. Identification of RNFL defect
2. Rate of progression of RNFL
3. Assessment of treatment effectiveness

Guided Progression Analysis™ for GDx

The new software which helps in investigating the progression is GPA™ **(progression analysis for GDx).** It helps to identify progression, determine its rate and assess treatment effectiveness. It measures and detects the progression based on three different parts of the analysis

1. Image change map
2. TSNIT change graph
3. Summary of parameter charts.

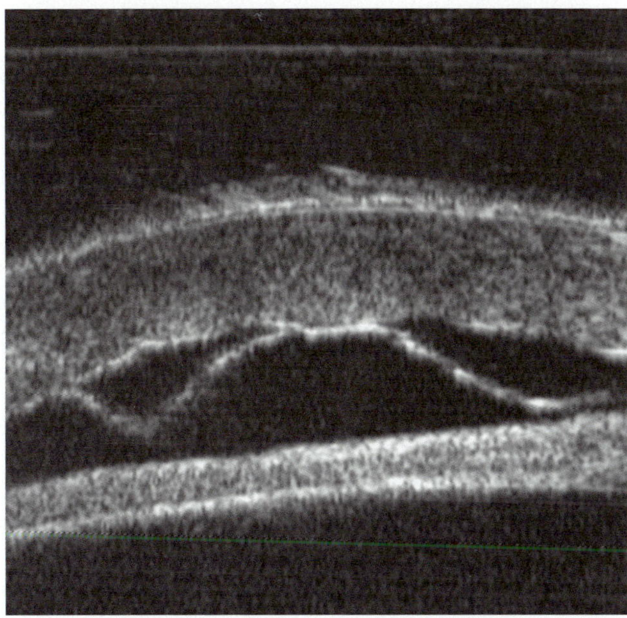

Fig. 31: Descemets membrane detachment

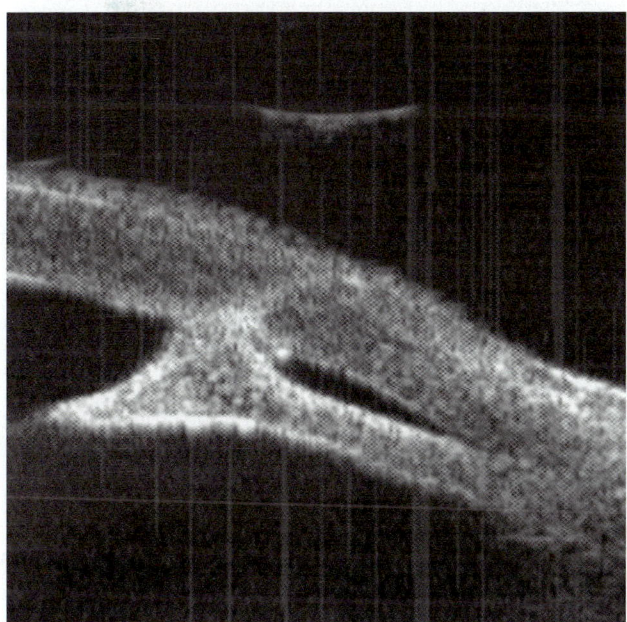

Fig. 32: Graft host junction synechiae

Image Change

Image change map recognizes the change in the reflectance image. The minimal cluster size considered is 150 pixels which is 2% of image area. Any significant change in the image is depicted on the progression map

It can detect narrower and deeper defects. This design has specificity of 95%

TSNIT Progression Graph

The ring around the optic nerve is divided into 64 equal segments and compared on follow-up. If 3 adjacent segments show significant change on follow-up the progression is indicated. This design also has 95% specificity to detect the defects. It can detect shallower and broader defect better as compared to other parameters.

Parameter Progression Chart

TSNIT average, superior average and inferior average are compared. On the chart regression line is drawn to show likely progression and $p < 5\%$. This design also has 95% specificity. This can detect diffuse changes in the RNFL better.

This parameter can also compare the rate of progression before and after treatment, thus helpful in guiding the treatment line.

Advantages of GDxVCC

- Easy to operate, good reproducibility
- Does not require pupillary dilatation, independent of the optical resolution of eye
- Does not require a reference plane
- Can detect glaucoma on the first exam, before standard visual field
- Comparison with age matched normative data base

Limitations

- Does not measure actual RNFL thickness (inferred value)
- Measures RNFL at different locations for each patient
- Does not differentiate true biological change from variability
- Limited use in moderate/advanced glaucoma
- Requires a wider data base from the Indian Population
- Affected by anterior and posterior segment pathology like:ocular surface disorders,macular pathology,cataract and refractive surgery, refractive errors (false positive in myopes), peripapillary atrophy (scleral birefringence interferes with RNFL measurement

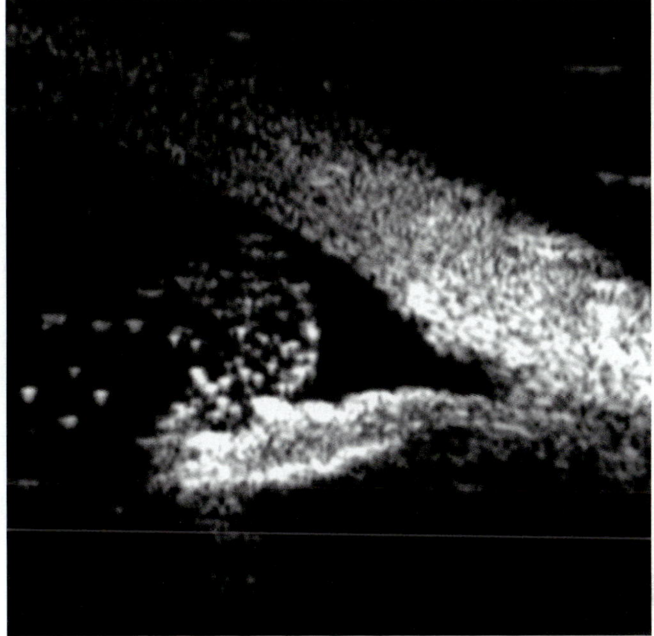

Fig. 33: Vitreous in AC, angle recession

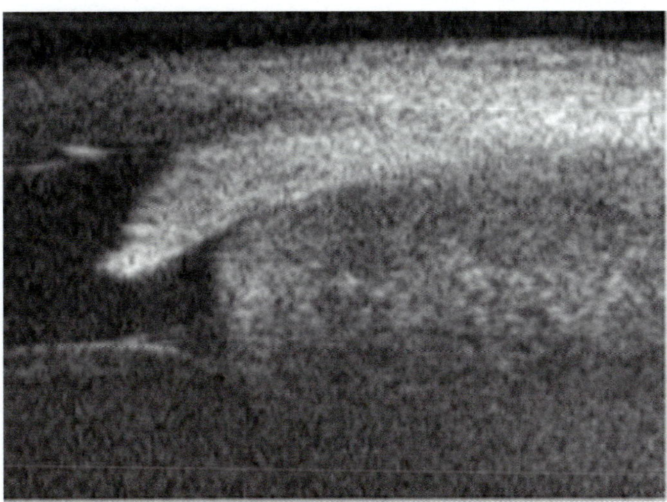

Fig. 34: CB melanoma

GDx-ECC: GDx—Enhanced Corneal Compensation

Retinal nerve fiber layer images obtained using enhanced corneal compensation show a stronger structure-function relationship with standard automated perimetry visual field sensitivity compared with variable corneal compensation. Scanning laser polarimetry ultimately depends on the strength of the retinal birefringence measurement relative to optical and digital noise. Sensitivity can be enhanced using a software algorithm (ECC) that measures the birefringence of the cornea and retina concurrently, as opposed to canceling out the corneal measurement with variable corneal compensation (VCC). This alternate method resulted in high-quality scans of all subjects. A baseline image, consisting of the mean of three scans, is used in the analysis. The computerized export of the temporal-superior-nasal-inferior-temporal (TSNIT) plots on the GDx ECC printout includes the mean RNFL thickness from 64 polar sectors (5.625 deg/ arc). The mean for each sector is computed along the 3.2 mm diameter measurement circle surrounding the optic nerve head. The mean RNFL thickness for the superior (0–180°) and inferior (181–360°)retinal region is computed separately by averaging the corresponding mean sectors.

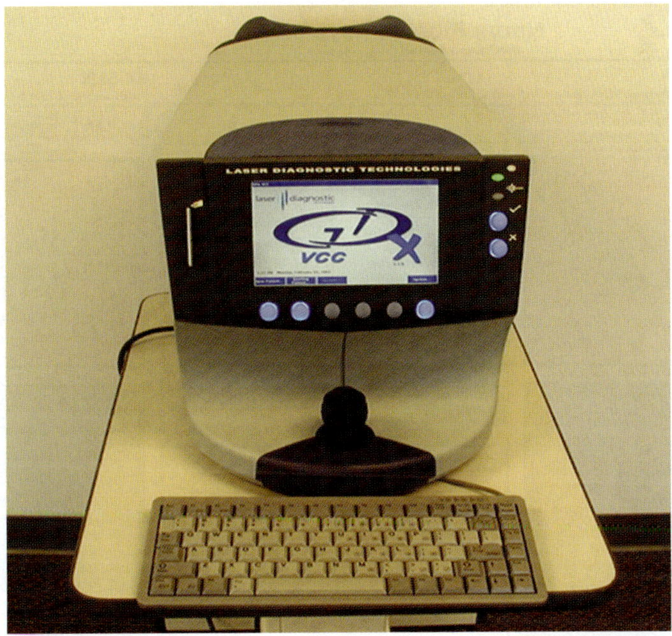

Fig. 35: GDx VCC

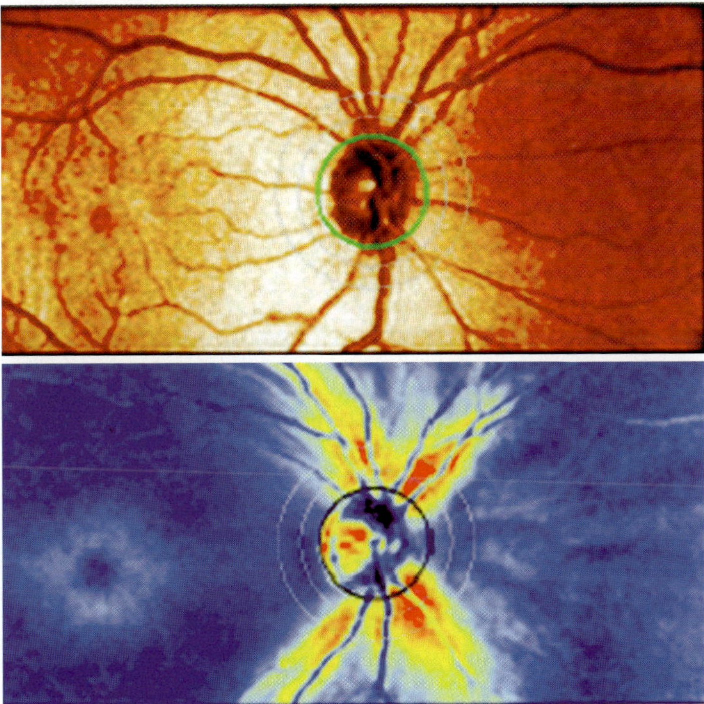

Fig. 36: Images generated by the GDx VCC: left image is the reflectance image, which is displayed as a colored intensity map (greater reflectance corresponds to a lighter color). The right image is the retardation map converted to RNFL thickness. The RNFL thickness is color coded based on the color spectrum, with thinner regions displayed in blue and green and thicker regions displayed in yellow and red

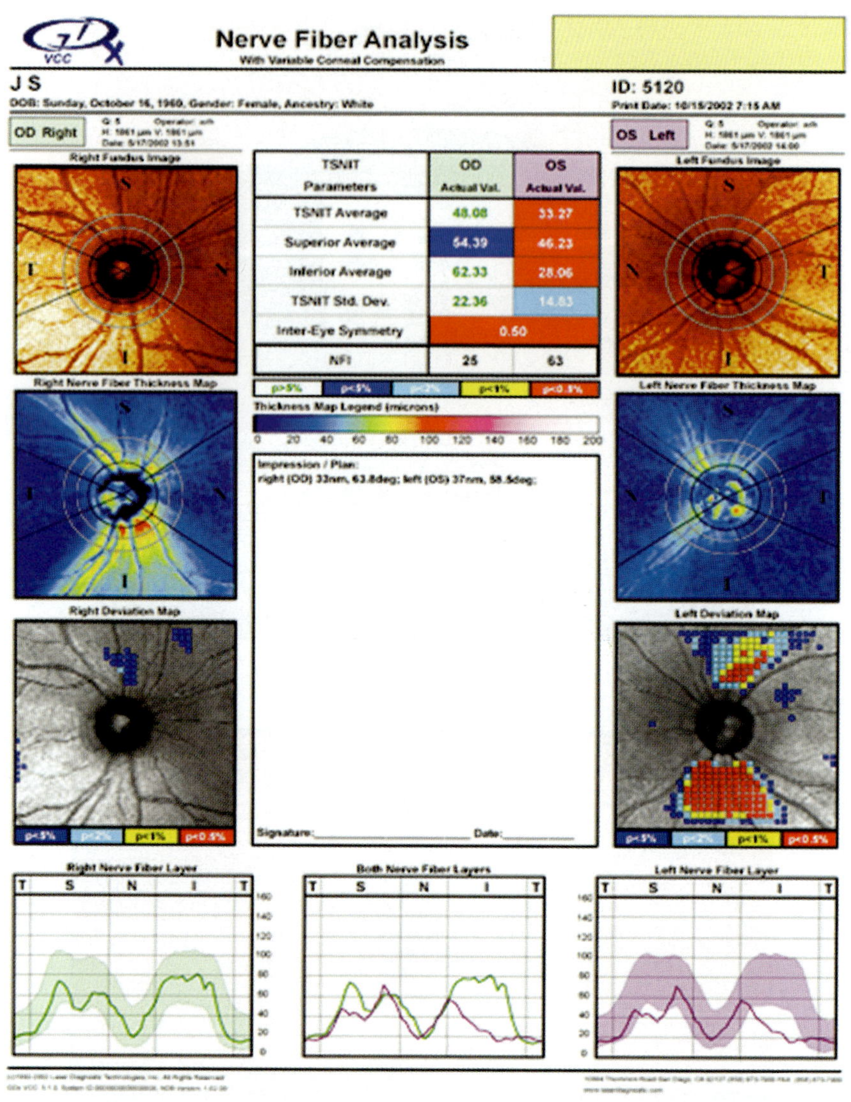

Fig. 37: GDx printout

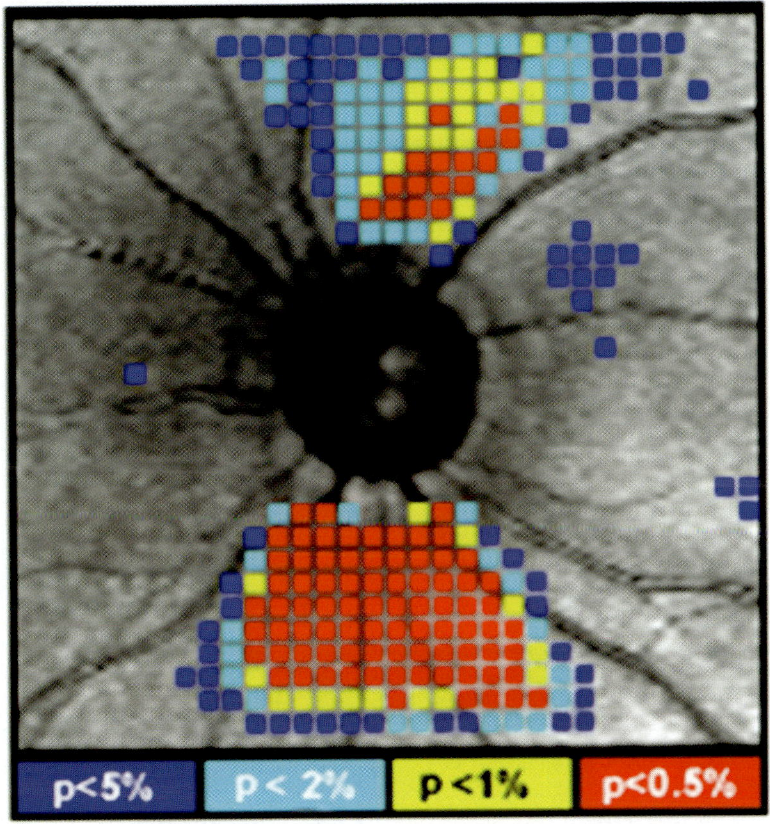

Fig. 38: Deviation map showing magnitude and area of RNFL thinning

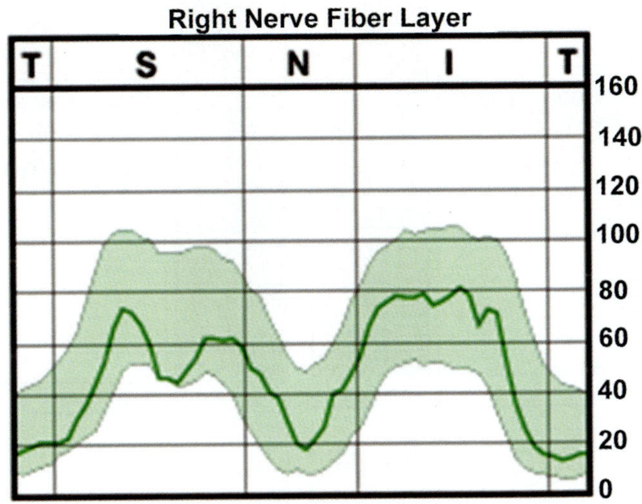

Fig. 39: TSNIT graph: typical double hump

TSNIT Parameters	OD Actual Val.	OS Actual Val.
TSNIT Average	48.08	33.27
Superior Average	54.39	46.23
Inferior Average	62.33	28.06
TSNIT Std. Dev.	22.36	14.83
Inter-Eye Symmetry	0.50	
NFI	25	63

p>5%	p<5%	p<2%	p<1%	p<0.5%

Fig. 40: RNFL parameters:1-30 normal, 31-50 borderline, > 50 abnormal

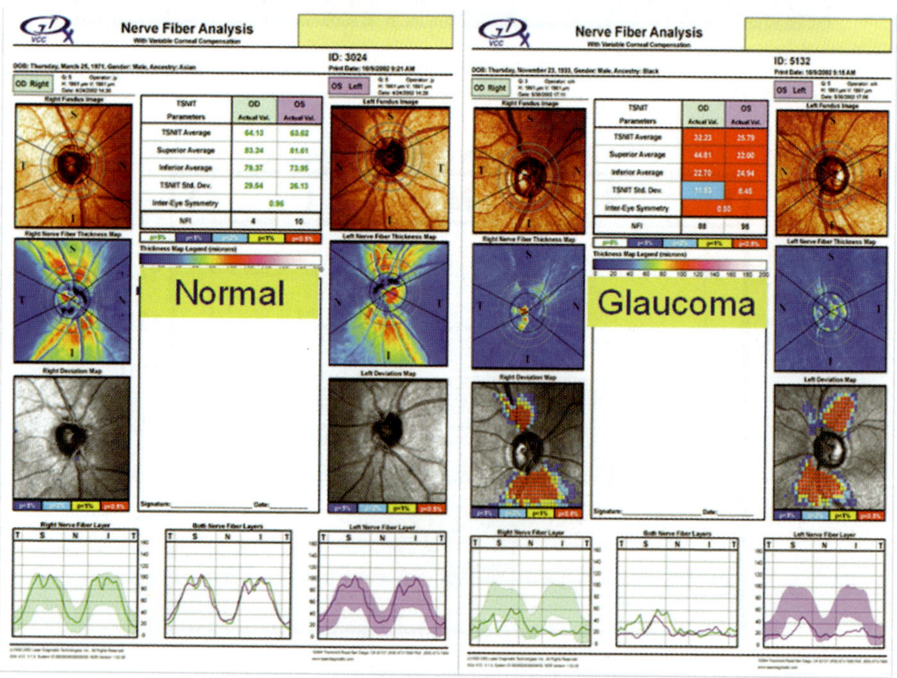

Fig. 41: Normal and glaucomatous GDx

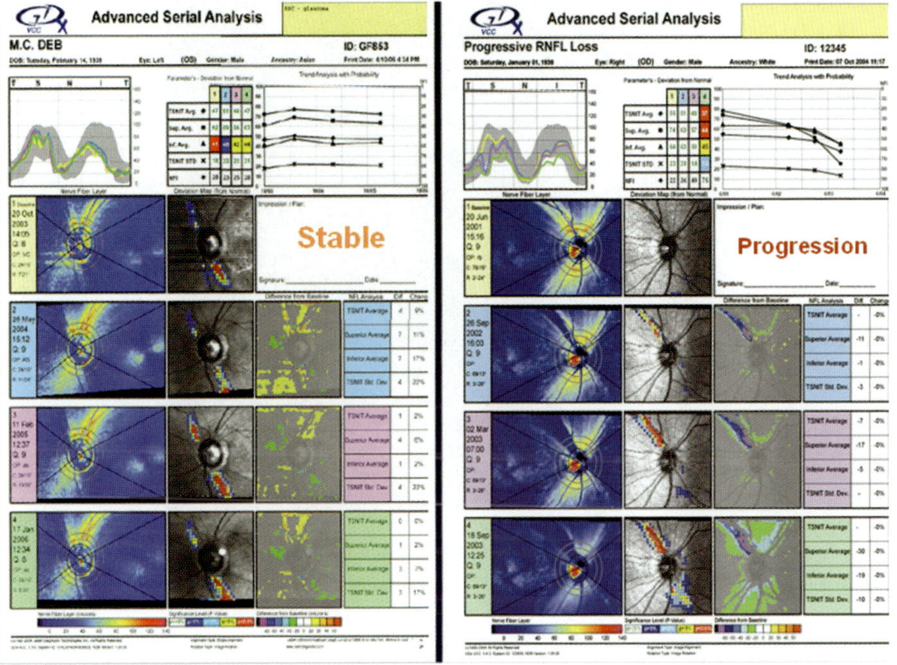

Fig. 42: Stable and progressive RNFL loss

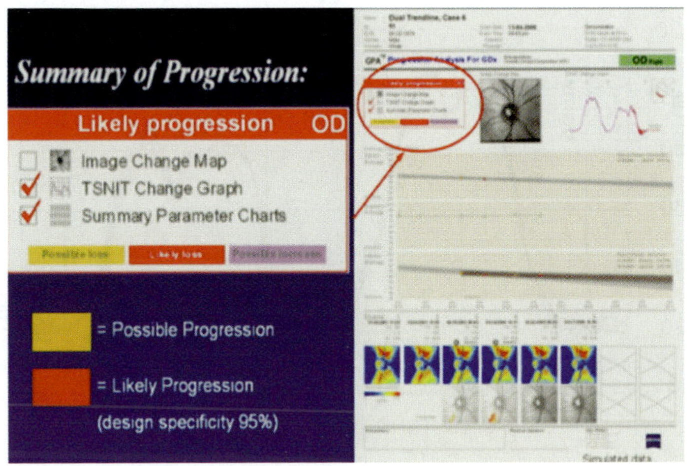

Fig. 43: GPA^{TM} – GDx progression analysis

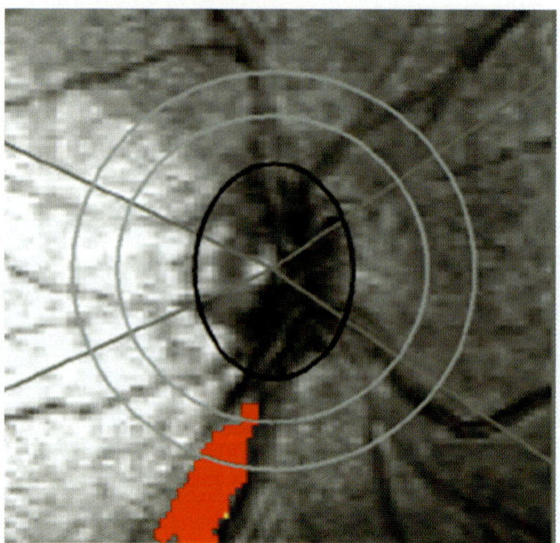

Fig. 44: Image change map

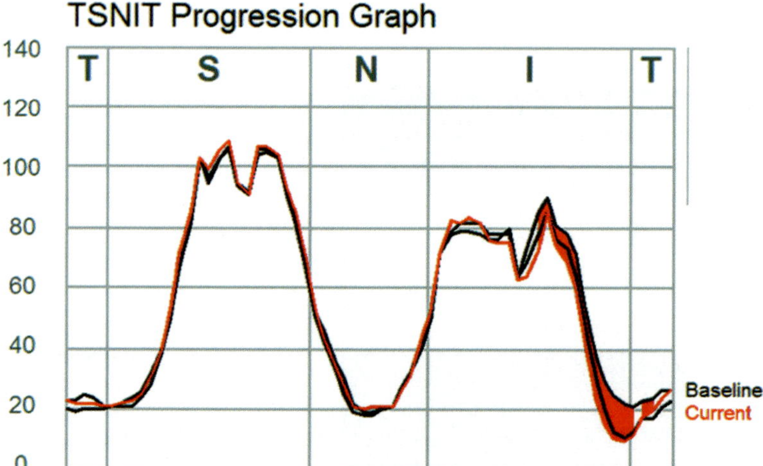

Fig. 45: TSNIT progression graph

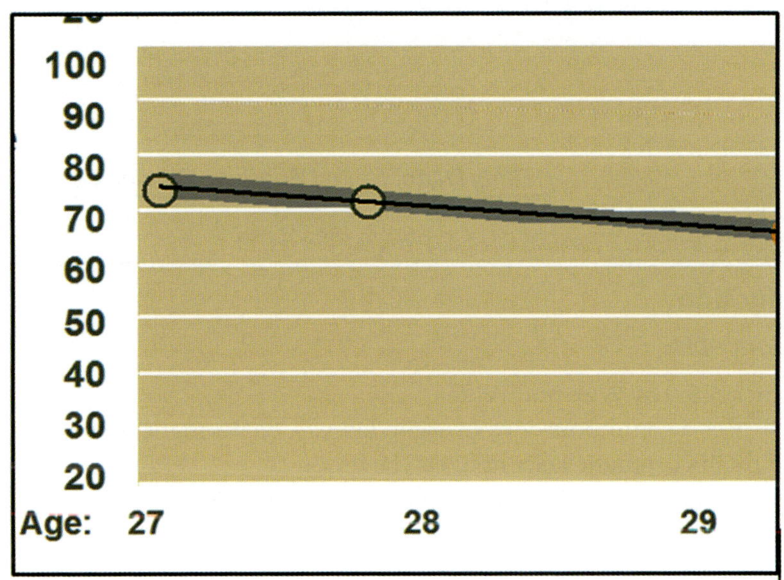

Fig. 46: Parameter progression chart

20

Laser Procedures in Glaucoma

Tanuj Dada, Shibal Bhartiya, Shalini Mohan (India)

ARGON LASER TRABECULOPLASTY (ALT)

Introduction

Key Concepts

- Term coined by Wise and Witter.
- ALT uses a continuous –wave argon laser. A bichromatic blue-green laser or a monochromatic laser light can be used.
- Alternatively, a krypton laser, frequency doubled Nd: YAG laser (532 nm) and diode laser can also be used.
- Diode laser causes less disruption of blood aqueous barrier, lesser perioperative pain and a reduced incidence of peripheral anterior synechiae (PAS) formation. Also it has the advantage of portability, lesser maintenance requirements and possible attachment with standard slitlamps.

Mechanism of Action

- Thermal energy produced by absorption of laser by pigmented trabecular meshwork causes shrinkage of collagen of the trabecular lamellae.
- This probably opens up intertrabecular spaces in untreated region and expands Schlemm's canal by pulling the meshwork centrally (*trabecular tightening*).
- Laser burns attract phagocytes that clean up the debris within the meshwork and allows aqueous to flow better.
- Laser destroyed endothelial cells stimulate the production of new, more viable endothelial cells with better outflow properties.

Indication of ALT

- Primary open angle glaucoma
- Exfoliation syndrome
- Pigmentary glaucoma
- Glaucoma in aphakia or pseudophakia
- To supplement maximal medical therapy to postpone filtration surgery
- As a primary treatment in patients with poor drug compliance
- Following trabeculectomy where additional lowering of IOP is required
- Before cataract extraction in patients with coexistent poorly controlled POAG.

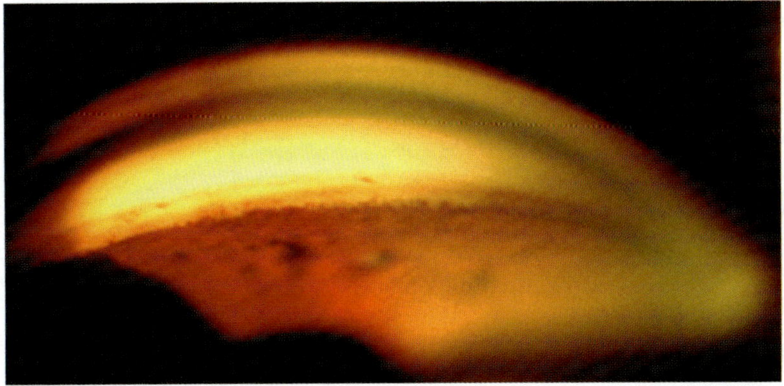

Fig. 1: Junction of pigmented and non-pigmented trabecular meshwork, where laser beam is aimed

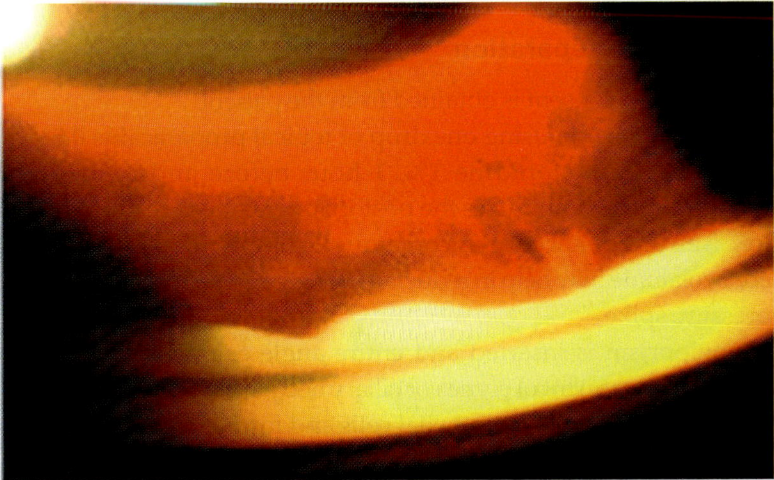

Fig. 2: PAS

Contraindications

- Closed or extremely narrow angles
- Corneal haze or diminished aqueous clarity
- Aphakia with vitreous in A/C
- Neovascular glaucoma
- Active uveitis
- Glaucomas with poor responsiveness, e.g. primary congenital glaucoma and angle recession glaucoma, etc.

Preoperative Work-up

- Routine total ophthalmic check-up
- Slit-lamp biomicroscopy : Corneal clarity, AC depth
- Intraocular pressure (IOP)
- Gonioscopy

Preoperative Preparation

- An informed consent is obtained from the patient.
- Topical anesthesia using one drop of topical proparacaine 0.5% .
- A drop of apraclonidine 1%, 1 hour before and immediately after trabeculoplasty minimizes the postoperative pressure rise.
- In cases of advanced glaucomatous cupping, intravenous mannitol or acetazolamide may help in reducing the magnitude of potential postoperative pressure spike.
- A gonioprism is inserted and entire angle examined carefully to avoid accidental treatment of cornea or ciliary body band with resultant downward migration of corneal endothelial cells and formation of peripheral anterior synechiae (PAS). In case of difficulty in lightly pigmented trabecular meshwork (TM), Schwalbe's line should first be identified by locating the apex of corneal wedge.

Gonioprism

A Ritch trabeculoplasty goniolens with antireflective coating on its front surface is usually preferred. It has two mirrors inclined at 59° for better view of inferior quadrant and two at 64° for the superior angle. It has a 17 D planoconvex button over two mirrors which provide X1.4 magnification reducing a 50 um laser spot to 35 um and increasing the laser energy by a factor of 2.

Laser Parameters

- Typical setting for ALT is 50 u spot size, 0.2 seconds duration and 750 – 1200 MW of power (avg. of 1000 mw).

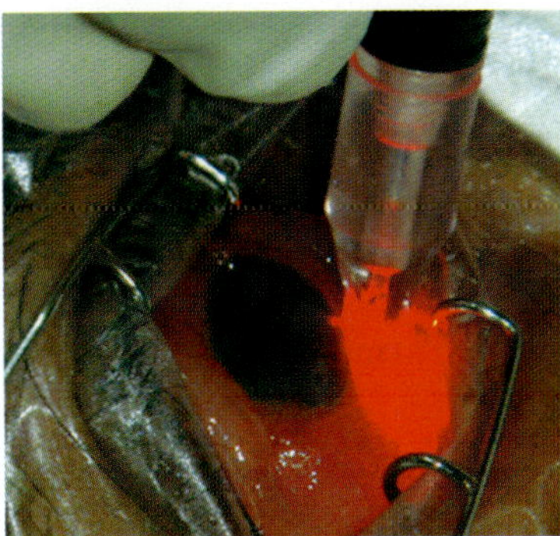

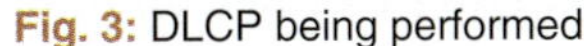

Fig. 3: DLCP being performed

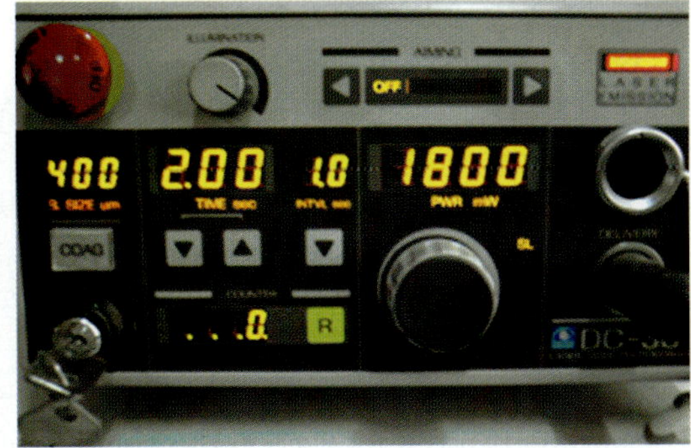

Fig. 4: DLCP machine (Nidek) showing the setting of the procedure. Power is kept at 1800, time duration is 2 seconds. Aiming beam has been kept off

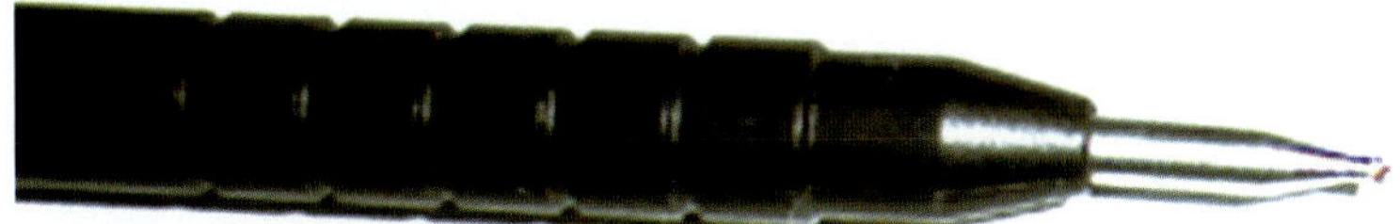

Fig. 5: DLCP probe (Nidek) which is to be placed over the ciliary body region after markeing with caliper

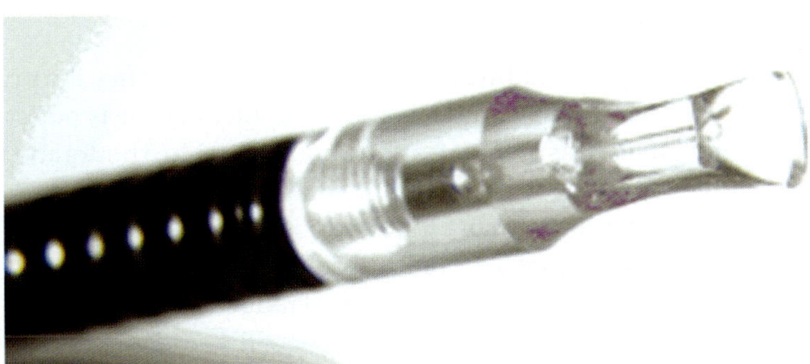

Fig. 6: IRIS G-probe (end on view)

- The power should be adjusted to produce a depigmentation spot or a small bubble at the treatment site.
- Power settings may be reduced in highly pigmented angles and vice versa for lightly pigmented TM.
- The variability of TM pigmentation in different quadrants require a change in power settings.
- Continuous refocusing of the aiming bean is essential to induce a circular burn.

Placement of Burn

The aiming beam is focused at the junction of pigmented and non-pigmented TM. The spot must be round and have a clear outline. This placement minimizes early post-laser pressure rise and PAS formation.

Ideal Reaction

Transient blanching of TM or appearance of minute gas bubble at the point of impact.

Number of Burns

- 180° or 360° of TM circumference can be photocoagulated in a single sitting or two sessions.
- 40 to 50 laser spots are applied in 180 degrees or 80 to 100 spots in 360° of the circumference.
- The burns (25) are regularly spaced from one end of the mirror to the other.
- The goniolens is then rotated clockwise for a 90° and a further 25 burns applied making a total of 50 burns extending in 180° of the angle.

Postoperative Management

- One drop of 1% apraclonidine is instilled immediately after the procedure or 1 tab of 250 mg acetazolamide is given if apraclonidine is not available.
- Subsequently, IOP measurement is done hourly for 1 to 3 hours and the next day.
- If there is no pressure rise, next follow-up is after 1 week. Meanwhile, all antiglaucoma medications are continued.
- IOP is reassessed after 4-10 weeks. A gradual reduction of medication is tried. If the pressure is still high, the remaining 180° of the circumference is treated.

Complications of ALT

- Elevated intraocular pressure
- Progressive visual field loss
- Iritis
- PAS

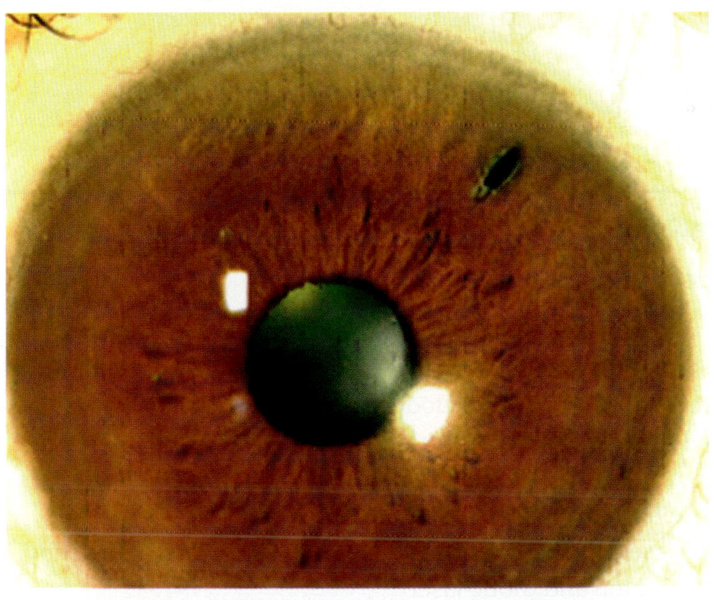

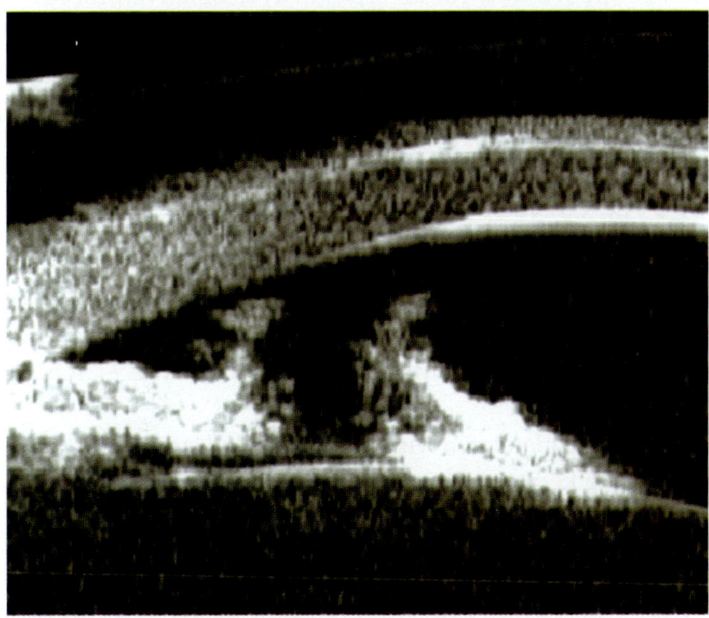

Figs 7 and 8: PI slitlamp and UBM view

- Hemorrhage
- Corneal edema
- Corneal abrasions and burns.

DIODE LASER CYCLOPHOTOCOAGULATION

Introduction

Key Facts

- Cyclodestructive procedures like surgical excision of ciliary body, cyclodiathermy, cycloirradiation, cycloelectrolysis, cyclocryotherapy, ultrasound, microwave cyclodestruction, and cyclophotocoagulation are generally used for refractory glaucomas.
- Beckman and Sugar first popularized the use of trans-scleral cyclophotocoagulation (TSCPC) by ruby laser in early 1970s
- Various lasers has been used for this purpose which includes ruby, Nd:YAG, argon, krypton and diode laser
- The therapeutic window for all types of cycloablative procedures is low. Therefore, too aggressive a treatment can lead to hypotony and phthisis and too little treatment will have no effect on IOP reduction. The variability in the location of the ciliary processes may account for the variable response to same degrees of treatment in different patients.

Indications for Cyclodestructive Procedures

- Refractive primary ACG, OAG
- Neovascular glaucoma (NVG)
- Post-traumatic glaucoma
- Aphakic/pseudophakic glaucoma especially with ACIOLs (anterior chamber IOLs)
- Severe congenital glaucoma with multiple failed surgeries
- Postpenetrating keratoplasty glaucoma
- Postretinal detachment surgery glaucoma
- Silicone oil induced glaucoma
- Inflammatory glaucoma
- Glaucoma with severe conjunctival scarring
- Failed trabeculectomy and drainage implants
- Medical condition precluding invasive surgery
- Patients' refusal to undergo invasive surgery
- Emergent situations (i.e. Acute onset NVG)

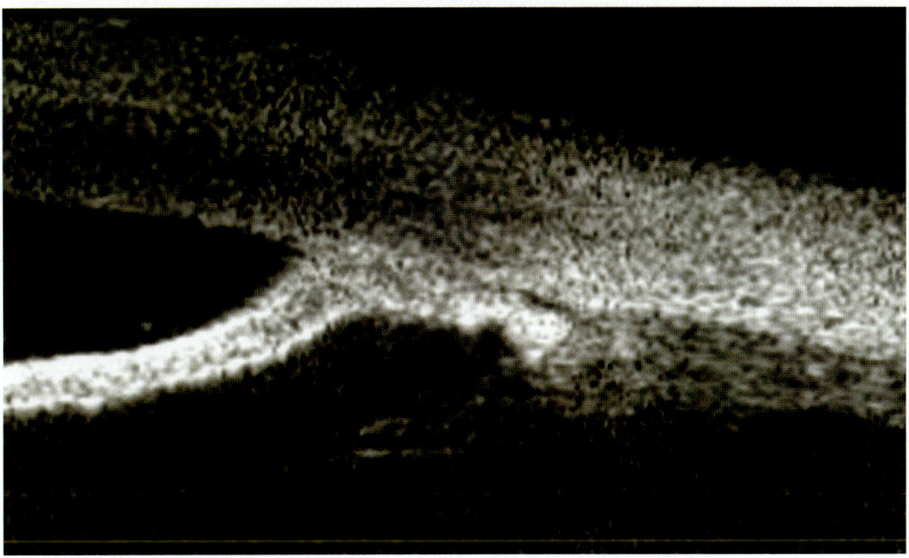

Fig. 9: PAS on UBM

Current Methods of Cycloablation

- Contact (transscleral) cycloablation
  - Cyclocryotherapy
  - Diode
  - Nd:YAG
- Noncontact cycloablation
  - Nd:YAG
  - Diode
- Transpupillary argon green cyclophotocoagulation
- Endolaser ablation
  - Diode
  - Argon

Mechanism of Action

Decreased Aqueous Production

- Destruction of the ciliary epithelium resulting in decreased aqueous production.
- Destruction of ciliary blood vessels and coagulative necrosis also contributes in decreasing aqueous production (ciliary body ischemia). Intraocular inflammation is also thought to be responsible for short-term hypotension.
- Creation of transscleral flow similar to cyclodialysis.
- Increased uveo-scleral outflow.

Increased Aqueous Outflow

Nd:YAG laser also produces a neuroepithelial defect resulting in increase outflow which is related to the extent of treatment. In an *in vitro* perfusion model, laser lesions placed 6 mm posterior to limbus had an equivalent effect on outflow to that of laser lesions directed towards ciliary process.

Technique

- An informed consent is taken from the patient
- The procedure is performed in the outpatient clinic under peribulbar local anesthesia and akinesia after proper cleaning with betadine under sterile condition
- The response of ciliary body destruction is gauged by the 'pop' sound

Settings

- 1500 mW for 2 seconds using 40 spots over 360^0
- The actual power setting is individualized after few spot applications by hearing a popping sound. The power is kept 50-100 wM below the appearance of popping sound

  The aiming beam is not needed in contact method and is kept off.

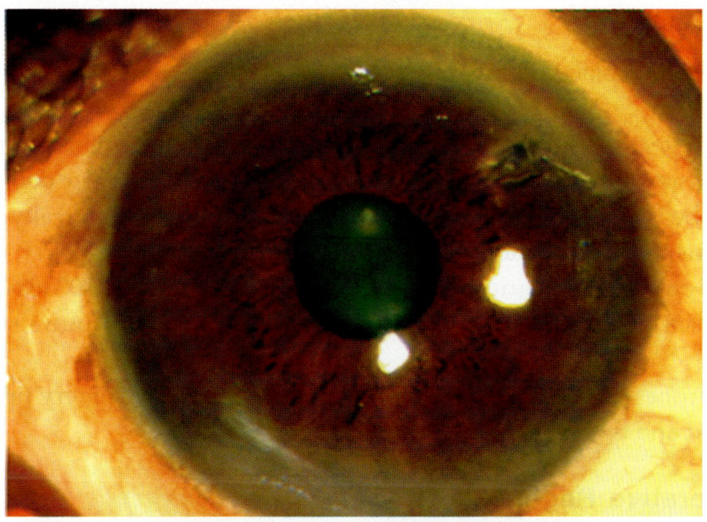

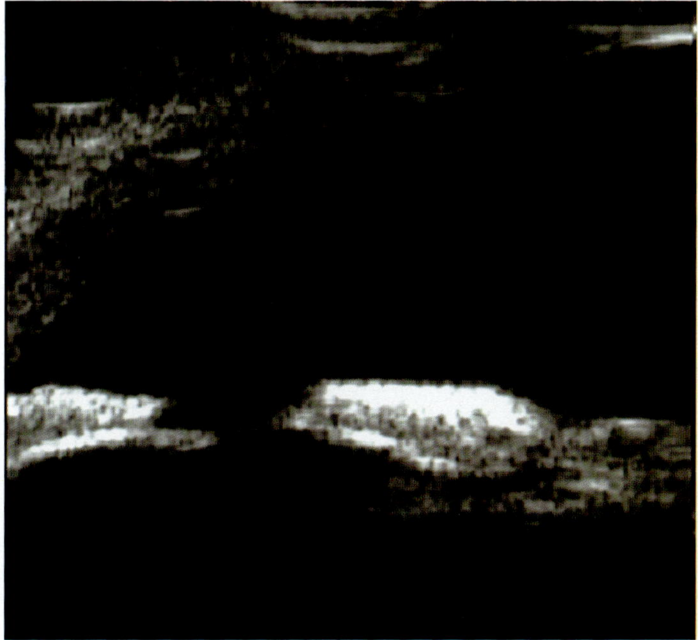

Fig. 10 and 11: Lamellar PI

Probe Placement

- The probe is placed 2 mm posterior to the limbus in the region of the ciliary body.
- The contact method can be performed using a G probe which has a small protrusion that indents the conjunctiva and sclera to optimize delivery. The G probe is placed with its edge at the limbus and is automatically centesed 1.2 mm posterior to the limbus in the region of the ciliary body.

Contiguous application of spots is done for about 270° leaving one superonasal quadrant. This is to leave the conjunctiva for future surgery if needed.

The probe is to be kept at limbus and the inner laser delivery tip with its protruded end is centred over the cillary body.

Postoperative Regimen

- At the end of the procedure eye is bandaged which is opened after 6-8 hours.
- Patient is prescribed with oral analgesic and anti-inflammatory agents along with anti-glaucoma medications for the time period the effect of DLCP appears.
- Topically antibiotic and steroids are prescribed for a week four times a day.
- At the follow-up, IOP is taken and gradually anti-glaucoma medications are tapered.

Complications

- Conjunctival burns
- Mild postoperative inflammation
- Atonic pupil
- Severe uveitis
- Loss of vision
- Hyphema and vitreous hemorrhage

Table 1: Treatment parameters for diode laser cyclophotocoagulation

	Noncontact	*Contact*
Energy	1.2 watts	1.5 watts
Duration	990 msec	1.5 seconds
Number	40 spots	25-30 spots
Circumference	360°	360°

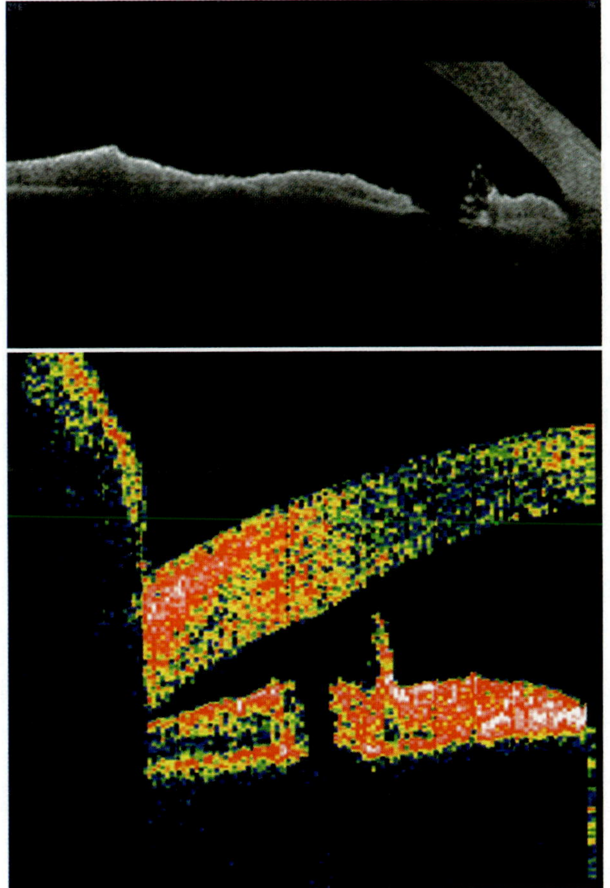

Figs 12 and 13: VISANTE and SL-OCT assessment of patent PI

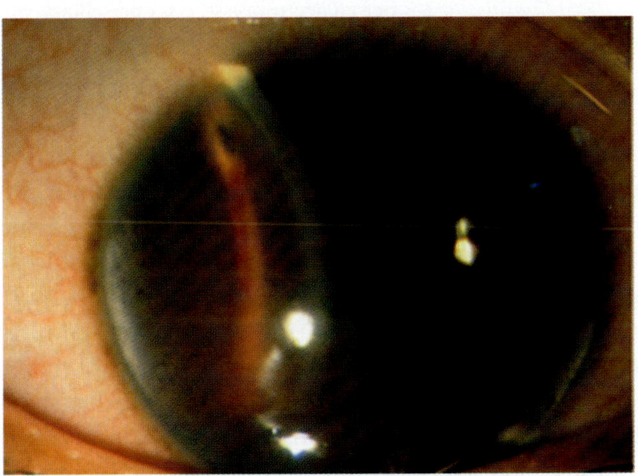

Fig. 14: Hyphema during PI

Endocyclophotocoagulation

ECP is a new technique to directly photocoagulate the ciliary body under endoscopic guidance. The ciliary body can be treated directly within the eye using argon laser light delivered through a 20 gauge fiberoptic probe placed through a pars plana port.

The endolaser probe uses an illumination source, 4, 5 lux video camera, and gives a 70 degree field of view. The optimal focal distance for the laser is 0.75 mm. A cotton-tipped applicator is used to indent the sclera and bring the ciliary processes into view through a dilated pupil. The end of the probe is placed about 3 mm from the ciliary body.

Newer endoscopic systems that incorporate a viewing fiberoptic as well as a laser fiberoptic are available, which permits the ciliary body to be visualized on a television screen. Endoscopic laser endocyclophotocoagulation can be performed at the time of cataract extraction or vitrectomy, for example, in a diabetic patient with neovascular glaucoma and a vitreous hemorrhage.

The two main approaches to reach the ciliary process are via a *limbal nor pars plana entry*. In limbal approach cyclophotocoagulation is done through a temporal and nasal limbal entry for nasal 180° and temporal 180° respectively. In pars plana approach after doing a limited three port anterior vitrectomy ECP probe is introduced through each superior port for opposite ciliary process treatment. The procedure can be done with argon or diode laser.

Table 2: Treatment Parameters for Argon green Laser Cyclophotocoagulation

	Endoscopic (limbal or pars plana)	*Transpupillary (slitlamp based)*
Energy	500-1000 mW	500-1000 mW
Duration	0.1-0.2 sec	0.1-0.2 sec
Number	3-5 per ciliary process	3-5 per ciliary process
Circumference	180-360°	Limited by view
Spot size	Fixed 20 gauge probe	50-200 um

The advantages of endoscopic cyclophotocoagulation include decreased energy requirement, inflammation and collateral tissue damage. While complications such as phthisis, chronic hypotony, and retinal detachment have rarely been reported, most ophthalmologists reserve ECP for cases of refractory glaucoma, in pseudophakic or aphakic patients, given a lack of established treatment parameters and an increased risk for endophthalmitis. Moreover, there is still no uniform agreement on the degree of cycloablation that needs to be performed in each sitting and when the procedure needs to be repeated. Till the time further studies clarify the missing questions it is advisable that 180 to 270 degrees of the ciliary processes should only be ablated in a single sitting.

IOP lowering following endoscopic cyclophotocoagulation takes anytime between 1-4 weeks.

Postoperative Management

These procedures unlike cyclocryotherapy are less painful.

- At the end of the procedure, subconjunctival corticosteroids are usually administered and patching done for approximately 6 hours.
- The patient should be placed on topical cycloplegics, antibiotics and corticosteroids, which are tapered as the inflammation subsides.
- Preoperative antiglaucoma medications glaucoma medications are continued until the effect of the procedure can be determined. The cholinergic drugs are avoided.
- Sometimes very strong analgesic is required and at times one may have to use narcotic analgesics.
- Follow-up at 1 hr, 1 day, 1 week, 1 month and then according to the response.
- Additional therapy should be considered if needed after one month. Interventions include drainage device, trabeculectomy, cyclocryotherapy and Enucleation.

Complications

- Pain
- Mild to severe iritis, synechiae and pupillary block
- Transient rise of IOP
- Hypotony
- Phthisis bulbi
- Conjunctival surface burn
- Lens and zonular damage
- Reduced accommodation
- Posterior capsule fibrosis in pseudophakia
- Pupillary distortion
- Corneal graft failure
- Scleral thinning and staphyloma
- Malignant glaucoma
- Macular edema
- Retinal detachment
- Serous and hemorrhagic choroidal detachment
- Intraocular hemorrhage
- Best corrected vision loss
- Sympathetic ophthalmia
- Endophthalmitis and panophthalmitis

- Treatment failure
- Inadvertent sclerostomy

Cyclodestructive procedures share similar risks, but they vary in degree of risk. The most troubling and common complication of these procedures is a decrease in visual acuity. This can result from a variety of causes, including hypotony, macular edema, and cataract. Due to risk of vision loss makes, cyclodestructive procedures are a last resort in patients with good vision. Less intense laser therapy on a repeated basis rather than a single high dose treatment is suggested to minimize complications of treatment.

LASER PERIPHERAL IRIDOTOMY (LPI)

Introduction

Key Facts

- Introduced in 1956, gained popularity with the advent of argon laser and, more recently, with the neodymium:yttrium-aluminum-garnet (Nd:YAG) laser.
- May be called iridotomy or iridectomy depending on whether a surgeon is opening a hole or destroying and removing iris tissue.
- Has replaced surgical iridectomy which is reserved for patients who cannot cooperate at the slitlamp or for those with severe inflammatory eye conditions that cause repetitive closure of the PI site with fibrin.

Mechanism of Action

Enables free passage of aqueous humor between the posterior and anterior chambers of the eye, which equalizes the pressures in between and lets the peripheral iris rest in a natural position,thus relieving the papillary block.

Indications

- Primary angle closure glaucoma (Pupillary block)
  - Acute angle closure
  - Subacute angle closure
  - Creeping angle closure.
- Fellow eye of patient with angle closure glaucoma
- Non-pupillary block angle closure
  - Plateau iris
  - Forward lens position
- Glaucoma suspect : Narrow and closed angle
  - Combined mechanism glaucoma
  - Reverse pupillary block in pigmentary dispersion syndrome or pigmentary glaucoma

— Nanophthalmos with angle closure
— Secondary glaucomas following cataract surgery, uveitis.

Contraindications

- Absolute
  — Visualization of iris not possible.
- Relative
  — Corneal pathology, corneal edema
  — Flat anterior chamber
  — Angle closure is caused by a non-pupillary block mechanism
  — Synechial angle closure, e.g. neovascularization or iridocorneal endothelial syndrome.

Preoperative Evaluation

- Routine total ophthalmic check-up
- Slit-lamp biomicroscopy: Corneal clarity,AC depth , presence of the crypts , pupil size
- Intraocular pressure (IOP)

Technique

- Informed consent is obtained from patient
- Pilocarpine 2% drops are instilled every 5 minutes times three in the procedure eye.
- A drop of apraclonidine or brimonidine may be given.
- Topical anesthesia is applied (0.5% proparacaine or 4% xylocaine)
- Patient and operator are adequately positioned the Q-Switched Nd-YAG laser. Patient's head may be secured with a head strap
- Abraham contact lens (+55 to +66 D) or Wise lens (+103 D) is applied after filling it with a coupling solution.

Laser Settings

- 3-10 millijoules per shot
- One to three shots per burst.
- Energy applied varies widely depending on the lasers calibration, precision of treatment focus, and thickness of the iris.
- Cone angles ranging from 13°, 15°, 18°. The larger the cone angle lesser the energy delivered per unit cone of cornea traversed and similarly the smaller energy passing on to unwanted structures posterior to iris.

Site

- Superior peripheral iris, usually at 11 o'clock or 1 o'clock
- Covered by the upper eyelid

- A more peripheral site as the anterior lens capsule is not directly adjacent to posterior surface of iris, therefore less chances of damage the lens
- Too peripheral means decreased visibility due to pannus
- Aim the spot in a crypt where the thickness is much less
- Beam is focused on the iris, the slitlamp is pushed forward toward the patient to defocus the beam slightly posteriorly (single spot separates into two or four spots, depending on the laser manufacturer), placing it deeper in the iris, in midstroma.

End Point

- Sudden outflowing of aqueous and pigment from posterior to the anterior chamber
- Sudden deepening of the anterior chamber
- The presence of retroillumination may not be a sure sign of total penetration.
- Visualization of the lens capsule.
- Before the contact lens is removed, patency of the PI is confirmed by disappearance of the aiming beam in the iridectomy and being able to see and focus on the lens capsule in the area of the PI (Figs 20.10 and 20.11).
- The contact lens is then removed, the patient is reassured and asked to wait for 1 hour for an IOP check.

Postoperative Management

- Continue previous anti glaucoma medications along with an additional anti-glaucoma agent for at least one week.
- A steroid antibiotic combination should also be started (in QID dosage) and continued for at least 3 to 4 days.
- Pilocarpine must be continued postlaser for around 10 days in order to keep the iris stretched and keep the iridotomy patent.
- Follow-up is usually in 1 to 2 weeks, at which time the PI patency is evaluated, IOP is rechecked and gonioscopy is performed to evaluate the angle for openness and occludability.
- Gonioscopy and dilation may be reserved for the patient's 6 weeks visit.

Complications

- Corneal epithelial burns
- Corneal endothelial burns
- Pupillary distortion, corectopia
- Iritis, inflammation
- Pigment dispersion, iris atrophy
- Hemorrhage

- Lenticular opacities
- Raised IOP
- Hemorrhage
- Lenticular opacities
- Retinal burns
- Monocular diplopia
- Posterior synechiae
- Malignant glaucoma
- Failure
- Late closure

21

Laser Surgical Treatment of Glaucoma by Excimer Laser with 193 nm Wavelength

KP Takhchidi, Nikolay N Ereskin (Russia)

INTRODUCTION

The initial application of excimer lasers has been oriented to the cornea and to refractive surgery. Today, different types of lasers have been used in the treatment of glaucoma (the Holmium laser, Erbium:YAG laser, Carbon dioxide laser and Excimer lasers).

All authors use well-known «traditional» methods of glaucoma treatment, but apply for this purpose the excimer laser with 193 nm wavelength: external trabeculoectomy, sclerostomy, transscleral sinusotomy, filtering sclerostomy, deep sclerectomy, NPDS, etc.

The argon fluoride excimer laser ablates the tissue with a high precision (1 micron per pulse) and without mechanical or thermal damage to surrounding structures and also has a cytostatic effect.

The current technology does not allow the 193 nm wavelength to transmit through the fiber optics, which limits the endoocular use of this laser.

We designed a special excimer laser unit with 193 nm wavelength for glaucoma surgery in 1999. It is possible to use this device in the standard operating room under the operating microscope. Portable in dimensions it has a special mobile manipulator to deliver the laser energy to the operating field. The laser beam works in «eraser mode» without the necessity of a special mask. The focal distance between the manipulator and the ocular tissues is about several millimeters, the beam area in the focal point is 0.5 × 1 mm .

This study was conducted to find out the effectiveness and longevity of non-penetrating glaucoma surgery (NPDS) with the use of excimer laser with 193 nm wavelength

PATIENTS AND METHODS

In a non-randomized prospective study there were 160 eyes of 154 patients aged from 18 to 88 years, between March 2000 and May 2005. The majority of patients had advanced and far-advanced stages of open-angle and narrow-angle glaucoma. Laser iridotomy was performed in 44 patients with narrow-angle glaucoma to enlarge the profile of the anterior chamber angle. Intraocular

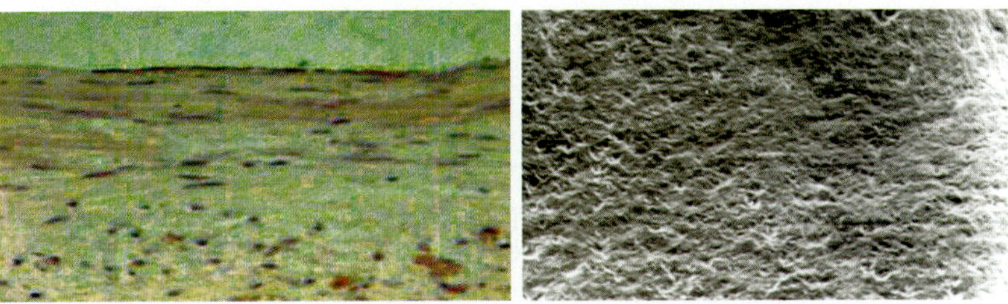

Fig. 1: Light photomicrograph and scanning electron microscopy of the stroma of rabbit cornea after excimer laser

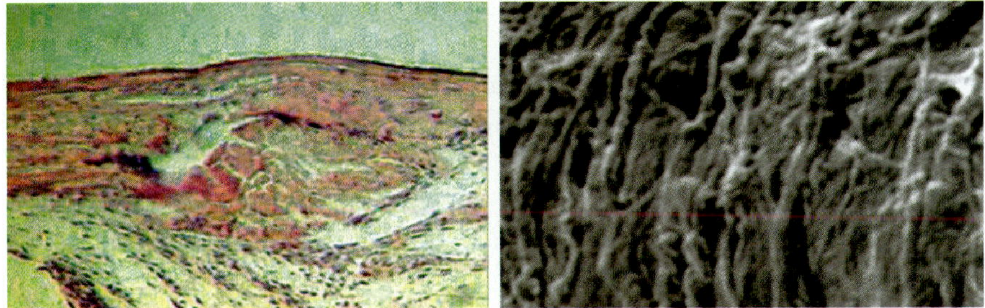

Fig. 2: Light photomicrograph and scanning electron microscopy of rabbit cornea after surgical incision

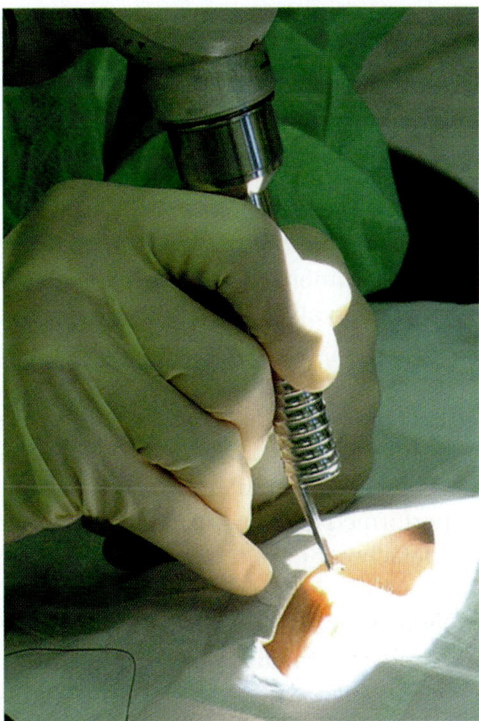

Fig. 3: A special mobile manipulator for a surgeon, that delivers the laser energy to the operating field of the eye

pressure (IOP) was recorded preoperatively and postoperatively at 1, 7, 14 days, at 1, 3, 6 and thereafter every 6 months.

SURGICAL TECHNIQUE

We describe a new technique of non-penetrating glaucoma surgery that uses the excimer laser to reduce the risk of perforation the trabeculo-descemet's membrane. With this technique the ablation is precise and homogeneous. The procedure can be performed with topical anesthesia. Excimer laser surgery consists of:

- Fornix-based conjunctival flap 2.0-2.5 mm in the upper quadrant;
- Minimal episcleral cautery;
- dissection of a superficial corneal groove;
- dissection of a 2.5 × 2.5 mm rectangular in half thickness lamellar scleral flap;
- Excimer laser ablation;
- Closure of scleral flap and conjunctival closure with a running 8.0 silk suture.

The deep layers of sclera were evaporated layer by layer with laser energy of a 150 mJ/cm^2 density until vessels of ciliary body appeared.

Then the Schlemm's canal was covered with a protector, and the deep layers of corneal stroma were removed by laser up to the Descemet's membrane until the moment of the aqueous humor drop appearance (energy density—50 mJ/cm^2).

Postoperative treatment consisted of antibiotics and dexamethasone drops instilled four times a day during 2 weeks.

RESULTS AND DISCUSSION

As a result of intrastromal excimer laser ablation (ISELA) the ophthalmotonus normalization was achieved in all cases independently of disease stages. The IOP averaged 10 ± 2 mmHg in the early postoperative follow-up. There were observed no cases of hemorrhagic or other complications, and the postoperative period was notable for a favorable course. All patients did not note any painful sensations both intra and postoperatively, in this connection this procedure may be transferred to the out-patient category. The B-scanning and ultrasound biomicroscopy were performed thoroughly in patients with hypotonia in order to reveal a choroidal detachment. As the rule, only edema and thickening of choroid by 50-100 µm took place in the first postoperative days that indirectly was evidence of aqueous humor resorption by vessels of ciliary body. The surgical technique supposes a creation of bypass between the Descemet's membrane and vessels of ciliary body which absorbability is 50 times more than in ordinary capillaries.

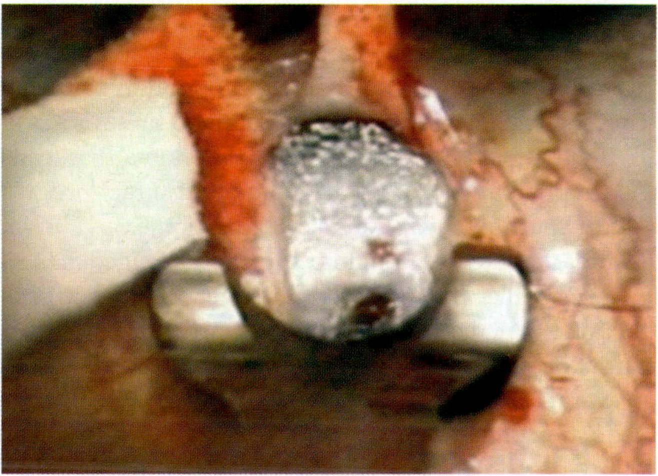

Fig. 4: The deep layers of sclera were evaporated by excimer laser until vessels of ciliary body appeared

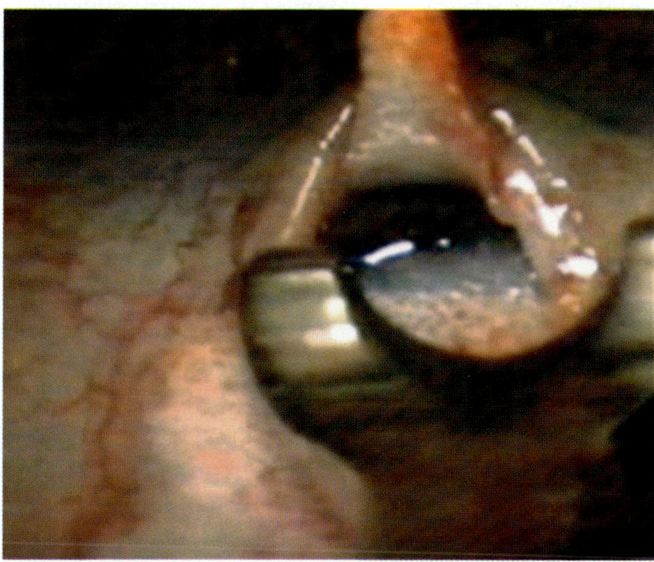

Fig. 5: The deep layers of corneal stroma were removed by excimer laser up to the Descemet's membrane until the moment of the aqueous humor drop appearance

In our opinion the normalization of intraocular pressure after the intrastromal excimer laser ablation is achieved owing to an improvement of uveal scleral outflow of aqueous humor, an elimination of Schlemm's canal collapse and a recovery of its functionally maintained sites. As a result there are no sharp IOP fluctuations in the direction of hypotonia that leads to proper complications (hyphema, choroidal detachment, cataract progression, etc.). Preoperatively the outflow facility index (C) did not exceed 0.04 mm^3/min/mmHg while after the intervention this index (C) averaged 0.32 ± 0.02 mm^3/min/mmHg, i.e. 7-9 times the increase. Moreover a tendency of the aqueous humor production (F) increase is revealed in a part of cases.

In the majority of cases (about 70% of eyes) an improvement of visual acuity is noted on an average by 0.1-0.2 obviously due to a decompression of optic disk fibers and a reduction of peripapillary edema that needs a further study. In the long-term follow-up the outflow facility index (C) decreased slightly, but remained within the norm (mean 0.20 ± 0.04 mm^3/min/mmHg) that provided a compensation of ophthalmotonus on a level of 17.0 ± 2.5 mm Hg.

In the long-term follow-up in patients with initial and advanced stages of glaucoma the IOP was compensated in all cases. In the group of patients with the far-advanced stage of disease the YAG laser descemeto-goniopuncture (DGP) in the intervention area was required within periods from 4 to 6 months in 16 eyes (10% of cases). It allowed to restore aqueous humor outflow pathways and to normalize the IOP.

Within the follow-up of 1 year and more a development of cystic filtering bleb was observed in 2 eyes. A monotherapy with the 0.5% Betoptic solution instillation one or two times was administered in 12 patients with far-advanced glaucoma.

CONCLUSION

Thus, the creation of a domestic specialized excimer laser unit with 193 nm wavelength allowed to develop practically a new safe technology of glaucoma surgery that cannot be performed using traditional knife surgery.

Small dimensions (portability), presence of manipulator for a surgeon, price of the unit differentiate it advantageously from other foreign excimer laser and also allow to adapt it in conditions of an ordinary operating room.

A new technology of glaucoma surgery (ISELA) is developed that allows to restore natural aqueous humor outflow pathways without a destruction of the Schlemm's canal, to return the greater part of aqueous humor to vessels of ciliary body. The procedure is especially efficient and safe in patients with initial and advanced stages of disease because allows to normalize ophthalmotonus and to maintain visual functions.

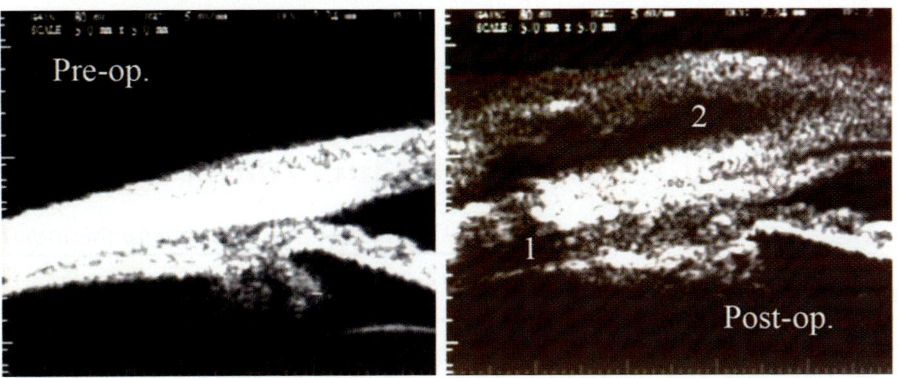

Fig. 6: Basic outflow pathways of aqueous humor in ultrasound biomicroscopy: 1- into the intrascleral space and vessels of ciliary body; 2 - into the flat filtering bleb

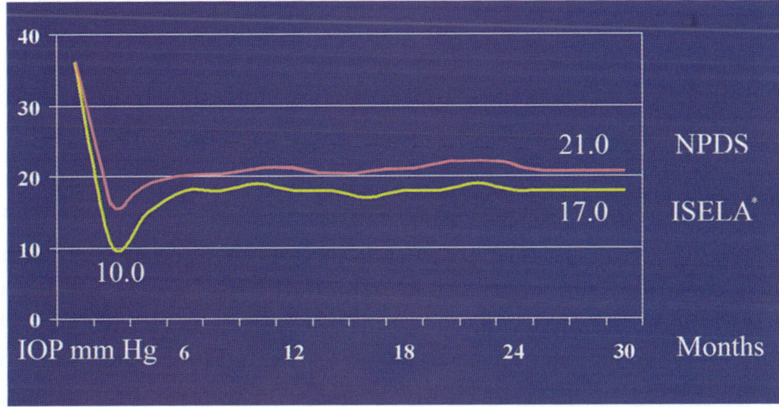

Fig. 7: IOP data after excimer laser treatment (ISELA) and NPDS

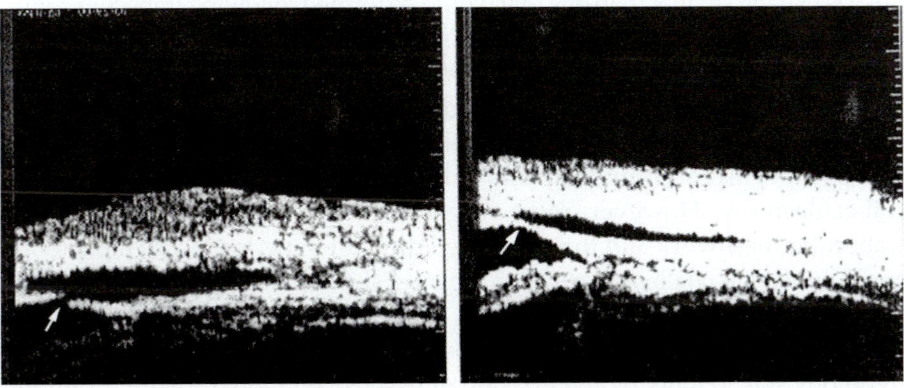

Fig. 8: The ultrasound biomicroscopy before and after the YAG-laser DGP (descemeto-goniopuncture) to create a microperforation in Descemet's membrane behind Schwalbe's line to improve filtration

22

Solid-state UV Laser for Minimally Invasive Glaucoma Surgery

JT Lin (Taiwan), Vivek Kadambi (India)

INTRODUCTION

The aim of surgical management of open-angle glaucoma is to create an alternate channel for drainage of aqueous humor from the anterior chamber of the eye by surgical techniques collectively called "filtration microsurgery", or to open previously blocked trabecular meshwork with the help of lasers. Various lasers have been used for photoablative filtration surgery including ArF laser (at 193 nm), XeCL laser (at 308 nm) and Er:YAG laser (at 2.94 μm). Conventional trabeculoplasty uses lasers such as argon laser (at 514/488 nm) and Nd:YAG (at 1064 nm). In this chapter, we introduce a UV solid-state laser (at 266 nm) for non-penetrating deep sclerectomy.

NPDS: AN EVOLUTIONARY TECHNIQUE

The ideal glaucoma surgery is that which can create adequate drainage to enable a controlled reduction of IOP without the risk of over-filtration while ensuring long-term patency of the filtration channel. Hence we believe that the model around which all glaucoma surgeries should be conceptualized is the non-penetrating deep sclerectomy (NPDS) or viscocanalostomy. In this procedure the intraocular pressure is lowered as fluid oozes through a permeable thin layer of tissue, the trabeculo-Descemet's membrane. A bleb may be formed, but it is usually smaller than one that would be formed following trabeculectomy. The main advantage of this procedure is that it minimizes the chances of over-filtration. This avoids the complications of filtration blebs and the shallow anterior chamber seen after trabeculectomy.

NPDS is fast gaining popularity among surgeons due to decreased incidence of postoperative complications when compared with conventional trabeculectomy. However, most surgeons find accurate dissection of the trabecular meshwork and the scleral bed difficult to perform. The meticulous tissue excision is challenging even to the most skillful and experienced surgeon. Additionally, it is commonly reported by surgeons, that once aqueous percolation starts to occur during the course of tissue dissection, a significant amount of hypotony sets in, making the excision of tissue even more difficult. From the variable reports of clinical success, it is clear that this technique has a long learning curve. Nevertheless, the potential opportunity to create a filtration

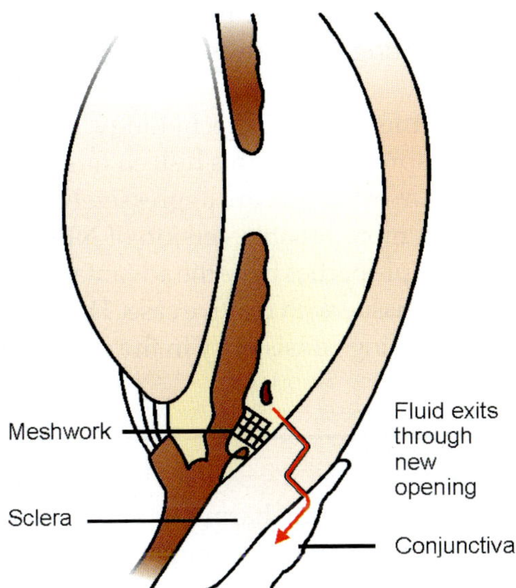

Fig. 1: Aqueous drainage through sclerostomy and then via subconjunctival route in NPDS

procedure, which successfully controls intraocular pressure in the absence of a prominent bleb, is prompting innovators to improve upon the technique of NPDS.

Accelerated advancement in laser technology in the late 90's has been responsible for the widespread use of this hi-tech modality in ophthalmology and it's no surprise that investigators are aggressively exploring the potential of lasers to help evolve a more reliable version of NPDS. Technically, Lasers with predominant *ablative* properties have the advantage of helping the surgeon remove precise amount of tissue with relative ease. This appears to be the critical factor responsible for ensuring consistency in the surgical technique.

UV-270

The UV-270 pulsed laser uses as it's source, the Nd:YAG laser crystal and nonlinear crystals to generate the 4th harmonic at a UV wavelength of 266 nm. It is very efficient in ablating tissues with high protein content such as cornea and sclera. The laser is delivered through a specifically designed articulated arm coupled to a handpiece, which delivers the UV laser energy via a focusing lens. The 3 nanosecond short-pulsed laser is focused to a spot size of about 0.6 mm on the treated area with energy per pulse of 5 to 7 mJ and operates at 10 to 20 Hz. Both, the pulse energy and frequency are adjustable. We note that this 3 ns pulse width is much shorter than the typical excimer laser (about 10 to 20 ns), Ho:YAG laser (about 200 microsecond) or Er:YAG (about 300 microsecond). Therefore it offers minimal thermal damage with effective tissue ablation. Furthermore, the focused UV laser spot may be as small as 0.3 mm if needed, an attribute, which is not available with IR lasers. Being *non-contact* in its operation the laser overcomes many disadvantages of the *contact fiber-based* lasers:

1. In the non-contact ablative systems, one does not encounter progressive decrease in the efficiency of ablation due to accumulation of coagulum at the end of the fiber tip.
2. There is no damage to the tips, which, in the fiber-based system, adds significantly to running cost.
3. Non-contact systems ensure better asepsis.

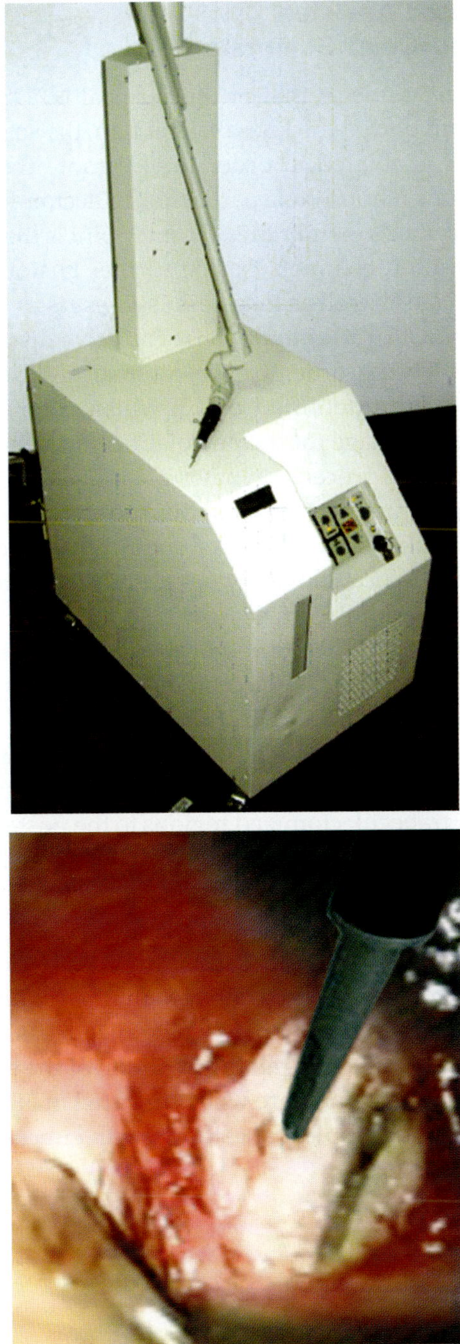

Figs 2A and B: UV-270 (A) UV-270 laser with the "articulated arm" delivery system (B) Handpiece of UV-270 demonstrating scleral ablation

Customized Laser Assisted Non-penetrating Deep Sclerostomy

The initial steps are same as that of the surgical NPDS procedure. After an initial 5 mm × 5 mm partial thickness scleral flap, the scleral bed overlying the canal of Schlemm is ablated in order to "De-roof" the canal. This ablative excision is carried on anteriorly as a partial trabeculectomy and further anteriorly to expose the Descemet's membrane. The endpoint is the visible percolation of aqueous. The filtration channels can be further customized to increase the efficiency of drainage as well as long-term success is as follows:

a. *Choroidal exposure:* An additional step of ablative dissection in the posterior part of the scleral bed in order to expose a small area of about 1 mm diameter of choroidal tissue (identified by brownish color) provides additional suprachoroidal drainage for the percolating aqueous humor.
b. *Collagen inserts:* The procedure may be combined with collagen implants sutured to the bed under the partial thickness scleral flap.
c. *Use of sodium hyaluronate:* A lake of sodium hyaluronate may be placed under the flap. Viscocanalostomy using sodium hyaluronate may also be for carried out for additive effect.
d. *Use of antimetabolites:* Judicious use of sponge soaked in 5-FU or Mitomycin placed over the scleral bed is advocated in select cases or at the discretion of the operating surgeon.
e. *Modified scleral bed ablation:* In order to facilitate the drainage of the percolated aqueous under the flap, the surgeon can conveniently create ablative grooves connecting the trabeculectomized regions to the posterior parts. Creation of such multiple drainage channels will also decrease the chances of closure of the drainage channel and the grooves will facilitate fixation of the collagen implant.

From the above description it can be appreciated that the surgeon can customize the type of ablative excisions to suit the requirement of individual cases. Hence we propose the name "Customized Laser Assisted Filtration Surgery" (CLAFS) to encompass all the variation of the procedures described. The multiple filtration channels are well illustrated in Figure 4. The procedure can be carried out under topical anesthesia with subconjunctival infiltration over the surgical site.

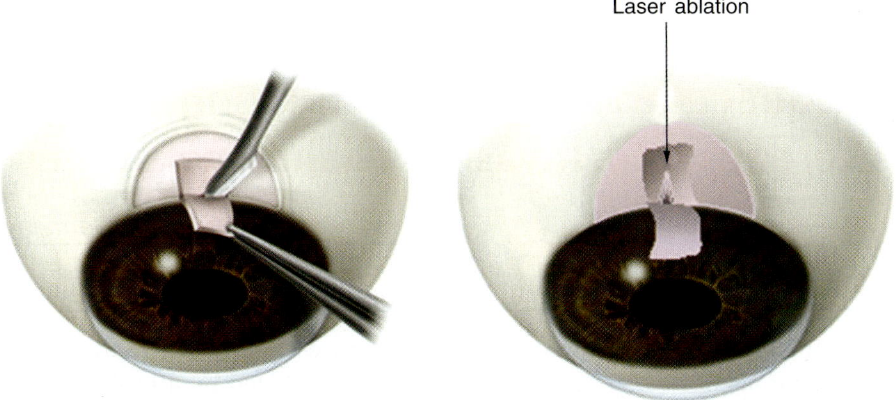

Figs 3A and B: CLAFS (A) Partial thickness scleral flap (B) laser ablation of scleral bed, trabecular meshwork and Descemet's membrane

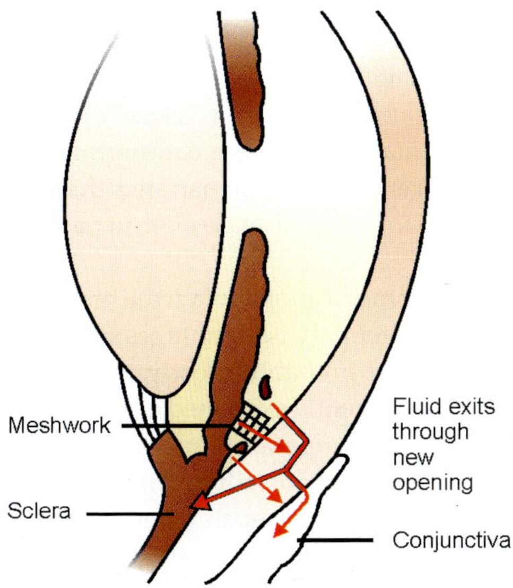

Fig. 4: CLAFS—Aqueous drainage through trabeculo-Descemet's membrane and then via subconjunctival as well as through suprachoroidal spaces

23

Trabecular Meshwork Ablation as an Alternative to Invasive Glaucoma Surgery

Mona Pache, Jens Funk (Germany)

INTRODUCTION

Open angle glaucoma is the second leading cause of blindness in the world. Glaucomatous optic neuropathy (GON) is characterized by a loss of retinal ganglion cells and their axons, associated by a tissue remodeling both of the optic nerve head (ONH) and the retina leading to the characteristic ONH cupping. Many glaucoma patients present with elevated intraocular pressure (IOP), most often caused by reduced outflow capacity of aqueous humor. The outflow resistance is localized at the level of the trabecular meshwork, or more precisely, at the juxtacanalicular meshwork and the inner wall of Schlemm's canal.

Data from several major studies available on this topic, such as the OHTS, EGPS, CIGTS, EMGT and the AGIS suggest that both development and progression of glaucomatous damage can be mitigated by lowering IOP. Moreover, the NTGS has clearly demonstrated that lowering of the IOP can slow down the progression of the disease even in patients with normal-tension glaucoma (NTG).

Topical IOP-lowering medication is often the first-line therapy for glaucoma, even though it harbors potential disadvantages such as local and systemic side effects, tachyphylaxis, and probably most important compliance problems. Friedman and co-workers recently examined a cohort of 1712 glaucoma suspects and 3623 diagnosed glaucoma patients and found that a large proportion of individuals requiring treatment are falling out of care and are being monitored at rates lower than expected from recommendations of published guidelines because they do not come for follow-up visits and do not ask for a refill of their prescribed glaucoma medication. Apart from this disappointing information, it has to be added that local medication is also not always sufficient if a very low individual target IOP is required. The CNTGS has shown that a 30% reduction in IOP is often only reached by surgical intervention. Another point is that the costs of medical control over a lifetime might also be prohibitive for some glaucoma patients.

Glaucoma surgery includes nowadays a number of potential therapies all aiming either to increase the outflow of aqueous humor or to decrease its production. Argon laser trabeculoplasty (ALT), for example, increases the

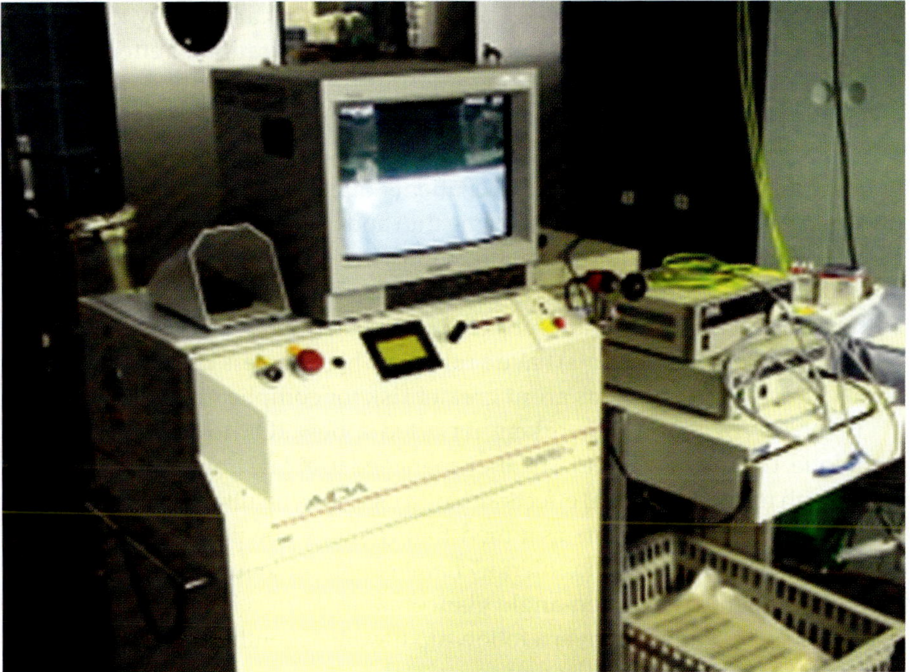

Fig. 1: The AIDA excimer laser (TuiLaser AG, Germering, Germany)

conventional outflow through the trabecular meshwork and is easy to perform. The procedure has however a limited efficacy and duration of effect, as ALT produces thermal effects with coagulation of the trabecular meshwork. A successfully performed trabeculectomy shows a much better efficacy, however a number of potential complications such as hypotony, suprachoroidal hemorrhage, and bleb failure exist. Patients often find the conjunctival bleb uncomfortable, moreover it can become thin and avascular, thus increasing the risk of bleb leaks, blebitis and endophthalmitis. In case of surgery failure, repeated operations can become necessary, however the chances for success decrease as both sclera and conjunctiva are subjected to repeated surgical insults. Glaucoma drainage devices (tube shunts) have a relatively high success rate in experienced hands, however the patients are at greater risk for complications.

In 1996, Vogel and co-workers reported a new IOP-lowering operation technique. Using an excimer laser, they managed to ablate trabecular meshwork tissue with minimal thermal effects and necrosis, thus resulting in only minimal scar formation. The authors assumed that it should be possible to create an open connection between the anterior chamber and Schlemm's canal. The group treated 6 patients with open-angle glaucoma. In 4 cases intraocular pressure was reduced by 11 mmHg over a follow-up time of 5 months. In 2 cases IOP rose by 2 mm Hg in spite of medication.

ERBIUM-YAG GONIOTOMY

Also in 1996, an endoscopic erbium-YAG laser system allowing effects on trabecular tissue comparable to those produced by a 308 nm excimer laser became available. In the following years, we could demonstrate a reduction in IOP with this laser system that was comparable to the excimer laser. We performed combined cataract surgery and erbium-YAG goniotomy in 24 eyes and compared the IOP results to a control group that underwent cataract surgery. In the combined surgery group, mean IOP dropped from 21.8 to 15.5 mmHg. IOP regulation was successful in 88% of these cases. In eyes that underwent only cataract surgery, the IOP reduction was less pronounced (mean IOP preoperative 20.0, postoperative 17.4, success rate 35%). The follow-up in this preliminary study was 4 months (mean 6.5 months, max. 12 months).

In another non-randominized clinical trial with a 3-year follow-up, we treated 20 eyes of 20 patients suffering from both glaucoma and cataract with combined phacoemulsification and erbium-YAG goniotomy and compared them to a control group that underwent cataract surgery. Main outcome variables were IOP, visual acuity, and number of antiglaucomatous drugs 1 year after surgery. The mean IOP dropped by 30% (23.5 to 16.3 mmHg) after 12 months in the laser-treated group and by 9% (19.8 to 18.1 mmHg) in the control group. After 3 years, the mean IOP in the laser group was 15.0 mmHg. The mean

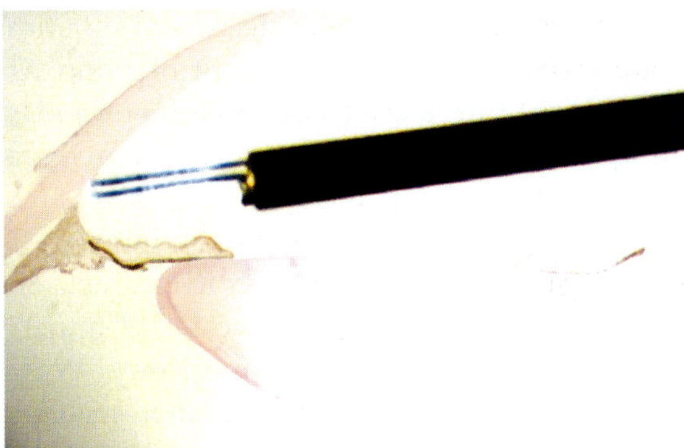

Fig. 2: Photomontage of the fiberoptic system contacting the opposite trabecular meshwork

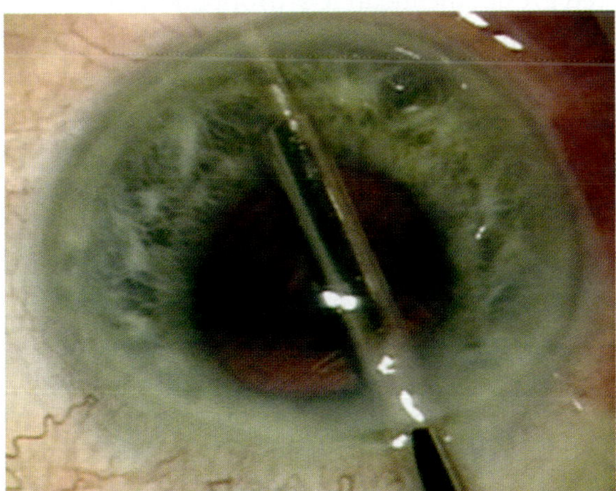

Fig. 3: Operative setting: the ELT probe has been inserted via a clear cornea incision and approaches the opposite trabecular meshwork

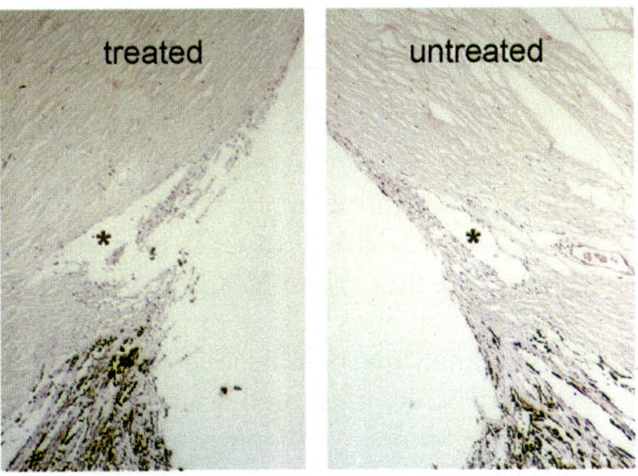

Fig. 4: Histology demonstrated that the wavelength of the AIDA laser ablates the trabecular meshwork without inducing thermal damage, thereby minimizing fibrous tissue healing reactions

number of antiglaucomatous drugs needed decreased significantly from 1.6 to 0.5 in the laser group and from 1.0 to 0.8 in the control group. Anterior chamber hemorrhage occurred in 12 eyes after laser treatment and resolved within 72 hours in all but 1 patient who was on warfarin sodium therapy. There were no cases of hypotony in either group.

We also aimed to compare the efficacy of erbium-YAG goniotomy to trabeculectomy, with both methods as adjuncts to cataract surgery. Fifty-nine eyes of 59 glaucoma patients with coexistent cataract underwent combined phacoemulsification and erbium-YAG goniotomy. We compared this prospective treatment arm to a retrospective inclusion-matched control group treated by trabeculectomy and cataract surgery in a single procedure. Primary endpoints were IOP, number of antiglaucomatous drugs, postoperative complications, hospitalization time and visual acuity 1 year after surgery. In the laser-treated group, the mean IOP dropped by 30% from 23.4 mmHg to 16.3 mmHg after 12 months. Without reoperation, treatment was successful in 71% of these eyes. In the control group, the IOP decreased by 33.5% from 22.7 to 15.1 mmHg. The success rate without reoperation was 46%. The number of antiglaucomatous drugs needed decreased from 1.48 to 0.48 in the laser-treated group and from 2.0 to 0.39 in the controls. Postoperative complications were more frequent in the control group, and postoperative visual acuity was as well. Hospitalization time was shorter in the laser group. It can be concluded from these data that the IOP-lowering effect of combined erbium-YAG goniotomy and cataract surgery is comparable to that of combined trabeculectomy and cataract surgery. Moreover, due to fewer postoperative complications, erbium-YAG goniotomy seems to be superior to standard fistulation surgery as the primary approach. To date, 3 years follow-up data of a small pilot group that underwent combined erbium-YAG goniotomy and cataract surgery are available; and the IOP-lowering effect has not diminished over this follow-up period.

EXCIMER LASER TRABECULOTOMY (ELT)

Background

In the meantime, the CE-certified AIDA excimer laser (TuiLaser AG, Germering, Germany) has become commercially availabl. We therefore switched from the erbium-YAG system prototype to the certified laser, assuming that it should have a comparable effect. Like the erbium-YAG laser, the AIDA excimer laser reestablishes the outflow of aqueous humor through conventional drainage pathways. By excising a defined area of trabecular meshwork, juxtacanalicular tissue, and the inner wall of Schlemm's canal via a fiberoptic probe delivering 308 nm XeCL excimer laser energy, aqueous outflow is reestablished. The creation of the openings through the trabecular meshwork and the inner wall of

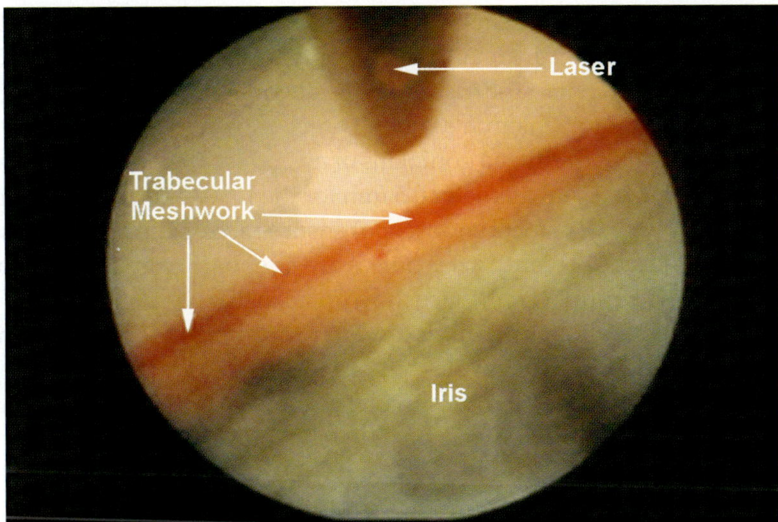

Fig. 5: ELT: Endoscopic view showing the fiberoptic delivery approaching the trabecular meshwork

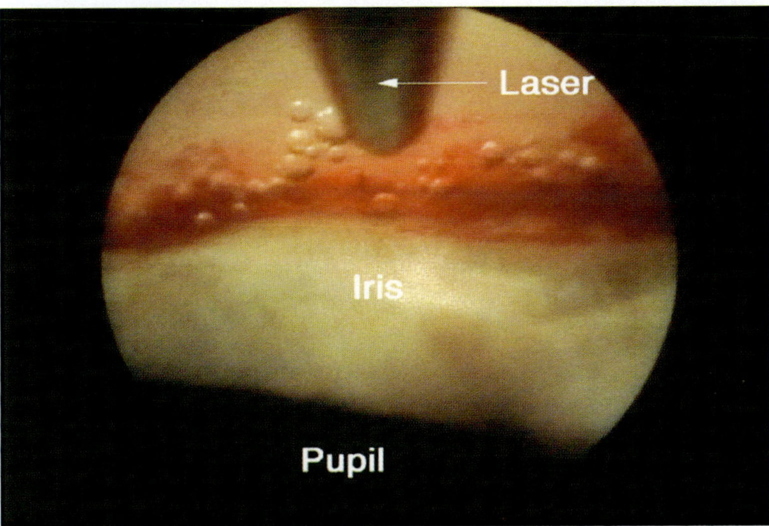

Fig. 6: ELT: Two trabeculotomies are already created. Note the retrograde bleeding from Schlemm's canal which we take as a sign of successful perforation

Schlemm's canal is accomplished by using the fiberoptic delivery system LAGO 200 or LAGO 200 ENDO. In detail, the fiberoptic system is positioned across the anterior chamber to contact the trabecular meshwork. Laser pulses remove tissue to create a fistula into Schlemm's canal. Direct viewing for positioning of the fiber is performed with either a goniolens or an endoscope. The small size of the delivery system (external diameter 0.5 mm for the LAGO 200, 1.3 x 0.95 mm for the LAGO 200 ENDO, coaxial endoscope) ensures access through a self sealing clear cornea incision. Twenty laser pulses are adequate to create a permanent opening into Schlemm's canal. Once the corneal incision is prepared, the actual procedure requires about three minutes. The procedure can easily be combined with cataract surgery. The wavelength of the AIDA laser - 308 nm - has been found to ablate the trabecular meshwork without inducing thermal damage, thereby minimizing fibrous tissue healing reactions.

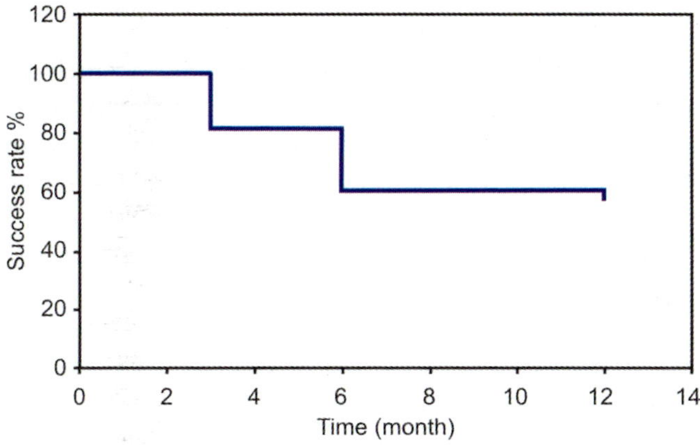

Fig. 7: ELT: Kaplan-Meier survival curve, preoperative IOP > 22 mmHg

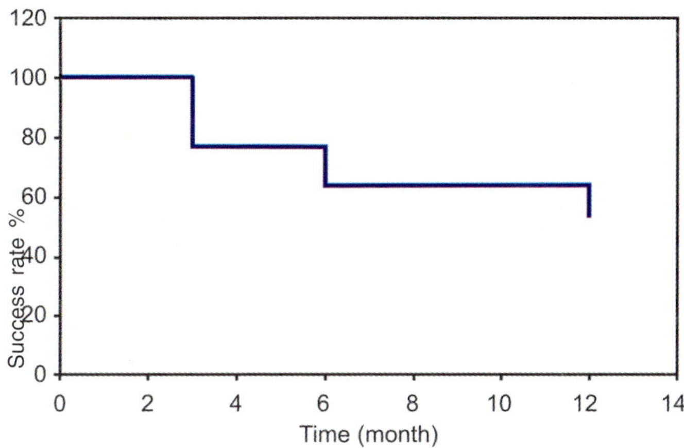

Fig. 8: ELT: Kaplan-Meier survival curve, preoperative IOP ≤ 22 mmHg

Surgical Procedure

ELT can easily be performed through a clear cornea tunnel incision as used for cataract surgery. We constrict the pupil with topical pilocarpine 2% or intracameral injection of acetyline chloride (i.e. Miochol®), then inject a viscoelastic gel (i.e. Healon) into the anterior chamber and insert the laser probe. We then advance the probe to the opposing chamber angle under gonioscopic or endoscopic visualization. The application of the laser pulses can be controlled when the probe tip is in contact with the trabecular meshwork. The probe tip is then repositioned such that ten trabecular meshwork perforations are created to the inferior 180°. Following removal of the probe (and endoscope), the viscoelastic is exchanged by BSS. Postoperatively, all eyes are treated with topical steroids 4x/d tapered over 3 weeks. In case of a persistent fibrin reaction, atropine 1% eye drops 2x/d can be added. In case of combined cataract + ELT procedure, we first perform cataract surgery followed by the ELT procedure, which takes about three minutes longer than cataract surgery alone.

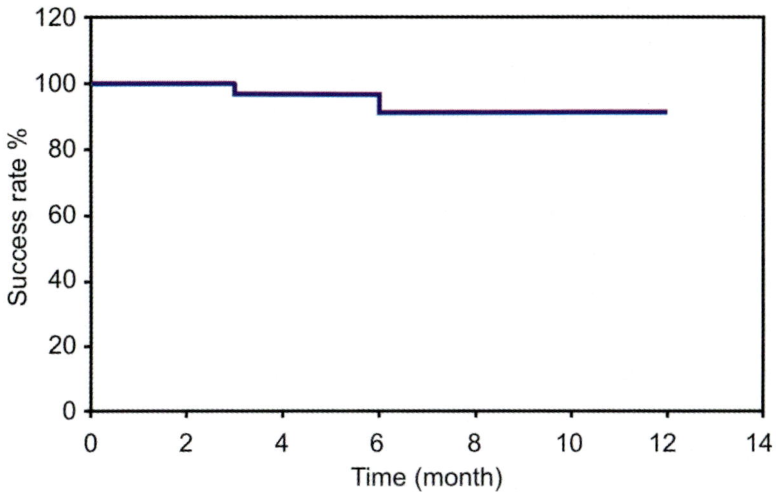

Fig. 9: ELT+Phako: Kaplan-Meier survival curve, preoperative > 22 mmHg

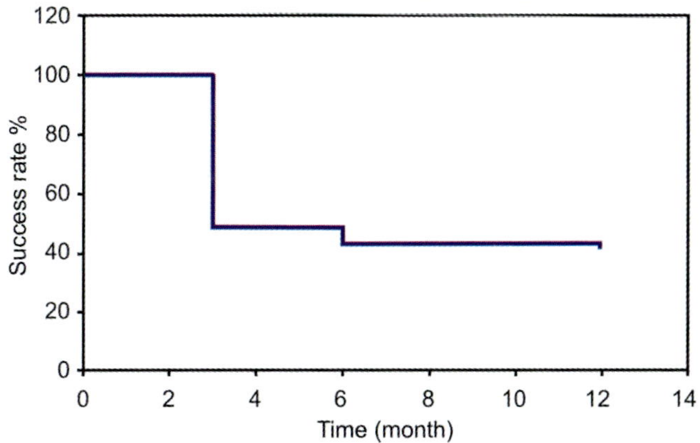

Fig. 10: ELT+Phako: Kaplan-Meier survival curve, preoperative ≤ 22 mmHg

STUDY RESULTS

Pooled data from a number of study groups have demonstrated that ELT is a safe and sufficient IOP-lowering procedure that can easily be combined with cataract surgery.

In our own clinic, we have retrospectively studied a group of 135 patients with open-angle glaucoma (n = 128) and ocular hypertension (n = 7) that were divided into two groups:

a. ELT as a stand-alone procedure (n = 75),
b. Combined cataract and ELT procedure (n = 60).

Both groups were further divided into 2 subgroups.

1. Preoperative IOP > 22 mm Hg,
2. Preoperative IOP ≤ 22 mm Hg.

Kaplan-Meier survival curves were calculated. Success criterion was 20% decrease of IOP in combinaton with IOP ≤ 21 mmHg and postoperative IOP-lowering medication ≤ preoperative IOP-lowering medication. Follow-up time was 1 year. For group

a. ELT,
   1. Preoperative IOP > 22 mm Hg,
   2. Preoperative IOP ≤ 22 mm Hg: Kaplan-Meier survival curves showed a success rate of 57% in subgroup 1 and of 41% in subgroup 2 For group
b. Combined cataract and ELT procedure
   1. Preoperative IOP > 22 mm Hg,
   2. Preoperative IOP ≤ 22 mm Hg: Success rate was 91% in subgroup 1 and 52% in subgroup 2.

Side effects of the ELT were rare

In two cases, an iris adhesion at the tunnel occurred, in 3 cases there was a fibroid reaction that responded very well to topical steroids. One patient developed an occlusion of the central retinal vein 5 month after surgery. IOP however was well-controlled at that time, indicating that there was no connection between the CRVO and the ELT procedure.

Our data indicate that ELT is not only a safe and efficient IOP-lowering procedure, but also that it is most effective in patients with a high preoperative IOP. The 2-year-follow-up data are now available for many patients, and it seems obvious that the IOP-lowering effect of ELT is conserved also after this longer period of time. We have a prospective multi-center study ongoing in this field and are looking forward to its result.

Due to its sufficient IOP-lowering effect and the minimal invasiveness of the procedure, ELT has become the therapy of choice for patients who suffer from cataract and glaucoma. We recommend the combined procedure in all cataract patients with an IOP of more than 22 mmHg without therapy. ELT as a stand-alone procedure is performed in patients whose IOP is above 22 mmHg despite maximally tolerated therapy. In patients with low preoperative IOP, such as patients with normal-tension glaucoma, ELT has proven to be less powerful. We assume that in such cases, the episcleral venous pressure limits the chances of success and prefer a trabeculectomy instead.

CONCLUSION

Excimer-Laser-Trabeculotomy is a promising IOP-lowering technique both as a stand-alone procedure and in combination with cataract surgery. It is especially suitable for patients with high preoperative IOP levels and can easily be combined with cataract surgery.

24

Non-penetrating Filtration Surgery with the CO_2 Laser

Ehud I Assia (Israel)

INTRODUCTION

Increased intraocular pressure (IOP) accompanied by evidence of damage to the optic nerve requires a life-long treatment to maintain the pressure at acceptable levels. The new generations and combinations of medical therapy are indeed highly effective, however they all require continuous instillation, at least once a day and often more, of eyedrops. Local side effects are significant and compliance is, therefore, a major problem in glaucoma medical therapy. Studies have shown that glaucoma surgery, namely trabeculectomy, is at least as effective as medications, and obviously does not require patients' compliance. However, surgery may be associated with numerous complications such as hypotony, shallow anterior chamber, endophthalmitis, leaking blebs and many others. Successful procedures are associated with a 3-fold increase in cataract formation, as this may occur in any penetrating ocular procedure.

Non-penetrating filtration surgery (NPFS) is, therefore, a very appealing option. Since the anterior chamber is not penetrated, the procedure is actually an extraocular operation. A success rate similar to conventional trabeculectomy without the complications of intraocular surgery seems to offer as an ideal solution. However, dissection of the scleral wall to over 95% of its depth until fluids effectively percolates, without penetration into the eye, requires very high skills and a long learning curve. Only a few highly experienced surgeons adopted this technique, which in spite of its obvious advantages did not gain a wide popularity. Also, several studies reported clinical results somewhat below the pressure reduction achieved by conventional trabeculectomy. Many modifications, such as placing spacers under the scleral flap, YAG laser goniopuncture and antimetabolites applications improved the efficacy of the procedure, however, not yet to the level of a wide acceptance. Attempts to apply laser technology to NPFS were previously reported, including excimer, holmium, and erbium:YAG lasers, however none was practically accepted.

In the last years we looked for surgical techniques that would make NPFS both a simple procedure, suitable for any anterior segment surgeon, as well as clinically effective. Utilizing some of the unique features of the CO_2 laser seemed theoretically optimal for this goal.

The CO_2 laser is very effective in ablating dry tissues, and is therefore widely used in general and plastic surgery. However, the far-infrared radiation of this

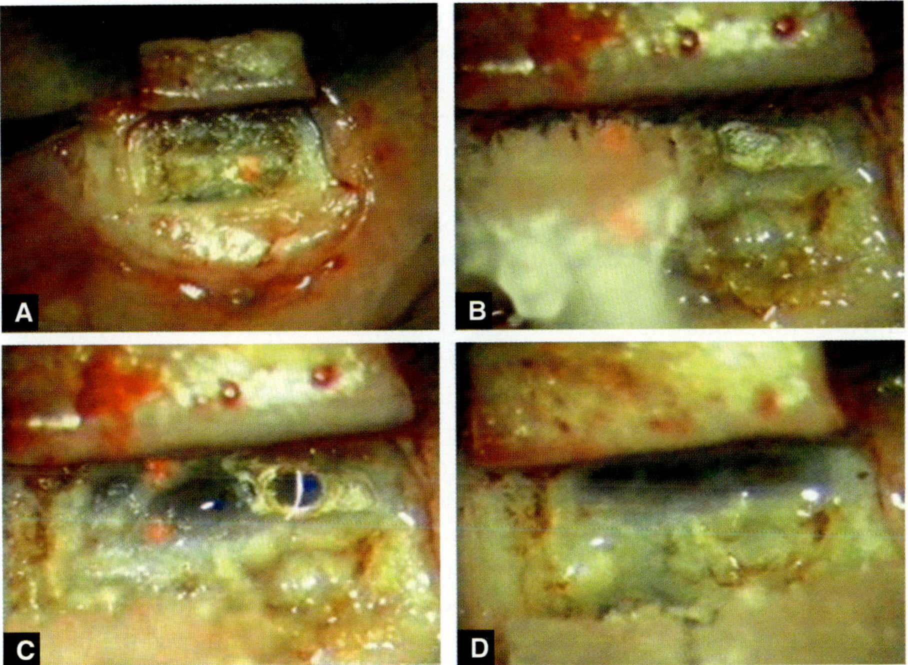

Figs 1A to D: Surgical procedure in a clinical case: (A) Before ablation – the red dots of the aiming beam indicate the scanned area, (B) The area over the trabecular meshwork/ Schlemm's canal on the upper right corner is partially ablated; however no fluid percolation is yet evident. The wetted sponge (on the left) protects the remaining tissue from the laser energy, (C) Aqueous fluid is seen emerging from the ablated zone on the right and center. The left side is still untreated, (D) Effective aqueous percolation is seen over the entire treated area. No perforation into the anterior chamber

laser is absorbed in water within a very short penetration depth and is thus ineffective when applied over wet tissues. We speculated that application of laser energy on the dried scleral tissue, over the trabecular meshwork, would cause a localized ablation of the sclera until fluid starts percolating through the thinned wall. When the aqueous wets the ablated area further laser applications would be ineffective, and would not cause any further tissue ablation (i.e. perforation). Thus, tissue ablation would cease "automatically" when the desired endpoint of the procedure is achieved, i.e. aqueous percolation without perforation into the anterior chamber. The surgical procedure is quite simple and does not require any specific skills other than creation of a scleral flap. Use of a scanning device may further assist surgery by predetermining and accurately controlling the shape of the ablated tissue block and the energy distribution.

The CO_2 laser that we used in our initial studies was the Kaplan PenduLaser 115® CO_2 laser system (Optomedic Medical Technologies Ltd., Or Yehuda, Israel). This is the smallest and the most portable and compact CO_2 laser in the market and it transmits a beam of 5-15 W through an articulated arm. A scanner was attached to the CO_2 laser to enable the surgeon to delimit the area to be treated and to provide even and regular distribution of the laser energy over this area. The laser probe was attached to the surgical microscope, thus maintaining the probe at a predetermined fixed distance from the ablated tissue when the microscope was in focus. In practice, tissue ablation is done while the surgeon is looking through the microscope, accurately targeting the scanner marks with the proper pattern and dimensions over the desired treatment location.

PRECLINICAL STUDIES

Initial studies were done on enucleated cow and sheep eyes at the Laboratory for Intraocular Microsurgery and Implants, Goldschleger Eye Research Institute, Sheba Medical Center, Israel, and at the Laboratory for Intraocular Microsurgery and Implants, Meir Medical Center, Kfar-Saba, Israel. The intraocular pressure was maintained at a constant predetermined pressure of 38 mm Hg by using anterior chamber maintainer (ACM) with the bottle placed at 50 cm above the tested eye. Following dissection of a scleral flap the tissue underneath was laser ablated until fluid was seen percolating in the treated area without evidence of penetration. These studies proved the validity and feasibility of the concept and help determine the laser parameters for clinical use.

The second set of experiments was done on rabbit eyes. Rabbits are known to be very reactive to any surgical procedure and even full thickness trabeculectomy is often closed and ineffective within days after surgery. Nevertheless, in order to investigate the pure effect of the laser treatment we did not use any tissue spacers, viscoelastic substances or antimetabolites to enhance and prolong the surgical effect. The IOP was measured by pneumotonometry and compared to the fellow, untreated eye. In one case perforation into the anterior chamber was accompanied by iris prolapse. In the rest of the cases the

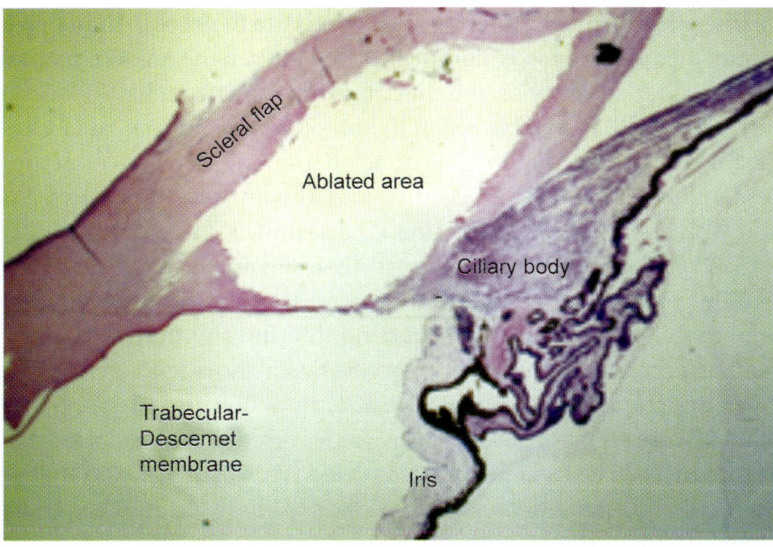

Fig. 2: Histopathology of a human cadaver eye after CO_2 laser ablation. The ablated area creates a "filtration pool". The trabecular-Descemet's "membrane" is only a few microns thick, but it is still intact. Note that in spite of the extensive tissue ablation, no damage is evident in the adjacent corneoscleral and uveal tissues

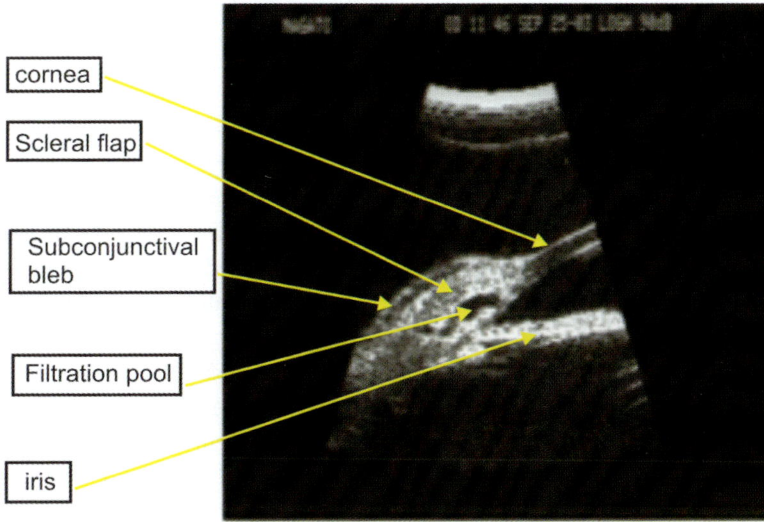

Fig. 3: Ultrasonic biomicroscopy of a clinical case. The filtration "pool" is open, even though no spacers were used. A thin active subconjunctival bleb is seen above the scleral flap. Compare with the histology on Figure 2

IOP decreased immediately after the laser surgery (a mean of 10 mmHg on day 1). The intraocular pressure was significantly lower than the fellow eye for the first 3 weeks. It should be emphasized that these rabbits did not have glaucoma and the pressure eventually stabilized at the preoperative normal levels.

The third set of experiment was done on human cadaver eyes at the Center for Research on Ocular Therapeutics and Biodevices, Storm Eye Institute, Medical University of South Carolina, Charleston, SC, USA (Director: David J. Apple, MD). A 4 × 5 mm scleral flap was dissected and laser pulses of moderate power (10 W) were applied over the exposed scleral wall. Since it was evident from the rabbit study that tissue charring interferes with the laser effect, the charred tissue was removed after every 5-7 laser shots with a wetted sponge. Upon approaching the trabecular tissue, or when the first signs of fluid percolation were seen, the laser power was lowered to 5 W and the application rate was reduced. The treated zone was dried with a sponge, and the next shot was applied only after a delay of 2-3 seconds to allow localized wetting by the percolating fluid. This way only the dry area was further ablated, whereas over the wetted area, where more ablation was not required, the laser energy was absorbed by the percolating fluid. If the treated area seemed to be too small, laser dissection of the tissue was extended laterally to a desired width until satisfactory aqueous percolation was achieved. Histopathological studies confirmed the deep ablation down to the trabecular meshwork and Descemet's membrane, leaving a micro-thin wall 30-50 μ thick, with no perforation. The neighboring structures, including the sclera, cornea, iris base, and ciliary body, were not affected and remained undamaged.

CLINICAL STUDIES

After completion of the preclinical studies that confirmed both the safety profile of the procedure and the potential efficacy for its clinical use, we proceeded to clinical controlled studies on patients with advanced glaucoma, uncontrolled with medications. Studies were done in 3 medical centers in Israel [Meir (Prof E. Assia), Carmenl (Prof O. Geyer) and Tel-Aviv Souraski (Dr S. Kurtz) Medical Centrs), 1 center in Johannesburg, South Africa (Dr E. Dahan) and at the L.V. Prasad Eye Institute in Hydrabad, India (Prof R. Thomas). Twenty-three patients were treated using the protocol determined in the preclinical studies. We decided that on our initial cases we would study only the net effect of the laser treatment and would not use any adjunctive treatment. Even though we knew that we might reduce the chances of low pressure and filter survival we did not use spacers under the external flap, apply antimetabolic agents to reduce tissue scarring, inject viscoelastics into the Schlemm's canal (viscocanalostomy) or perform YAG laser goniopuncture in failed cases.

Surgical procedure succeeded in all cases and the pressure dropped dramatically on the first postoperative day from a mean of 27.4 to 5.2 mm Hg.

There was no case of flat anterior chamber or any significant postoperative complication. In one eye prolapse of the iris base into the treated area was seen on gonioscopy and the iris was surgically repositioned. The mean pressure after the first week was 11.3 mmHg; however, from the two-week visit on, two distinct groups were evident: those patients whose IOP was low at the two-weeks visit maintained a low pressure thereafter (half of the cases), whereas increased pressure at two weeks was usually associated with long-term elevated pressure that required additional medications, and in 3 cases re-operations.

The clinical studies confirmed that the CO_2 laser can effectively ablate the dry tissue without tissue perforation by a relatively simple procedure. Satisfactory fluid percolation was achieved in all cases and no significant complications were seen in any of the eyes. The immediate postoperative results indicate that by applying the laser alone, long-term pressure drop without medications can be achieved in half of the cases. The late failure in the other cases is probably secondary to the localized tissue heating, which causes tissue irritation and inflammatory reaction. Anterior synechia and localized fibrosis were typically seen in the failed cases. The optimal laser parameters that would provide the desired tissue effect with minimal heating still need to be determined. We speculate that by using adjunctive therapy, such as placing spacers and applying mitomycin C under the scleral flap, frequent application of local steroids and using external lasers for suturelysis and goniopuncture will increase the success rate of the procedure.

SUMMARY

The CO_2 laser assisted NPFS utilizes the unique qualities of this far-infrared laser, i.e. the ability to ablate dry tissue and the almost complete absorption by water. This promising procedure enables accurate dissection of the scleral wall and un-roofing of the Schlemm's canal without penetration into the anterior chamber. The technique is therefore practically extraocular, relatively simple and requires only a short learning curve. Further modifications of the surgical procedure, and more controlled clinical studies are still required.

VIDEO

A clinical case of CO_2 laser assisted non-penetrating filtration surgery.

A large area under the scleral flap is first ablated in order to create a filtration "lake". Then, the scanner pattern is narrowed to create a slit over the area above the trabecular meshwork. Treatment is applied until fluid easily exits through the thinned wall. Note that when the treated area is wet, repeated laser application are not effective and the remaining scleral "membrane" is not perforated. Two 10-0 nylon sutures are used to close the external flap and a single suture is sufficient to close the conjunctiva. Anterior chamber maintainer was used in this case to maintain constant intraocular pressure, however it is not necessary in a routine case.

25

Selective Laser Trabeculoplasty

Madhu Nagar (UK)

INTRODUCTION

Glaucoma is a multifactorial disease characterized by increased intraocular pressure resulting in damage to the optic nerve and retinal nerve fibers. It is one of the leading causes of blindness but visual loss in most cases is preventable and can be treated with medications and surgery. The aim of glaucoma treatment is to preserve visual function with a minimum of side effects at an affordable cost. The best "neuro-protector" available is the "lowering of intraocular pressure" and this is still the treatment of choice in attempting to arrest or retard the loss of retinal ganglion cells. Effective medical treatment for glaucoma was first introduced in the later part of nineteenth century. In recent years, more and more drugs have been developed for the treatment of glaucoma and it is now possible to achieve low target IOP with drops; however, safety issues and the tolerability of glaucoma treatment cannot be ignored. The burden of daily treatment, including cost, inconvenience, possible side effects and quality of life are factors that the doctor and patient should discuss as they lead to noncompliance or poor compliance and hence progression of disease despite early diagnosis and prompt treatment.

Laser treatment of the trabecular meshwork for glaucoma has become a widely accepted treatment modality since Wise and Witter first introduced Argon Laser Trabeculoplasty in 1979. Many articles have since been published on the evidence base of the clinical effectiveness of Laser Trabeculoplasty using Argon lasers, solid state double neodymium lasers Dye Lasers and Diode Lasers. The laser wavelengths used in the majority have been those provided by the continuous wave Argon lasers (ALT), with wavelengths of either 488 nm (blue) or 514 nm (green) or green only 514 nm. The parameters used include a spot size of 50 μm and pulse duration of 200 msec, producing powers between 700 and 1000 mW, titrated by the expected visible reaction on the trabecular meshwork (TM). This energy absorption by the TM produces thermal coagulation effects detectable by most histopathology techniques. Clinically, this energy absorption produces a drop in intraocular pressure in approximately 90% of patients treated through 360°. The efficiency decreases by 5 to 10% per year following treatment. ALT causes inflammatory changes sufficient to induce peripheral anterior synechiae and trabecular scarring. The mechanism of action of LTP/ALT is unknown to date although scientific speculation indicates that the likely mechanisms are either mechanical, by postcoagulative collagenous

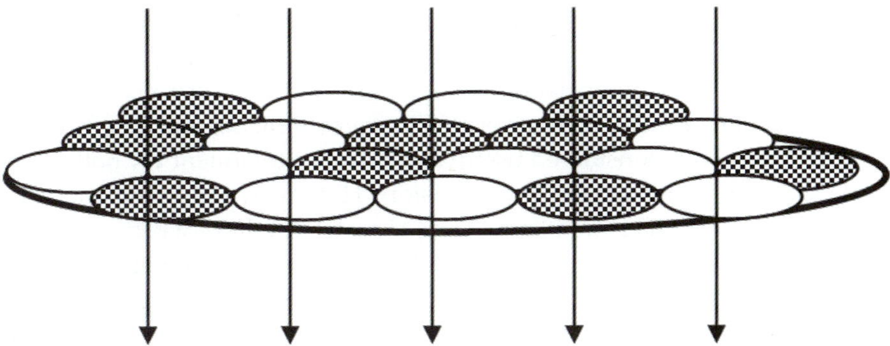

Fig. 1: Schematic drawing of the laser irradiation passing through a mixed cell culture of pigmented and nonpigmented TM cells

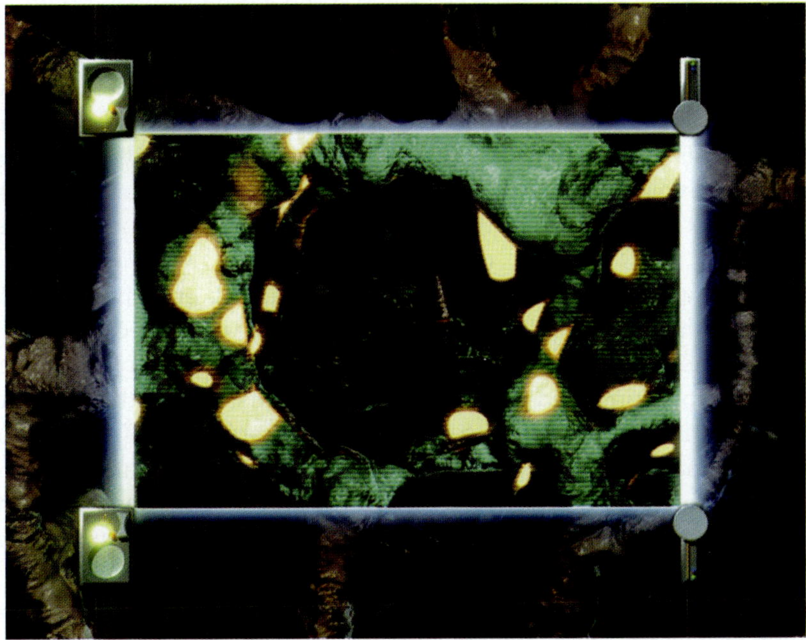

Fig. 2: Melanin-laden pigmented TM endothelial cells

contracture stretching the TM open, or ultrastructural, by TM endothelial renewal following laser induced TM endothelial loss. In vitro studies have confirmed coagulative damage at the edge and base of ALT craters as well as disruption of collagen beams, associated fibrinous exudates, lysis of endothelial cells and nuclear and cytoplasmic debris. In view of the great potential benefit of this form of treatment, in terms of effectivity, compliance and quality of life, ALT/LTP has been considered useful as a primary treatment for both open-angle glaucoma and ocular hypertension. However, following the early conclusions of the Glaucoma Laser Trial, the later results of which were very positive, many glaucoma specialists felt that, in view of the damage to the TM from ALT, the use of this treatment modality was best restricted to an intermediary role between failed medical treatment and surgery: certainly repeat treatment (repeat treatment over previously treated TM, i.e. more than 360° treatment) should be entertained only if surgery is delayed for a short period of time after determination that medical therapy has failed.

In the search for a less invasive form of laser treatment for the trabecular meshwork, Mark Latina and co-workers in 1995 defined a new means for delivering exactly this. The group studied the effect of delivering differing forms of laser energy to selective targets in the TM (the pigmented cells). They noted that by irradiating cell cultures of pigmented and nonpigmented TM cells with laser parameters that confined the energy absorption to the pigmented cells only, using pulse durations between 10 nanosec and 1 microsecond, coagulative damage was avoided, hence potentially preserving the structural integrity of the meshwork while still having the biological effect of intraocular pressure reduction.

Selective laser trabeculoplasty (SLT) is a safe and effective out-patient procedure with minimal and transient side effects. The presumed theory of SLT action is that it selectively targets melanin-laden pigmented cells of the trabecular meshwork: nonpigmented cells and connective tissues are believed to be unaffected. It is a safe alternative to argon laser trabeculoplasty and studies have shown that SLT provides effective reduction in intraocular pressure also in eyes that had previous argon laser trabeculoplasty (ALT) treatment. One of the greatest roadblocks to successful glaucoma treatment is compliance with medical therapy, which can be overcome by SLT.

The conclusions drawn from this study led to the development of a commercial laser system, the Selecta 7000 for selective irradiation of the pigmented TM cells (Selective Laser Trabeculoplasty—SLT), initially produced by Coherent and later Lumenis. A number of clinical studies have demonstrated SLT to be a safe alternative to argon laser trabeculoplasty. It reduces the IOP by the required 20-30% in about 80% of the patients. The studies have shown that SLT provides effective reduction in intraocular pressure also in eyes that had previous argon laser trabeculoplasty (ALT) treatment. It is less traumatic to the

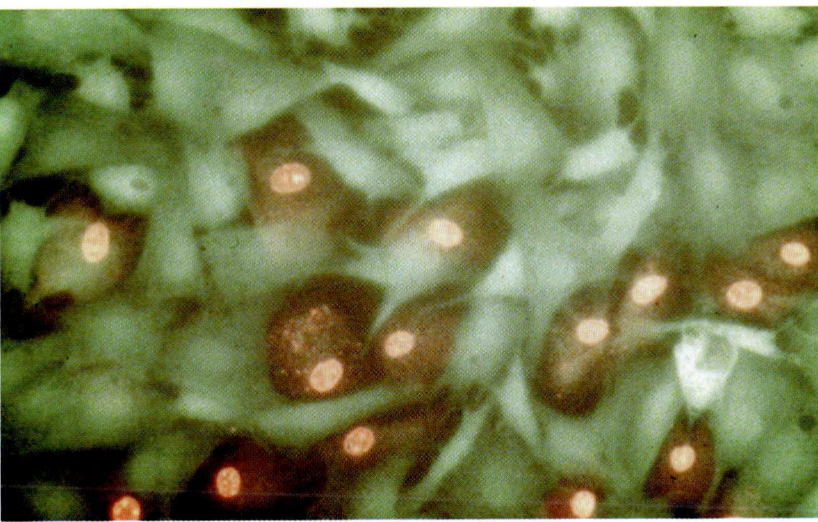

Fig. 3: Photomicrograph of the TM using fluorescent viability/cytotoxicity assay after irradiation with SLT. Only the pigmented trabecular cells exhibit nuclear staining (orange fluorescence - which indicates cell death) and absence of green cytoplasmic staining (green fluorescence). The nonpigmented TM cells were not affected by the SLT energy, as shown by the cytoplasmic

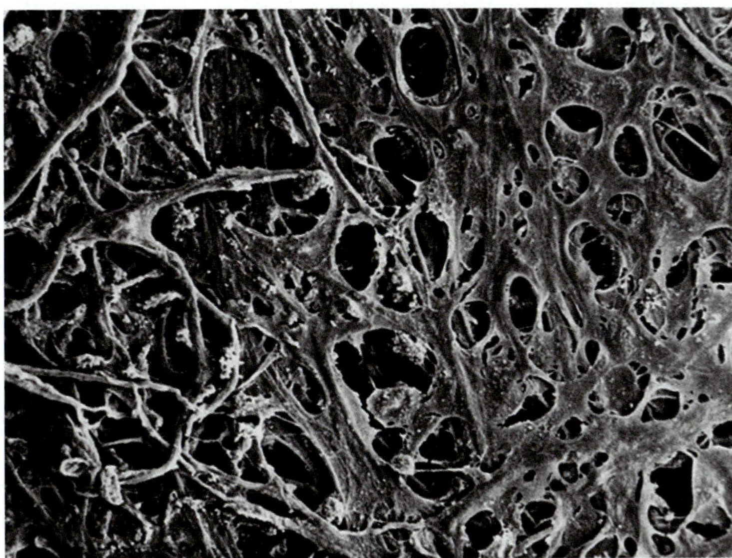

Fig. 4: Electron micrograph of the TM after SLT demonstrating minimal damage to the trabecular beams (SLT works by using a specific wavelength to irradiate and target only the melanin-containing cells in the trabecular meshwork, without incurring collateral thermal damage to adjacent nonpigmented trabecular meshwork cells and underlying trabecular beams). As quoted by Theresa R Kramer MD, Associate Professor of Ophthalmology, Emory University, Atlanta, Georgia: "SLT appears to cause no coagulative damage to the human TM, and less structural damage to the TM compared with ALT"

eye than ALT, which has been the standard laser procedure. There are some indications that the SLT treatment can be successfully repeated.

MECHANISM OF ACTION

SLT selectively targets the pigmented cells of the trabecular meshwork without producing collateral thermal or coagulative damage to the adjacent structures. There is no evidence of photocoagulation or scar formation with SLT, yet it significantly lowers intraocular pressure. It is derived from selective photothermolysis that is based on three principles:

1. The absorption of laser energy by intracellular targets must be greater than that of surrounding tissues.
2. Its wavelength must match the absorption wavelength of the target.
3. A short pulse is required to generate and confine heat to the pigmented targets.

(When all these parameters are present, target specificity is independent of focusing).

There is no mechanical effect or heat induction causing structural changes of the trabecular meshwork, so the mechanism of action for lowering IOP is believed to be a biological response. Selective laser trabeculoplasty works at a cellular level without any of the mechanical effects of ALT. Selective disruption of pigmented cells induces a response resulting in intraocular pressure reduction. There occurs an activation and recruitment of monocytes which turn to macrophages. The macrophages engulf melanin granules, clear them from the trabecular meshwork tissues when they leave the eye and return to circulation via Schlemm's canal, which increases aqueous outflow (research conducted by Jorge Alvarado MD et al. Injury to pigmented trabecular meshwork cells also results in the release of at least three specific cytokines that may play an important role in the function of the trabecular meshwork. These cytokines are Interleukin-1 alpha and beta (IL-1 alpha and beta) and tumor necrosis factor- alpha (TNF-alpha). These are believed to act as growth factor for trabecular cells causing cellular proliferation and extracellular modeling which further invigorates TM filtering and outflow. The precise pressure lowering mechanism of SLT, like that of ALT, has not been conclusively determined.

This should be contrasted with the effects on the trabecular meshwork after Argon Laser Trabeculoplasty.

LASER AND DELIVERY SYSTEM

The procedure is performed with a Frequency Doubled, Q-Switched, Nd: YAG Laser which delivers 532 nm wavelength of laser light with a pulse duration of 3 nanoseconds and a spot size of 400 μ. Systems are available from Lumenis and Laserex.

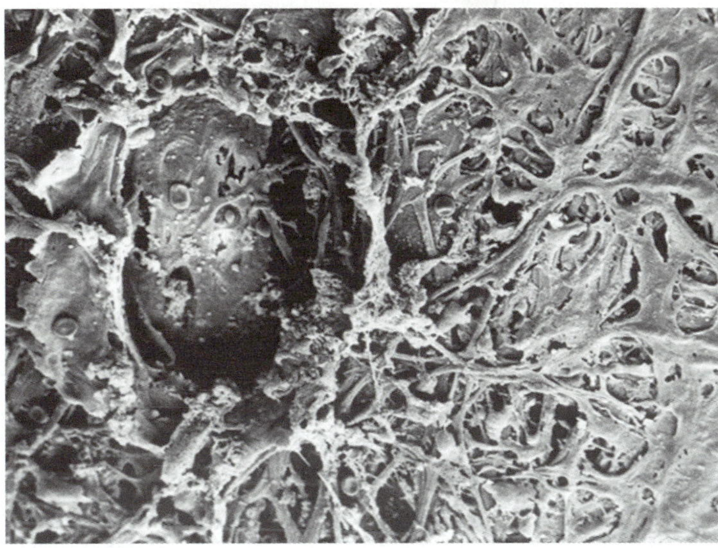

Fig. 5: Electron micrograph of the trabecular meshwork following argon laser trabeculoplasty (ALT). The damage to the trabecular beams in considerably more than the damage following selective laser trabeculoplasty (SLT)

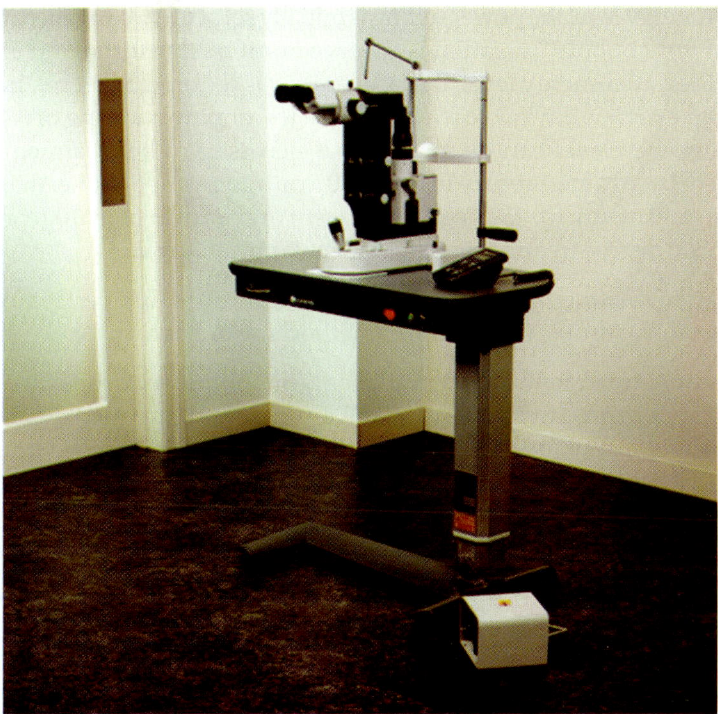

Fig. 6: The selecta duet which delivers both Q-switched 1064 nm Nd: YAG laser for photo disruption and Q-switched 532 nm frequency doubled laser for SLT

TANGO LASER FROM LASERX

The SLT Laser delivery parameters are as follows:

1. Solid state Nd:YAG laser (1064 nm), frequency doubled, producing a wavelength of 532 nm.
2. The Laser is Q-switched producing short pulse durations (3 nanoseconds)
3. The spot size is 400 µm diameter.
4. 40 to 50 contiguous applications per 180°.
5. Power range 0.4 to 1.2 mJ (no visible endpoint).

OPERATIVE TECHNIQUE

The technique of treating patients with SLT is very much similar to that of conventional ALT. The pulse duration of 3 nsec is too short for melanin to convert the electromagnetic energy to thermal energy and hence no heat is liberated. The large spot size covers most of the anteroposterior diameter of the trabecular meshwork and low fluence (energy per unit area) is achieved, which avoids the mechanical and coagulative disruption seen with ALT. 100 times less energy is used as compared to ALT.

The energy level is titrated to the degree of trabecular pigmentation. The greater the pigmentation, the lesser is the energy requirement. To determine the optimum energy level the power setting is initially set at 0.8 mJ, and then increased by 0.1 mJ until bubble formation is observed or if bubble formation is already noted at the initial energy level, the laser energy is reduced by 0.1 mJ. In heavily pigmented eyes it is advisable to start with a lower power setting of 0.4 mJ and then the energy level can be increased if necessary. The treatment is then completed by placing approximately 50 contiguous spots over half of the trabecular meshwork for 180 degree treatment or approximately 100 contiguous spots for 360 degree treatment of the trabecular meshwork.

Preoperative treatment: It is a simple outpatient procedure performed under local anaesthetic drops, for example amethocaine or benoxinate.

Postoperative treatment: Nonsteroidal anti-inflammatory drops three to four times a day for three to five days may be prescribed. If patients are on anti-glaucoma medication prior to SLT, the prescription is maintained unchanged following SLT or the drops may be washed off prior to SLT.

The wash off time needed for a topically administered drug to completely lose its effect varies greatly:

• Beta blockers	2-5 weeks
• Sympathomimetics	2 weeks
• Direct acting miotics	1-3 days
• Indirect acting miotics	1 month
• Topical CAI	1 week
• Oral CAI	1 week
• Prostaglandins	4-6 weeks

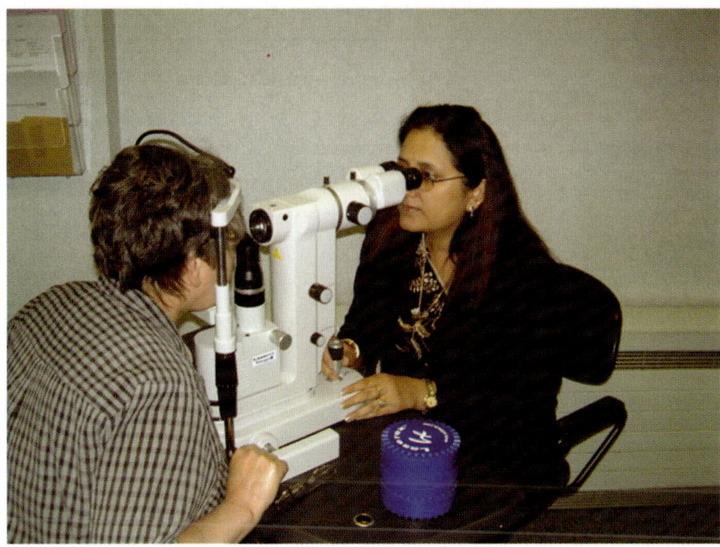

Fig. 7: The Tango also delivers both Q-switched 1064 nm Nd: YAG laser for photo disruption and Q-switched 532 nm frequency doubled laser for SLT

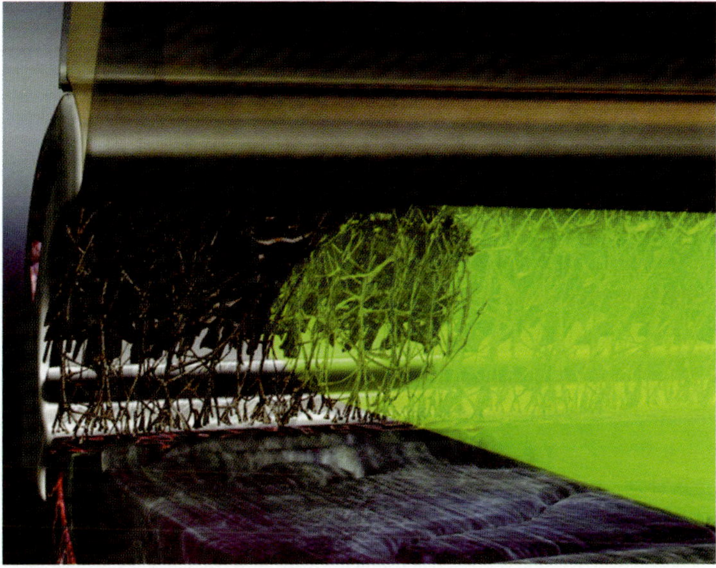

Fig. 8: A schematic of the relative size of a 400 μm spot size on the trabecular meshwork (Note that an eye with white-to-white measurement of 12 mm has a trabecular distance of approximately 39 mm, permitting a maximum of 98 contiguous applications, or 49 applications per 180°

INDICATIONS AND CONTRAINDICATIONS

The indications for treatment with SLT are similar to the indications for Argon Laser Trabeculoplasty (ALT):

- Newly diagnosed open-angle glaucoma (OAG) patients
- OAG patients uncontrolled on medical treatment
- OAG patients poorly compliant with medical treatment
- OAG patients intolerant to their glaucoma medications
- Patients with previous failed ALT treatment
- SLT has been shown to work well in patients with pseudoexfoliation and pigmentary glaucomas.

Trials are ongoing using SLT on chronic angle-closure glaucoma patients after iridotomy.

SLT is currently contraindicated in patients with:

- Inflammatory/uveitic glaucomas
- Primary or secondary narrow angle glaucoma
- Congenital glaucoma
- Poor visualization of the trabecular meshwork.

ADVERSE EFFECTS

Adverse effects are minimal and transient. They include mild discomfort during treatment, an IOP spike a few hours post-SLT, increased anterior chamber activity for a few days following the procedure. No case of persistent iritis has yet been reported. Vision is blurred for five to ten minutes after laser delivery and patients may suffer from sore eyes for 3-5 days post-laser treatment. Occasionally, patients do complain of headaches or precipitation of migraine. No induction of peripheral anterior synechiae is observed.

BENEFITS OF SLT

- SLT results in a biological response that increases aqueous drainage and reduces IOP
- It avoids the adverse reactions from medications
- It does not cause adverse scarring of the trabecular meshwork
- It may reduce the need for lifelong use of expensive eyedrops and other medications
- It may reduce or eliminate the inconvenience of always having to take glaucoma medications.

CLINICAL TRIALS

In 1998, a pilot clinical study was conducted to evaluate the intraocular pressure lowering effect of SLT in 53 open-angle glaucoma patients whose intraocular

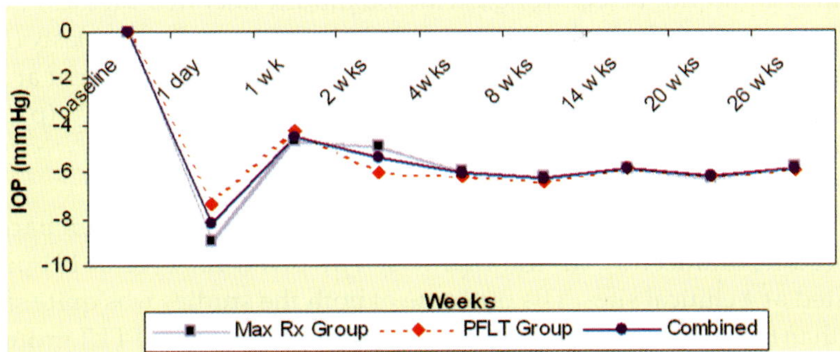

Fig. 9: Mean reduction of intraocular pressure in SLT treated eyes (Max Rx – OAG uncontrolled by maximum medical therapy; PFLT–uncontrolled OAG with a previous history of ALT treatment; Combined – all SLT treated patients in the study)

pressures could not be controlled with maximum tolerated medical therapy (Max Rx group) or who had a previous failed argon laser trabeculoplasty (PFLT). Seventy percent of the patients responded with an IOP reduction of at least 3 mm Hg. At 26 weeks of follow up, the mean IOP reduction was 23.5% ($p < 0.001$) for the Max Rx group, 24.2% ($p < 0.001$) for PFLT group and 23.8% ($p < 0.001$) for both groups combined.

The promising results of this study led the investigators to embark on a prospective, multicentre clinical trial which involved 101 eyes in 101 patients recruited at 4 clinical sites. The outcome of both the studies was quite similar: more than 66% of the patients who had a previous failed ALT (PFLT group) had an IOP decrease of 3 mm or greater after treatment with SLT.

Another clinical study from the UK "A randomized, prospective study comparing 90°, 180° and 360° SLT with Latanoprost 0.005% for the control of intraocular pressure in Ocular Hypertension and Open Angle Glaucoma" also demonstrated the safety and efficacy of SLT in lowering IOP. This study demonstrated a greater IOP lowering response with 360° and 180° SLT laser application compared to 90°. The results of 360° SLT treatment was comparable to standard medical treatment: with 360^0 SLT, 80% of eyes achieved 20% or greater IOP reduction and 60% achieved 30% or greater IOP reduction.

Investigators in other countries have also demonstrated the safety and efficacy of SLT in lowering the IOP.

Table 1: Safety and Efficacy of SLT in Lowering IOP

	Latina et al 1998	*Latina et al 2001*	*Melamed et al 2003*	*Nagar et al 2005 (360^0)*
Type of study	Prospective clinical trial	Prospective clinical trial	Prospective clinical trial	Prospective clinical trial
No. of Eyes treated	53 eyes	101 eyes	45 eyes	44 eyes
Duration of follow up	6 months	24 months	18 months	12 months
Mean IOP decrease after SLT	23.8%	17.2%	30%	>20% in 80%, >30% in 59%

SUMMARY

Selective Laser Trabeculoplasty was developed as an alternative to Argon Laser Trabeculoplasty in the treatment of OAG. By selectively targeting only the pigmented TM cells and avoiding collateral thermal damage to surrounding cells and structures, SLT avoids permanent scarring of the TM as occurs with ALT. Hopefully, this translates clinically into a procedure that avoids the disadvantages of ALT: immediate postoperative IOP elevation, degradation of IOP lowering in the long-term and relatively poor efficacy with sometimes deleterious results when retreating previously treated TM.

Selective laser Trabeculoplasty is a safe and effective means of lowering intra ocular pressure. The effect is sustained over a period of 2 to 5 years of follow-up period as shown by various studies. Q-switched Trabeculoplasty does not cause collateral thermal damage, so it is repeatable and is an option for failed ALT patients. The procedure is indicated in medically uncontrolled OAG and OHT patients, newly diagnosed OAG and OHT and also in patients with uncontrolled IOP who had undergone previous ALT. The IOP reduction is immediate, seen on day one in most of the patients though there may be few Late or Slow responders demonstrating reduction of IOP in period of 4 to 12 weeks. IOP reduction may also be observed in the untreated contra lateral eye (if only one eye is treated) and that supports the biological response theory of Jorge Alvarado.

In a nutshell, SLT will prove to be a useful tool in lowering IOP in newly diagnosed patients as a first line treatment and will also be of value in known glaucoma patients already on medical treatment but who are either non-compliant or who have developed intolerance or tachyphylaxis to anti-glaucoma drops. Noncompliance is an important cause of visual loss in patients with glaucoma. The latest diagnostic techniques (which attempt to detect glaucoma prior to any visual loss) and treatment advances (which attempt to hold the disease at its current stage and prevent further optic nerve damage) are of no benefit in medical management if the patient is not compliant. Reasons for Poor/Non Compliance are asymptomatic disease, active social life, old age, arthritis, senile dementia to name but a few and **SLT is the answer.**

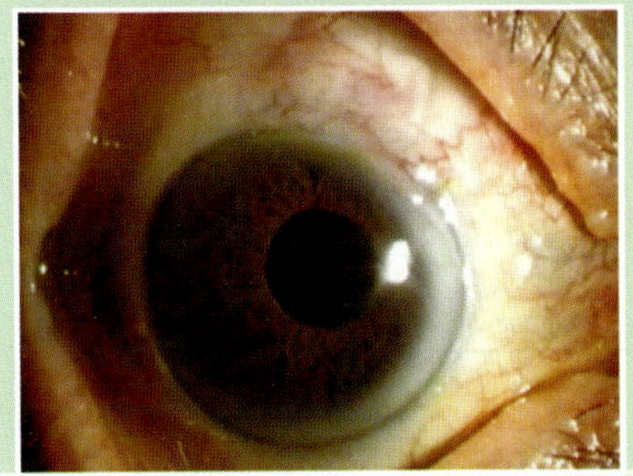

SECTION

2

SPECIAL GLAUCOMA SURGICAL TECHNIQUES

26

Drainage Implant Surgery

Keiki R Mehta, Cyres K Mehta (India)

INTRODUCTION

Virtually all of glaucoma filtering operations required to maintain patency of a drainage fistula, a great number of alternate materials have been implanted in the eyes consisting of the lens wires, there is made of silver gold platinum or even polypropylene which were placed to form a track or fistula. Unfortunately, most of the procedures were unsuccessful in maintaining a plate and fistula. Never devices utilized tubes which drained into external reservoir is.

All modern drainage implant devices have the same basic design, namely a plastic tube which extends from the anterior chamber to a plate disk or encircling element under the content driver or the daemons gaps. This shape and the size of the device may differ, however, the fundamental basics remain the same. The only a variant being that it either has an open tube implant, i.e. valved implants or would tube implants.

In virtually all the implants the double tube shunts aqueous from the anterior chamber to an encapsulated space which forms are round the plate the fibrous capsule composed of densely compacted collagen fibres which develops three to five weeks after implantation. Unlike the typical thin limbal filtering blebs with conjunctival microcysts, the vaults of the encapsulated cavity are thicker, more vascular, and less permeable to aqueous humor. The capsule at thickness and volume determine the rate of aqueous humor outflow and the extent of intraocular pressure lowering. The generally the larger the plate surface area, the lower the intraocular pressure.

Valveless Shunts

Valveless shunts include the followings:

- Molteno implant: This implant looks like a water dish, with a high ridge around the side. The surgeon places the tube at the limbus and connects it to a plate positioned on the globe surface.
- Baerveldt implant: Multiple fenestrations through the plate allow fibrous connections to form between the front and back parts of the cyst that usually encapsulates the shunt. This leads to fewer complications.
- Schocket encircling tube: This shunt consists of a 30 mm elastic tube sutured into the grooved portion of a silicone gutter. It shunts aqueous to an equatorially encircling silicone band, resulting in posterior drainage.

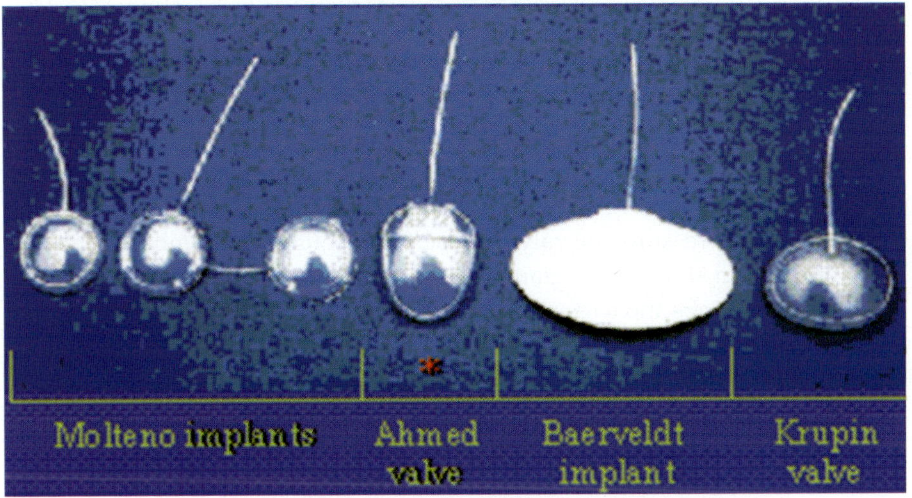

Fig. 1: Glaucoma drainage devices

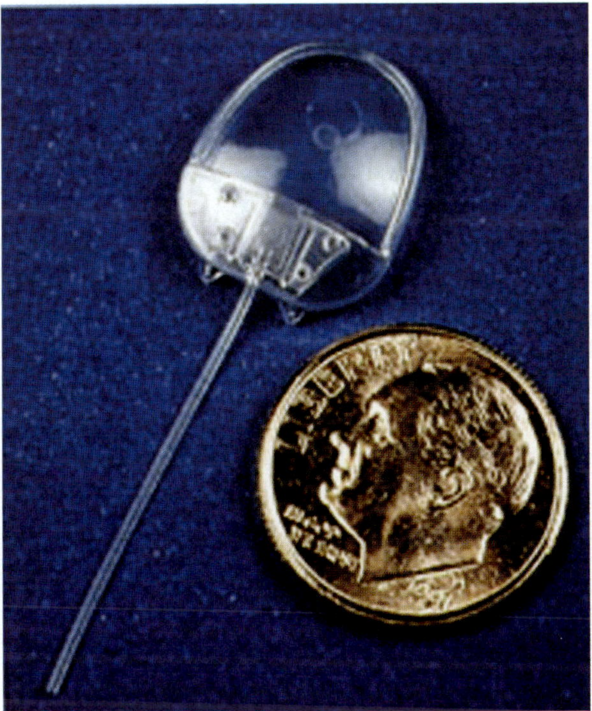

Fig. 2: Ahmed Glaucoma valve

Valved Implants

Valved implants include the followings:

- Krupin eye valve with disk (the Krupin disk). This shunt incorporates a slit valve to minimize early postoperative hypotony.
- Ahmed glaucoma valve: This features two flexible leaflets that open when IOP rises to 12 mm Hg and close when IOP falls to 8–10 mm Hg. By closing at the lower pressure, the valve helps prevent anterior-chamber collapse.
- White pump shunt: This glaucoma pump-shunt consists of an inlet tube anchoring wings and a reservoir bounded by two unidirectional valves that lead to an outlet tube. This differs from other shunts that use a large plate as the reservoir tube shunt surgery is an efficacious way to lower IOP in complicated glaucomas.

All glaucoma shunts work by a similar mechanism. Aqueous flows through the tube into an encapsulated space surrounding the equatorial plate and passively diffuses through the surrounding bleb walls.

Indications

Shunts are indicated in patients with complicated glaucoma who are unresponsive to conventional filtering procedures in which 5-fluorouracil or mitomycin-C is used or when the filtering procedures are unlikely to succeed or are technically difficult. Complicated glaucoma's may include those associated with aphakia, pseudophakia, failed filters, penetrating keratoplasty, and retinal surgeries, as well as neovascular and pediatric glaucoma.

Dr Heuer, in his opinion has three specific indications for aqueous shunts

1. Eyes in which trabeculectomy with mitomycin-C has already failed and that had no identifiable, correctable complications.
2. Eyes with neovascular glaucoma and active anterior segment neovascularization in which IOP is too high to wait for regression of neovascularization and peripheral retinal photocoagulation adequate to achieve regression cannot be administered.
3. Eyes with active or recurrent moderate-to-severe uveitis.

Glaucoma shunts fall into two categories

- Non-restrictive flow devices, which require temporary tube occlusion to prevent hypotony while the episcleral plate is encapsulating.
- Restrictive flow devices, which allow immediate aqueous drainage.

The Molteno implant (IOP Inc.), one of the most widely used non-restrictive flow devices, is the prototypical drainage device. It has a silicone tube attached to one or two polypropylene plates. Numerous reports have been published about the Molteno implant, but direct comparisons among the studies are difficult because they differ as to the types of glaucoma included and the outcomes measures used. The original design (shields) consisted of a single plate of thin

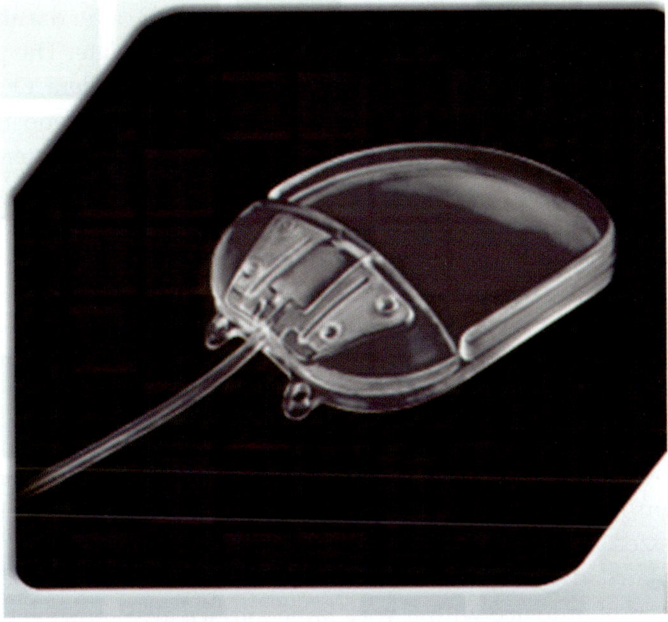

Fig. 3: The popular S2 Ahmed model

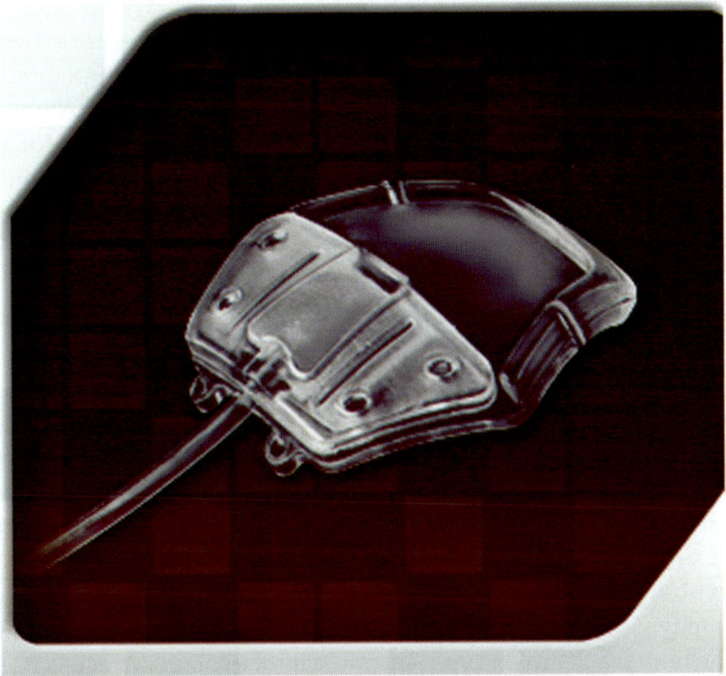

Fig. 4: The S3 model used in children

acrylic with a diameter of 13 mm. A silicone tube of 0.63 outer dia and 0.30 mm innerr diameter connected to the upper surface of the plate. The plate had a thickened rim which is perforated to allow suturing to the sclera. Over a period of time, to enhance the filtering surface are a double plate Molteno implant was developed. In a randomized trial (Hueur, the dual plate gave better results). In another modification, is a dual chamber, single pate implant in which the V shape enclosed a area around the opening of the silicone tube. This pattern helped to address to some extent the problem of hypotony. Implants with larger surface areas control IOP better than those with smaller surface areas, although studies with the Baerveldt implant suggest there may be a limit beyond which further increases in size do not provide greater IOP reduction.

The Baerveldt Implant

It is an non-restrictive flow device, consists of a thin silicone tube attached to a thin barium impregnated silicone plate. The device is available in 250 and 350 mm^2 sizes.

"The main advantage of this implant is that it allows single-quadrant implantation of a device with a very large surface area, however, it may be associated with higher rates of strabismus than implants that do not come into contact with the extraocular muscles."

Problems with IOP elevation: The main disadvantage of non-restrictive devices is that IOP elevations often occur during the first month after implantation. The restrictive devices, such as the Krupin (Eagle Vision Inc.) and Ahmed (New World Medical) implants, were designed to allow immediate flow of aqueous while reducing the risk of hypotony, Dr. Lloyd explained. While their manufacturers describe them as valves, some studies suggest that in physiologic conditions, they act more as flow restrictors than true valves that open and close in response to pressure changes.

The Krupin-Denver valve with disc is composed of a silicone tube attached to a 184 mm^2 silicone disc. Flow restriction is achieved by the horizontal and vertical slits in the distal end of the tube.

The concept of a one way valve that opens at predetermined pressure to avoid the postoperative complication of hypotony was first introduced by Krupin and his associates in 1976. The original Krupin-Denver valve was composed of an internal supramid tube cemented to an external silastic tube. The valve effect was created by making slits in the closed external end of the silastic tube. Though initially encouraging the fibrosis closed the subconjunctival portion of the valved tube leading to failure. In a modification, it was attached to a Schroket type silicone scleral explants which is its present modification.

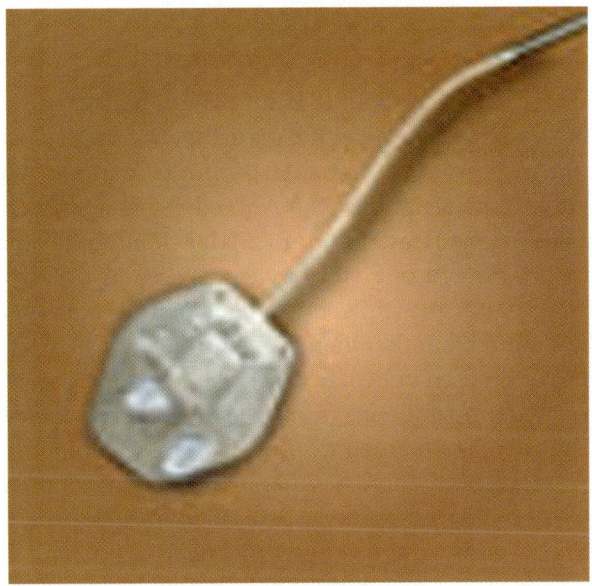

Fig. 5

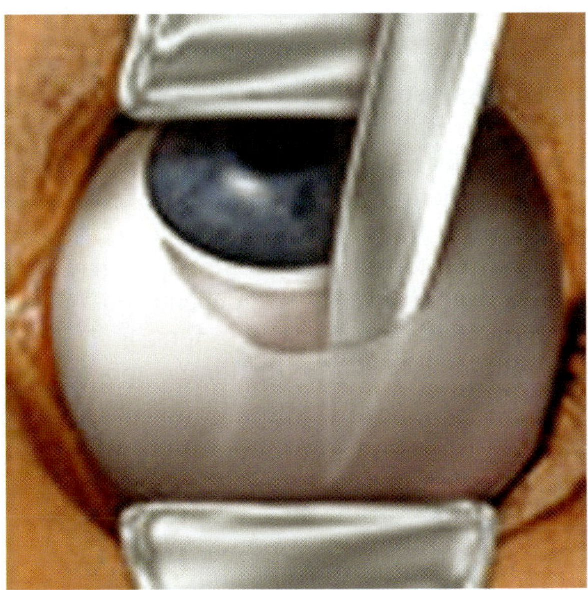

Fig. 6

The Ahmed Valve

The Ahmed glaucoma valve is composed of a silicone tube attached to one or two polypropylene plates, each about 184 mm^2. The valve is made of thin silicone membranes in the anterior portion of the plate that open and close in response to pressure changes. The inlet is wider than the outlet, which creates a pressure differential that allows aqueous flow the Ahmed™ Glaucoma Valve (AGV™) utilizes a specially designed, tapered trapezoidal chamber to create a Venturi effect to help aqueous flow through the device. As demonstrated by Bernoulli's equation of hydrodynamic principle, the inlet velocity of aqueous entering the larger port of the Venturi chamber increases significantly as it exits the smaller outlet port of the tapered chamber. In an AGV™ this increased exit velocity greatly helps in evacuating aqueous from the valve, thereby helping to reduce valve friction. The valve is designed to open at a pressure of 8–10 mm Hg.

The Ahmed™ Glaucoma Valve has no obstruction in its path of fluid flow. For the fl ow to be non-obstructive, a particle large enough to pass through the lumen of the tube, will easily pass through a much larger opening of the Venturi-Flow™ chamber. The elastic membranes help to regulate fluid flow valved all times, consistently by changing their shape. The tension on these membranes is responsible for reducing hypotony.

Potential Shunt Risks

Some of the potential risks associated with both restrictive and non-restrictive shunts are wound leak, flattening of the anterior chamber, hyphema, inflammation, corneal edema, cataract, strabismus, tube blockage, tube or plate erosion, aqueous misdirection, choroidal detachment, retinal detachment, and phthisis.

Tube shunts are valuable for managing complicated glaucoma but they are associated with risks. The reduction of IOP depends not only on the surface area of the shunts, but also on undetermined factors.

Valved devices allow early IOP reduction postoperatively, but initial hypotony or elevated IOP can occur. Success rates achieved with all aqueous shunts decline over time (Lloyd).

Aqueous Shunts in Pediatric Group

Aqueous shunts are the next step for patients whose glaucoma is not controlled with other techniques. Wilson who has a great deal of experience in Pediatric valves mentions that he uses shunts in preference to trabeculectomy in aphakic patients who require a contact lens, or in patients with chronic uveitis. Eyes with shunts seem to tolerate more inflammatory debris than eyes with trabeculectomies in his opinion.

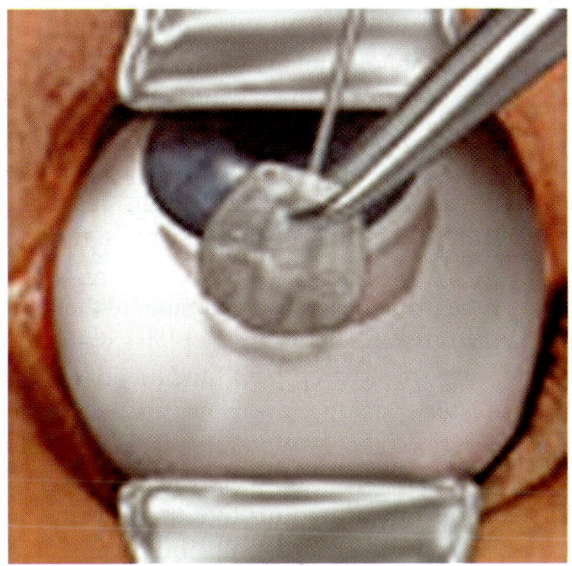

Fig. 7

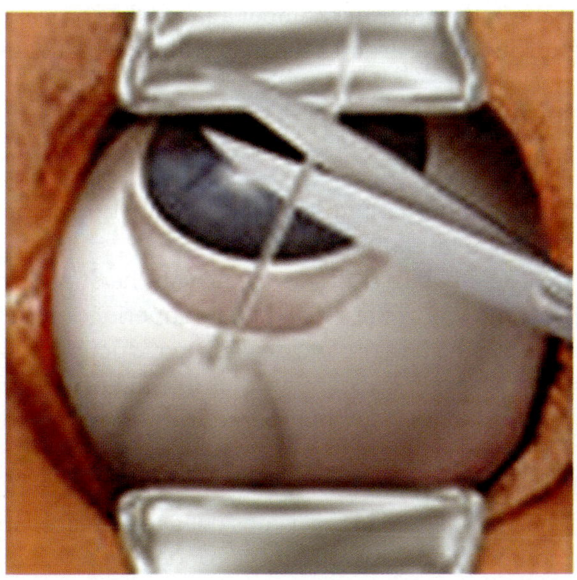

Fig. 8

Wilson prefers the 250 mm^2 Baerveldt shunt in patients under one year of age and the double-plate Molteno shunt in older patients. The latter causes less diplopia than the 350 mm^2 Baerveldt, whose wings protrude under the adjacent muscles, effectively shortening them. The Ahmed valve is a popular alternative with surgeons who are not as comfortable with ligating the tube and adding venting slits. The smaller reservoir area, which results in a higher final IOP if only one plate is used, and the bulk of the first plate in a small orbit are disadvantages.

Wilson ties off the tube from the anterior chamber to the first plate with an 8-0 polyglactin (Vicryl) suture and between the plates with a 6–0 polyglactin suture. This results in a safer, staged drop in IOP and less inflammation, allowing a thinner bleb over the later opening plate. He advises that whichever shunt you choose, the reservoir should not be placed too far posteriorly, as it is likely that you will be back later removing the thickened capsule of scar tissue overlying the reservoir. Wilson does not use adjunctive mitomycin-C for the initial implantation, because he has not seen a definite improvement in results.

Aqueous shunts are much more problematic in pediatric patients than in adults. Some of the problems common in children are inflammatory membranes that encase the internal tube and block the inner ostium or pull the iris over it, migration of the tube in the anterior chamber against the cornea or into the iris, and build-up of fibrous tissue around the plates limiting aqueous filtration

Surgical Technique

Basic Principles

Irrespective of the type of implant utilized these basic surgical principle apply in general to all drainage implant devices.

The conjunctival fornix based flap is created in the superior temporal or superior nasal quadrant. It is preferential that the superior or nasal quadrant be avoided especially with the larger plate designs to reduce the risk of inducing strabismus. Some of the larger bulkier implants like the Ahmed implant when placed in the supero nasal quadrant may come within 1 mm of the optic nerve (Leen et al).

The surgical exposure should be adequate as it has to extend beyond the equator of the globe. Radial relaxing incisions need to be placed in one or more quadrants of the conjunctival flaps. Small eyes or deeply set globes can best be handled by isolating the two rectii muscles and passing traction sutures to position the eye. Spatulated needles with 8/0 silk sutures are threaded through the anterior position holes of the external plate and the plate is then sutured to the sclera such that the anterior part of the plate positions itself 9 to 10 mm posterior to the limbus. Some implants with thin plates such as the Molteno can be fitted under larger adjacent rectii muscles. In the case of the Ahmed implant which has a large anterior posterior dimensions in may be advisable not to extend the anterior border of the plate more than 8 mm behind the limbus.

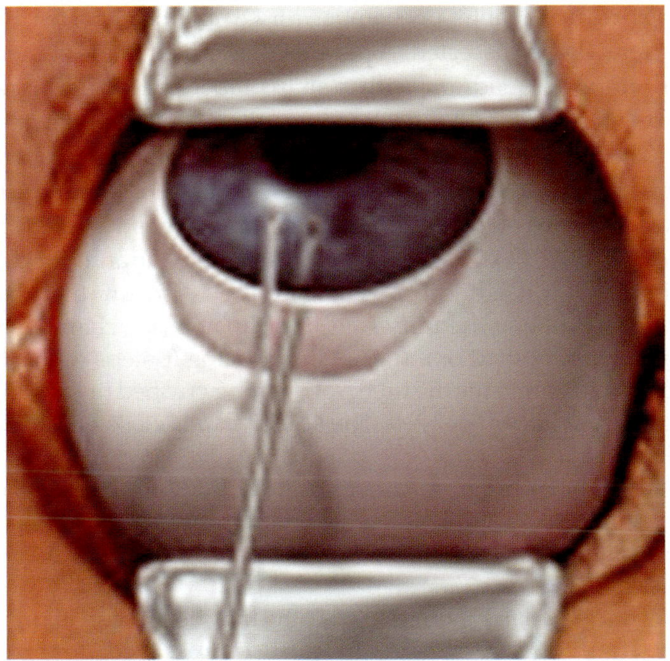

Fig. 9

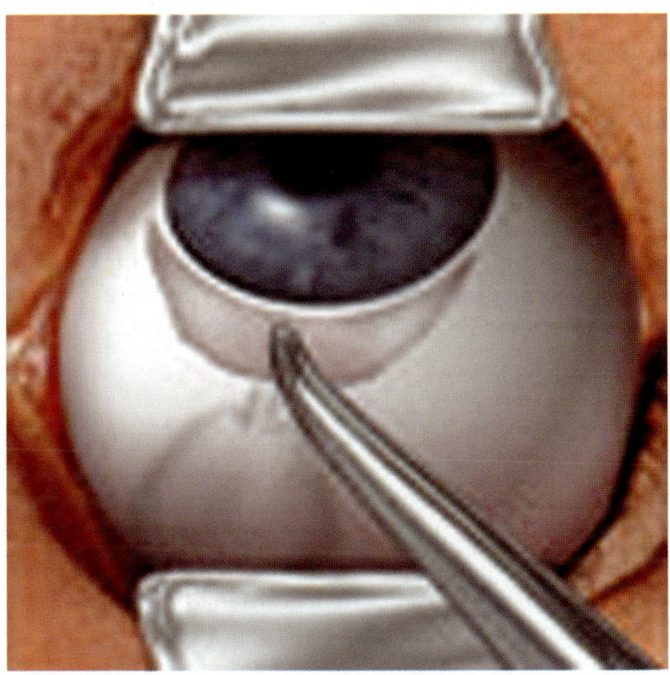

Fig. 10

For inserting fit to do the anterior chamber, a 6 × 8 millimeter partial thickness limbal based scleral flap is dissected. A paracentesis is next made at the limbus in the inferior temporal quadrant with a sharp tapered blade. The anterior chamber is next entered beneath the sclera flap with 21–23 G needle parallel to the iris plane. The angle at which the needle enters the anterior chamber is critical since it is important that the tube, which will pass along the needle track will vault between cornea and iris without touching either structure. The tube is cut bevel up to permit its extension 2–3 millimeters into the anterior chamber. With valved implants it is advisable to irrigate BSS to ensure that the valve opens properly. The tube is then inserted into the anterior chamber via the needle track using nontoothed or a special introducing forceps with a built in groove (Ahmed) which prevents the tube from getting crushed or kinked, and is secured to the sclera with 9–0 or 10–0. The scleral flap is closed and the valve checked that it is stable.

Non-valved implants often, to prevent undue hypotony, and excessive filtration, has its tube with a slip knot on the ligature. After the fibrous capsule had the opportunity to form (6–8 weeks), the ligature is opened up under topical anesthesia.

Dissection of a scleral flap for burying the tube may be difficult in previously operated eyes. It strongly recommended to use preserved donor cornea, sclera,dura or pericardium (Tanzgrafti) (Smith et all) to cover the tube.

Postoperative Care

Topical 1% perdnisolone 4–6 times a day under antibiotic cover (Gatifloxacin or maxifloxacin) qid tapered over 6 weeks is usually adequate.
Cycloplegics are not used.

Complications

Although the standard complications of hyphema, choroidal detachment, choroidal hemorrhage, or malignant glaucoma can occur after any glaucoma filtering surgery, glaucoma drainage operations typically are associated with a special groups of intraoperative and postoperative problems.

Hypotony

Until the fibrous capsule is properly formed, valve less implant s will have a tendency to develop hypotony. The best way is to temporarily diminish the flow by narrowing the lumen with an ligature which may be opened at a later time. Often the earlier days it is the leakage around the tube which causes the problem. The patient must be given an empty shield (no gauge below) to wear for a period of a month after the surgery to prevent inadvertent pressure on the eye from a pillow or straying fingers.

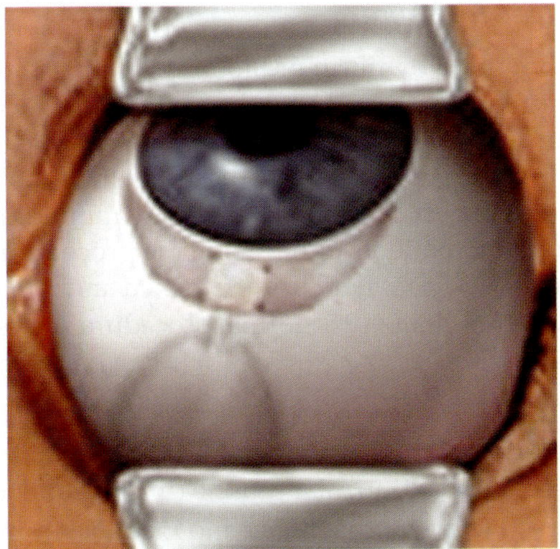

Figs 5 to 11: Show implantation of the S3 valve

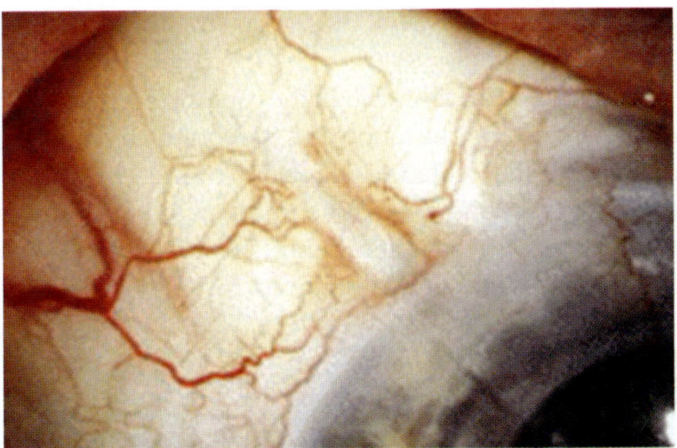

Fig. 12

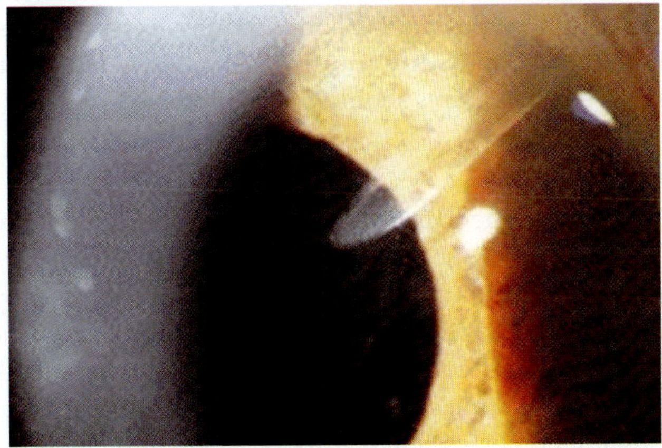

Figs 12 and 13: Show the Ahmed valve in eye with tube in the anterior chamber

Elevated Intraocular Pressure

The tube may be occluded by fibrin or blood if the operation is not perfectly clean and if the surgeon has nor cleared the lumen with BSS prior closing up. Though a variety of techniques have been promulgated from using 30 G needles to the use of laser, to rhythmic pressure on the globe, the simplest is to simply go in, flush the tube and repost it back. Takes hardly minutes and the patient is happy. It is wise to tell all patients undergoing the procedure that occasionally the tube in the first 6 week does tend to get chocked and it may be necessary to flush it out. That way they realize it is normal procedure and not a complication.

Ocular Motility Disturbance

Implants with the larger plates, especially when implanted in the inferonasal quadrant tend to interrupt extraocular muscle function and lead to strabismus and diplopia. Corrective measure will need to include removal, repositioning of the implant or its replacement with an smaller implant or transfer to the superotemporal quadrant.

Tube or Plate Extrusion

The tube or the plate may extrude through the conjunctiva particularly if relaxing incisions had been made and the tenon and the conjunctiva improperly closed. Late extrusions can best be treated with a scleral preserved patch over the tube. It is imperative that if repairs once done to the position of the tube or a flap repositioning or an preserved scleral emplacement, the tenon be properly positioned and closed over the area repaired. Simply closing the conjunctiva will invite a future erosion.

Problems of Tube Migration

At a later stage whether inadvertently or by rubbing or trauma the eye, the tip of the tube may come in contact with the iris or the cornea. This should be immediately treated, by repositioning and trimming. Typically it tends to occur if the plate had not been properly sutured to the sclera. Hence at the time of repositioning the scleral sutures should be re-enforced.

Results of Implants

In a large study of the Molteno implant, Dr. Lloyd and colleagues reported that after 5 years of follow-up, success rates declined with time for patients with different types of glaucoma who received one or two plates. Success rates remained higher in the patients who received two plates. In another study conducted by Heuer and colleagues, aphakic and pseudophakic patients received either single- or double-plate Molteno implants. After 2 years of follow-up, the investigators reported that the double-plate implants provided about

50% higher success rates than single-plate implants. However, the single-plate implants were associated with fewer complications, Dr. Lloyd noted.

In 50 patients with mixed glaucomas in whom the Krupin-Denver shunt was used, Krupin and colleagues reported a mean IOP of 8.3 mm Hg on the first postoperative day. After 25 months, the mean IOP was 13.1 mm Hg, and the patients were using a mean of 0.8 medications. On the first postoperative day, four eyes had an IOP greater than 30 mm Hg resulting from tube blockage and 12 eyes had an IOP less than 5 mm Hg.

In a smaller study of the Krupin device in patients with mixed glaucomas, Fellenbaum and colleagues reported similar initial postoperative IOPs and a success rate of 66% at 12 months postoperatively. Large studies have only been conducted on the single-plate Ahmed implant. Coleman and colleagues reported a 78% success rate at 12 months and a mean IOP of 14.4 mm Hg in 60 patients with mixed types of glaucoma; 13% of eyes had an IOP less than 5 mm Hg and 10% had tube blockage on postoperative day 1. After 4 years, the cumulative probability of success was 76% when patients with corneal complications were not included as treatment failures, and 45% when they were. Another study by Huang and associates showed a comparable success rate at 24 months.

In patients undergoing penetrating keratoplasty in whom the Ahmed device was implanted, the success probability was 51.5% at 20 months, with 75% of the grafts remaining clear. In young patients with glaucomas in whom the Ahmed device was implanted, the success rate was 60.6% at 24 months.

SUMMARY

Drainage implants have been successful in maintaining the patency of the fistula in glaucoma filtering surgeries. Though implant designs differ, a proper surgical technique with an very meticulous closure and keen attention to tube patency will lead to fairly successful results in cases where all other surgeries have failed.

27

Pneumatic Trabeculoplasty: A Noninvasive Glaucoma Treatment

Guillermo Avalos-Urzua (Mexico)

Currently, glaucoma is defined as a disturbance of the structural or functional integrity of the optic nerve that causes characteristic atrophic changes in the optic nerve, which may also lead to specific visual field defects over time. This disturbance usually can be arrested or diminished by adequate lowering of intraocular pressure (IOP). The generic term glaucoma should only be used in reference to the entire group of glaucomatous disorders as a whole, because multiple subsets of glaucomatous disease exist.

People who maintain elevated pressures in the absence of nerve damage or visual field loss exist, they are considered at risk for glaucoma and have been termed glaucoma suspects or ocular hypertensives. POAG is a major worldwide health concern, because of its usually silent, progressive nature, and because it is one of the leading preventable causes of blindness in the world. With appropriate screening and treatment, glaucoma usually can be identified and its progress arrested before significant effects on vision occur.

Following keratomileusis *in situ* and lamellar keratectomy in 1990, the author detected a decrease in the IOP of some patients. At first it was thought that this IOP dropping was due to modification of radial curvature or thickness of the cornea. Later, it was supposed that suction was the lowering pressure mechanism, so in 1995 the application of the suction ring was started in a group of ocular hypertensive patients with no eye surgery antecedents. Intraocular pressure was measurably lower in a significant number of cases. This has also been seen in laser-assisted in situ keratomileusis (LASIK). It has been proposed that the decrease in IOP may be a real event.

The mechanism may well involve stretching of the zonule which stretching produces some form of change in the trabecular meshwork either physiologically through chemical mediators, or through a mechanical opening of the trabecular pores.

Pneumatic trabeculoplasty (PNT) is a noninvasive treatment, performed in an ophthalmologist office, which has been demonstrated to reduce the intraocular pressure (IOP) in patients with primary open-angle glaucoma (POAG), pigmentary glaucoma and ocular hypertension (OH).

The Ophthalmic International PNT device consists of a suction ring, a vacuum pump, and connecting tubing. The suction ring is made of disposable plastic. This ring is connected to a vacuum pump via three-way silicone tubing, which in turn connects to a single tube attached to the pump inlet.

The pump is preset to deliver a maximum vacuum pressure corresponding to 65 mm Hg within the eye. The pump also provides a digital timer which counts down the treatment time selected by the user. The ring is supplied

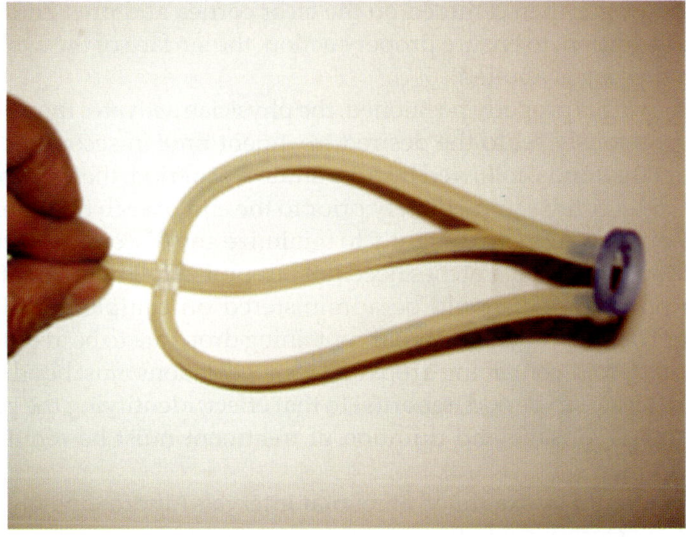

Fig. 1: Tubing of suctions

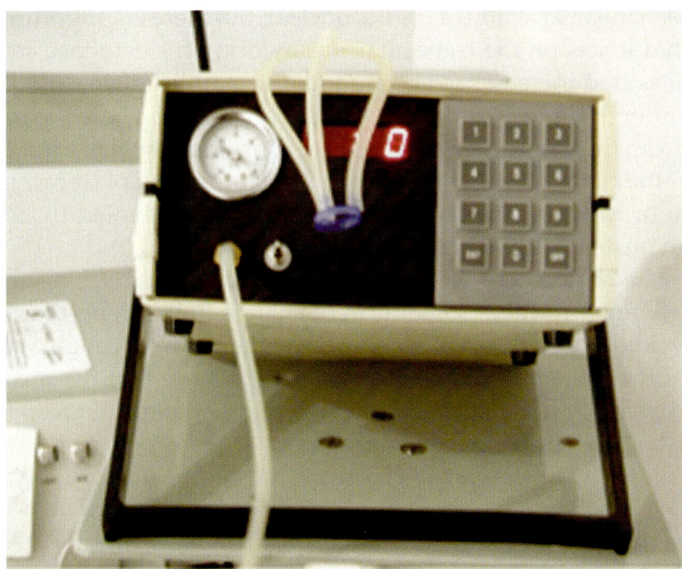

Fig. 2: Suction unit

sterile, while the other components, which do not contact the patient, are supplied no sterile.

To use the device to perform the PNT procedure, the physician first administers topical anesthesia to the patient. The patient is then placed in a supine position, and the eyelids are spread either manually (a speculum can be used but is not recommended). The ring must be positioned to clear the upper eyelid. The ring is then centered on the clear cornea and pressed downward slightly. In addition, to ensure proper suction, the surface of the eye should be wet when the ring is applied.

Once the ring is properly positioned, the physician activates the pump which has been previously set to the desired treatment time in seconds. Suction is applied for 60 seconds, followed by a 5-minute rest period, then repeated for an additional 60 seconds. Immediately prior to the end of each treatment period, the ring should be depressed slightly to minimize any discomfort to the patient when suction is released. Patches need not be applied following treatment, but one drop of antibiotic should be administered on completion of the PNT procedure. Tobradex or other steroid containing drops are to be avoided during this study. If steroid-containing drops and/or medications must be administered during the follow-up period, report(s) to that effect, identifying the patient, the eye(s) involved, dosage and duration of treatment must be remitted to the Medical Monitor.

Patients should be examined at regular intervals (approximately every 3 to 4 months) to determine whether additional treatments are needed to maintain IOP control. Preliminary trials have shown that a repeat of the procedure at 1 week provides a more profound and lasting decrease in IOP.

The mechanism of action of PNT is unclear, but there is supporting evidence to show that it acts on the trabecular meshwork. This evidence comes in the form of measured increases in accommodative amplitude in early presbyopic patients undergoing PNT, albeit of a temporary nature. There is corroborating evidence from the studies of Schachar and Thornton in which expansion of the sclera over the cilliary body either by means of implanted plastic ring segments (Schachar) or radial incisions (Thornton) was accompanied by a measured decrease in post-surgical IOP.

As we stated before the mechanism may well involve stretching of the zonule which stretching produces some form of change in the trabecular meshwork either physiologically through chemical mediators, or through a mechanical opening of the trabecular pores. Additional evidence that the mechanism of action involves improvement in outflow is that patients who respond well to latanoprost also seem to do well with PNT.

There is no evidence that PNT causes any form of cyclodialysis and no cases of PNT have shown either flare or cells post-treatment.

Clinical trials have demonstrated that approximately 75% of POAG patients will demonstrate a PNT response. Of these patients, approximately 50% will eliminate their need for medication and the remainder will demonstrate a reduction in medication requirements.

Pneumatic trabeculoplasty, when used in combination with antiglaucoma medication, was evaluated in two studies: a feasibility study involving 177 patients, and a separate efficacy study involving 317 eyes.

Both studies were nonblinded, single-armed, and nonrandomized; the primary efficacy end-point in each study was a decrease in intraocular pressure (IOP) compared with baseline. The first study reported a mean drop in IOP of

6.3 mm Hg across the entire group. The second study showed a mean IOP after PNT treatment level at least 1 mmHg less than the pretreatment mean; except at 3, 6, 9, and 12 months, when it was at least 2 mmHg less than the initial mean IOP. The lesser reduction observed in the second study can be explained by the fact that a number of the patients were at least partially controlled by antiglaucoma medications at enrollment, and, as a result, the group had a lower starting IOP than those enrolled in the first study. In both studies, a clear trend to less medication was observed when PNT was added to a patient's treatment regime. The ability of PNT to reduce IOP and medication requirements, along with its relatively benign safety profile, supports the use of PNT as part of a glaucoma patient's treatment regimen.

Adverse Events

Adverse events reported following PNT are generally mild in nature and resolve within a few days. Patients receiving PNT typically experience transient 'gray-out' of vision sometimes associated with multicolored light patterns during the application of the vacuum ring. These phenomena typically vanish with 30-40 seconds upon release of the vacuum. Patients may experience some mild ocular discomfort (conjunctival hyperemia and conjunctival hemorrhage) following the PNT procedure. This discomfort will typically resolve, without treatment, within a few hours but may last as long as a day or two. Long-term side effects are absent following PNT.

Considerations for Reduction in Antiglaucoma Medication

Generally speaking, reduction of antiglaucoma medications can begin three weeks following the PNT repeat application. Given the numerous variations in antiglaucoma medication regimes, it is not possible to recommend a single specific medication reduction strategy.

Substantive Equivalence of PNT and ALT

Argon laser trabeculoplasty is the procedure probably closest to being equivalent to pneumatic trabeculoplasty in its affect and possible mode of action. Clinical data show that, overall, PNT produces the same or similar reduction in IOP with fewer serious side effects and has the advantage of being both totally non-invasive and repeatable with high success rates in repeated treatment.

PNT lowers IOP in glaucoma patients at least as well, if not better than ALT and with much greater safety since no complications such as those reported to occur following ALT.

CONCLUSION

PNT can produce a significant reduction in IOP; reduction in IOP can be permanent; it is repeatable with similar or greater effect; can reduce or eliminate medication dependency; there is no damage to optic nerve fibers; does not accelerate/produce VF changes; may improve VA in some patients.

28

Combined Phacoemulsification and Deep Sclerectomy with T-Flux®

Pascal Rozot (France)

INTRODUCTION

The association of a primary open-angle glaucoma (POAG) and a cataract has led many ophthalmic surgeons to perform combined procedures, to treat the two diseases at the same time, in spite of the well-known hypotensive effect of catatact extraction alone, which seems to be limited in duration, rarely exceeding one year in actual glaucoma patients. Intraocular pressure (IOP) results were improved when going from extracapsular extraction to phacoemulsification, probably because of the reduction of the size of the incision, leading to less postoperative inflamation, but significant complications from hypotony were sometimes encountered after trabeculectomy associated to phacoemulsification. The combined procedure with deep sclerectomy and placement of a non-absorbable, hydrophilic acrylic drain (T-Flux®, IOL Tech Laboratories) is a safe procedure which can provide a sustained IOP reduction in glaucomatous eyes requiring cataract extraction.

SURGICAL TECHNIQUE

The combined surgery begins with cataract removal using phacoemulsification through a 2.8 mm clear corneal incision followed by implantation of a foldable intraocular lens (IOL). Then the anterior chamber is refilled with the rest of the ophthalmic viscoelastic device (OVD) used for phacoemulsification, in order to begin sclerectomy on a firm eye. The conjunctiva is opened at the limbus using Vannas scissors; a superficial (one third of the sclera) 4.5 × 4.5 mm scleral flap is dissected quite anteriorly using a disposable crescent knife.

Then a trapezoidal profound flap is pre-cut with a disposable 15° blade and dissected with the crescent knife. At this step, it is particularly important to enter directly into the Schlemm'canal at the end of the dissection. Next, mitomycin-C at concentration 0.2 mg/ml is applied for one to two minute, this time being used: first, to check the permeability of the two openings of the Shlemm's canal with a trabeculotome, or a Rycroft cannula, and secondly to remove the trabeculum of the inner wall of the Shlemm's canal using the disposable capsulorhexis forceps. This step is facilitated by the absence of aqueous outflow through the surgical wound from the trabecular area, as the

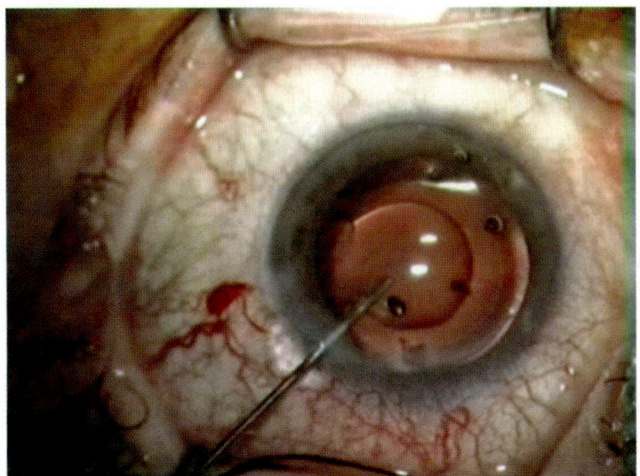

Fig. 1

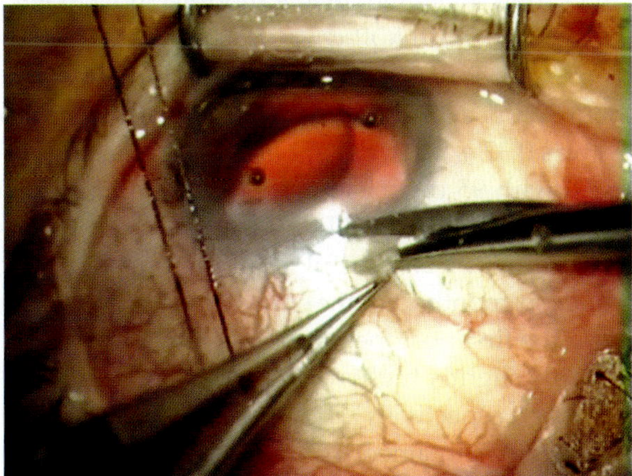

Fig. 2

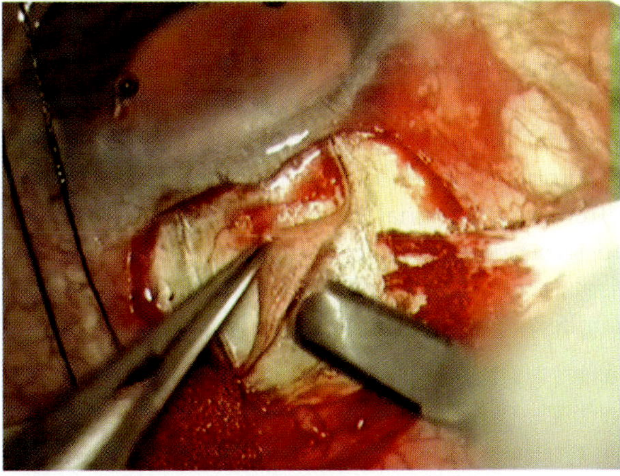

Fig. 3

the anterior chamber is filled with the OVD ("dry technique"). After having carefully rinsed the mitomycin-C, the non-absorbable, hydrophilic acrylic drain is placed beneath the superficial scleral flap and embedded into the deep sclerectomy to create a permanent drainage space. No suture fixation of the is required, as the two lateral tips of the device enter the Shlemm's canal, preventing any migration. There is also no need for suturing of the superficial flap; only two 10/0 Vicryl sutures are placed to close the conjunctiva at the limbus. Finally, the OVD is completely aspirated beneath and below the IOL with the I/A cannula.

Personal Study

Here is presented a retrospective study of 200 consecutive eyes of 158 patients aged 72 ± 11 were operated on between September 2001, and November 2003. Follow-up for the group averaged 26 ± 8 months and ranged from 16 to 41 months. Prior to surgery, mean IOP was 19.2 ± 4.4 mm Hg and patients were using an average of 1.4 ± 0.9 glaucoma medications, with at least one medication being used in about 80% of eyes. The preoperative best distance corrected visual acuity (BCDVA) was 0.37 ± 0.24 ; the spherical equivalent was – 3.5 diopters ± 6.4 (–26 to +6 D) with 95 myopes > –1D (47.5%) and 34 hyperopes >+1D (17%). About one half of the eyes had POAG.

The surgery was initially successful in all but one eye, which went on to trabeculectomy after six months. For the entire group, mean IOP was reduced to 13.1 + 6 mm Hg on the first postoperative day, remained at 13.6 mm Hg at 12 months, and was only slightly higher at 24 and 36 months (15.2 ± 3.3 mm Hg and 15.1 + 3.3 mm Hg, respectively).

IOP control has been maintained without the need for goniopuncture in any eye and with minimal use of topical hypotensive medication. At the last available visit, medical therapy was being used in only 36 (21%) of 171 eyes. That treatment consisted of a single agent in 19 eyes, a betablocker plus a prostaglandin in 16 eyes, and 3 medications in a single eye. The postoperative BCDVA was 0.67 ± 0.30, with a mean postoperative equivalent of –0.74 diopters ± 1.38. 71% of the eyes gained at least 2 lines of visual acuity; 4.5 % lost least 2 lines of visual acuity. The only complications encountered were: a malignant glaucoma treated by posterior vitrectomy; a retinal detachment in 12 diopters myopic patient, which required two procedures to flatten the retina. There was no case of migration or displacement of the drain, neither under the conjunctiva nor inside the anterior chamber.

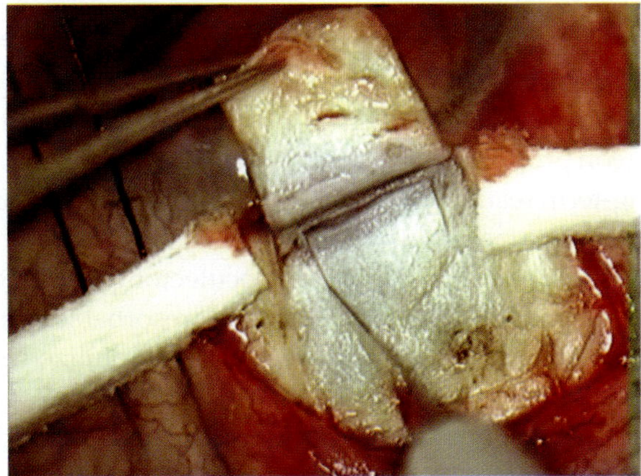

Fig. 4

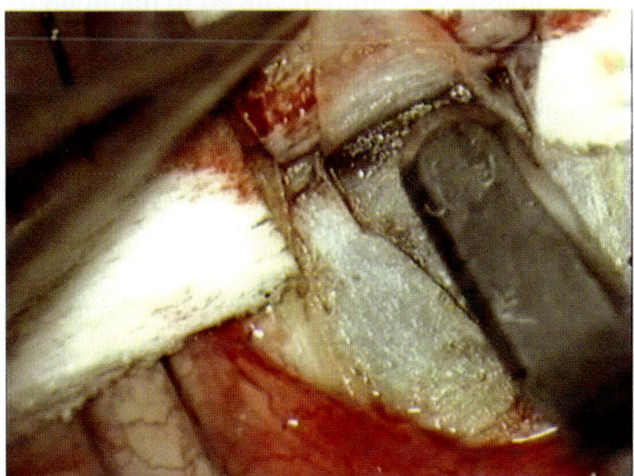

Fig. 5

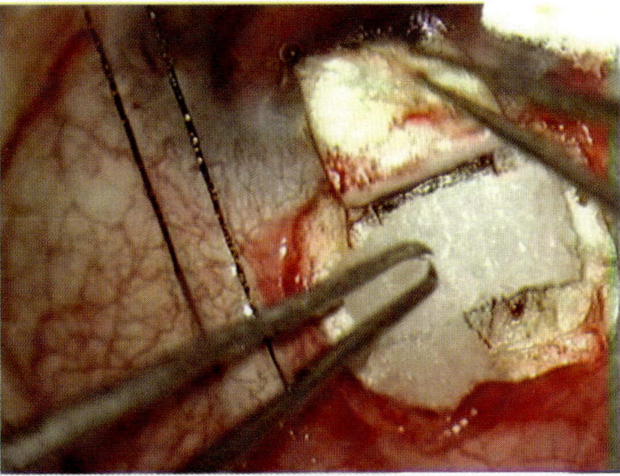

Fig. 6

CONCLUSION

Since its first description in 1989, deep sclerectomy (DS) has regularly evolved to attain a reproducible surgical method, which is not yet stereotyped, as every ophthalmic surgeon propose his own technique. The IOP results are fairly good, even though long-term results are sometimes deceiving. The main advantage of DS is the absence of postoperative hypotony with its well-known complications; it also give less astigmatic change than trabeculectomy. From the beginning, many authors have proposed the adjunction of resorbable drainage devices, such as collagen, as Aquaflow® processed from lyophilized porcine scleral collagen or reticulated hyaluronic acid (SK-Gel®). Histopathological evaluation confirmed that the presence of a drain could form a smooth and regular intrascleral space to prevent collapse of the scleral flap over the site of the DS. More recently, a non resorbable drain made of hydrophilic acrylic material and designed by E. Dahan has been commercialized to maintain more durably an wide opened intrascleral space. With this drain, Ates et al showed IOP success rates comparable to viscocanalostomy, with few complications. As it has been recently proved that the adjunction of mitomycin-C could give better IOP results without increasing the complication rate, it appears logical to use this drug to reduce a possible postoperative fibrosis around this foreign body represented by the acrylic drain.

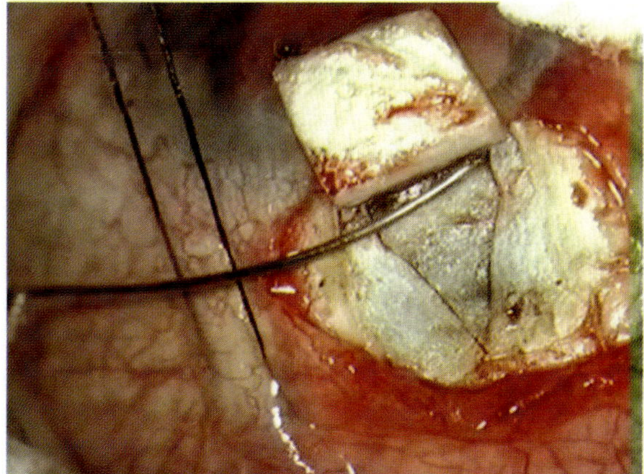

Fig. 7

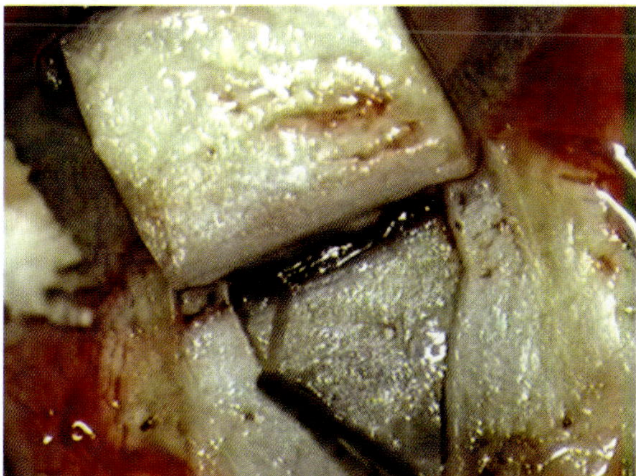

Fig. 8

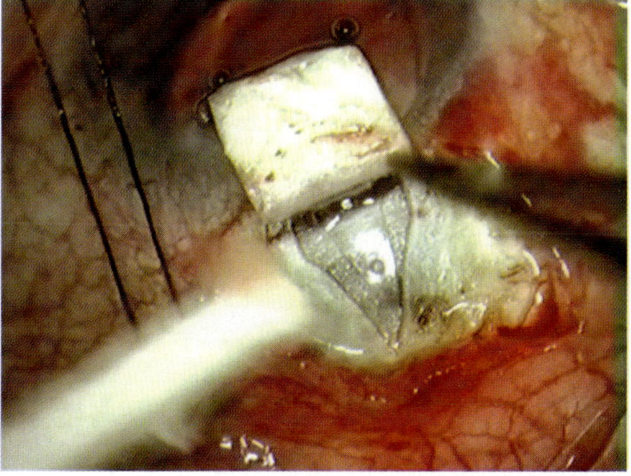

Fig. 9

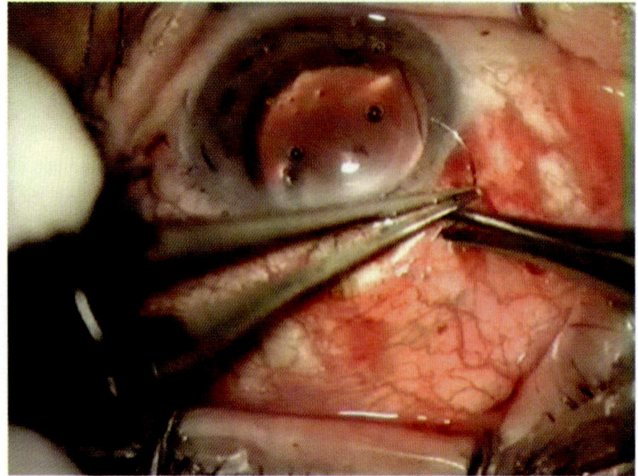

Fig. 10

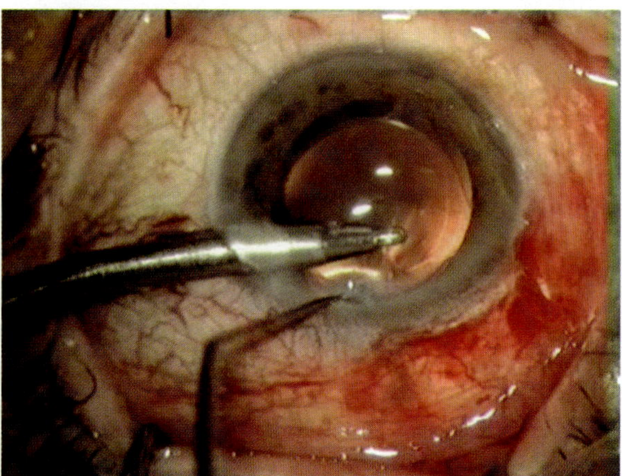

Figs 1 to 11: Various surgical steps of combined procedure

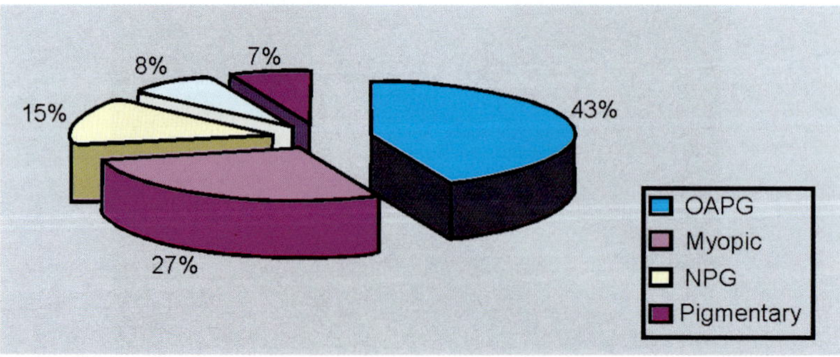

Fig. 12: Graphic presentation of various clinical glaucoma in study

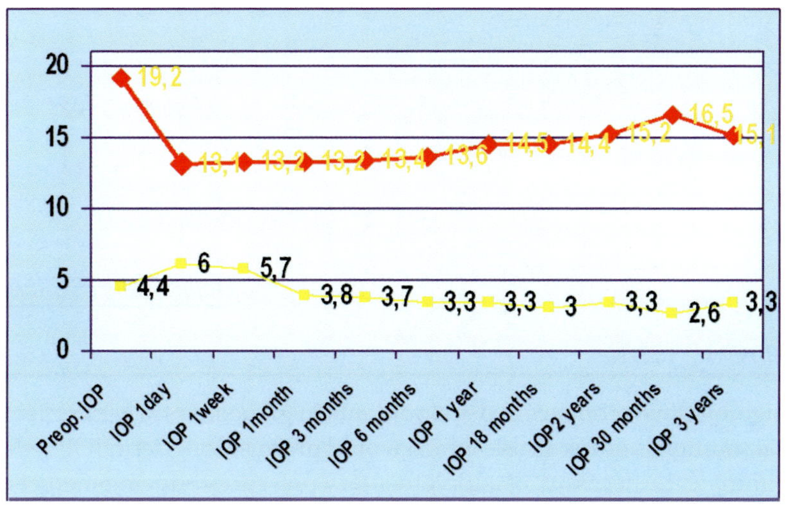

Fig. 13: Preoperative and postoperative IOP control chart at various durations

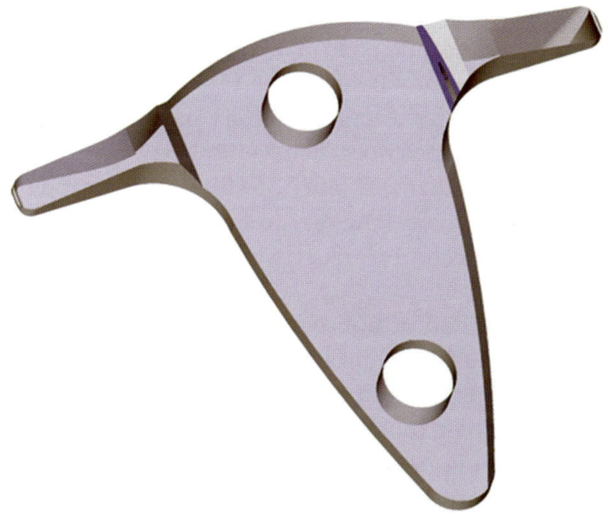

Fig. 14: Non-resorbable Hydrophetic acrylic drain

29

Sclerothalamotomy Ab Interno: A Minimally Invasive Surgical Option for Glaucoma

Bojan Pajic (Switzerland)

INTRODUCTION

The ongoing devote on recent developments in glaucoma surgery reflects that an ideal solution is not available which would promise long-term IOP reduction and eliminate the necessity of supplementary pressure-reducing medication at low complication rates. Trabeculectomy, first described in the sixties is probably the most widespread approach in glaucoma surgery presently. The intention of trabeculectomy is to bypass the resistance of trabecular meshwork by channeling aqueous humor directly to the Schlemm's canal. In literature the success rate of trabeculectomy ranges between 32 and 96%. On the other hand, postoperative complications like hypotony and choroidal detachment are reported up to 24%. Variation of success rates may be explained by different criteria of surgical indications, selection of cases, various diagnoses, the various degrees of surgical experience and variations in postoperative medical treatment. Failure of pressure regulations is associated with the assence of a filtering bleb and depends on the duration of follow-up involved. It has become evident that successful reduction in IOP following trabeculectomy is clearly related to the presence of a filtering bleb.

The more recent method of non-penetrating deep sclerectomy, was first described by Fjodorov in the eighties. This techniques tries to achieves an improved uveoscleral outflow and therefore is not depending on the presence of a filtering bleb. Koslov expanded this method by introducing a collagen implant. Literature on non-penetrating deep sclerectomy indicates a success rate of 58 to 74% without collagen implant and 74 to 90% with collagen implantation.

In 1976, Benedikt described that the exposure of the ciliary body (i.e. a form of penetrating sclerectomy) was leading to successful long-term IOP regulation in 27 of 38 cases involving hemorrhagic, aphakic and irreversible angle-closure glaucoma after initially failed filtering surgery. This technique was the basis for later development of perforating deep sclerectomy, a method which has been used since 1985 was described previously as *"sclerothalamectomy."* Bypassing of the trabecular meshwork is an alternative for aqueous humor outflow from the anterior chamber to the Schlemm canal. It is the principal mechanism for

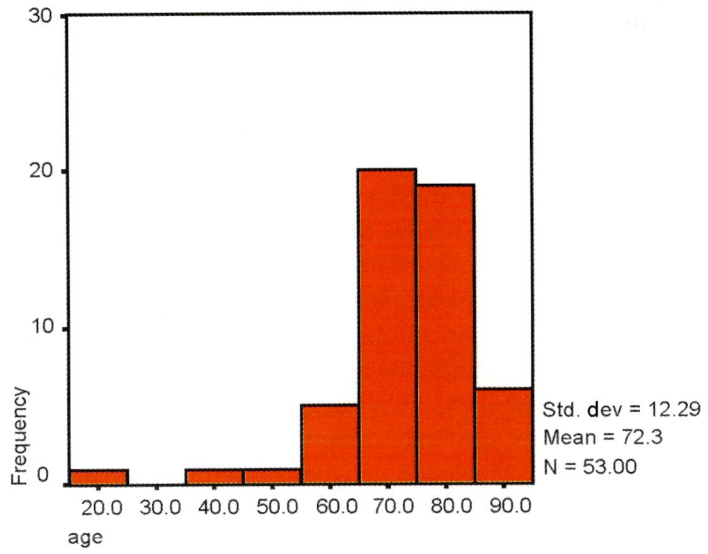

Fig. 1: Mean age

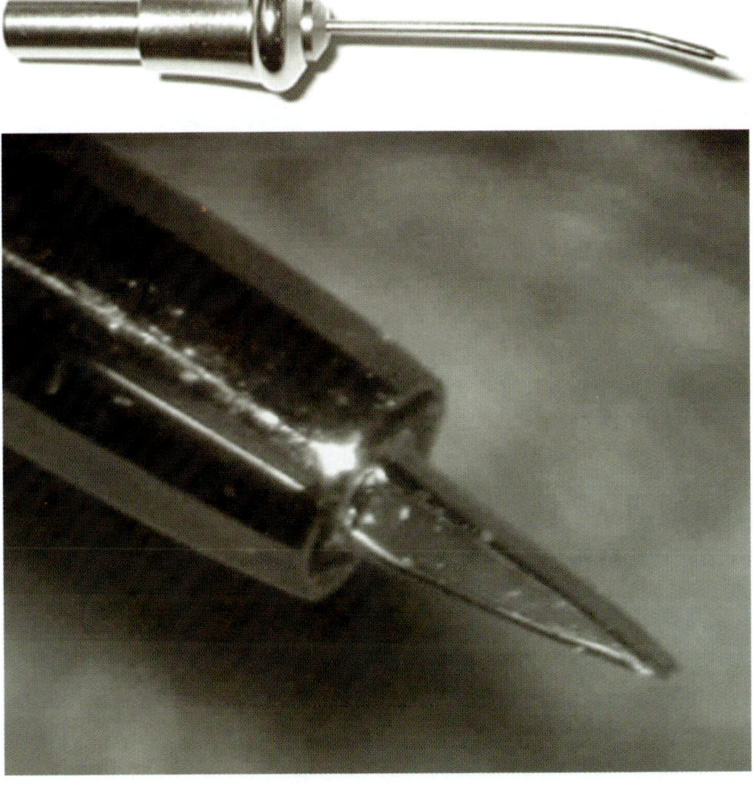

Figs 2A and B: STT glaucoma tip (Oertli Reference VE 201750)

non-penetrating glaucoma surgery, in particular, for deep sclerectomy and viscocanalostomy. These surgical procedures provide effective IOP reduction as well as the elimination of typical filtration bleb complications. So far clinical application of these procedures has been limited by technical difficulties to perform this kind of surgery and a poor predictability of pressure reduction.

The concept of trabecular meshwork bypass as a surgical principle for glaucoma treatment evolved from the discovery that pathologic outflow resistance is caused primarily by the juxtacanalicular conjunctival tissue of the trabecular meshwork and, in particular, by the inner wall of the Schlemm canal. A further publication in this area indicates that 35% of the outflow resistance arises distally to the inner wall of the Schlemm canal.

Spiegel et al have described a new surgical technique involving the use of an implanted tube, the so-called trabecular meshwork bypass tube shunt, which should provide a direct connection between Schlemm canal and the anterior chamber. This surgical technique avoids technical difficulties of non-penetrating deep sclerectomy, especially the delicate microperforation of the trabecular meshwork in order to ensure the permeability of the Descemet's membrane. Furthermore, these techniques avoid the disadvantages of filtration blebs.

All surgical procedures for glaucoma involving the creation of external access may be complicated by the risk of fibroblast proliferation and failure of filtration. The novel procedure published offers a chance to avoid some of the above-mentioned disadvantages. We refer to this technique as *sclerothalamotomy ab interno*.

PATIENTS AND METHODS

Before beginning the clinical study phase, the tips used for the STT ab interno procedure were developed using a large number of pigs' eyes. The high-frequency diathermic technique was already very well known in the application for capsulorhexis in cataract surgery. It was important to create a design for optimal application of the STT probe in the iridocorneal angle and to evaluate the charcteristic of the achieved deep sclerotomy. By virtue of this results the STT ab interno probe development as describe below.

53 sclerothalamotomies ab interno in 53 patients were carried out in primary open-angle glaucoma between 1 April 2002 and 31 July 2002. Main inclusion criterion into this study was an insufficient response to medical treatment of IOP. Data were documented according to a prospective study protocol. Mean age of patients were 72.3±12.3 years (range: 15-92 years) patients (32%) were female, 36 patients (68%) male. In 25 cases (47.4%) the right eye in 28 cases (52.6%) the left eye was treated. There was no patient who received bilateral surgery. Snellen visual acuity was 0.7 ± 0.3 (range 0.1 to 1.0) preoperatively. In 5 cases a moderate cataract was observed which didn't have influence on the visual acuity.

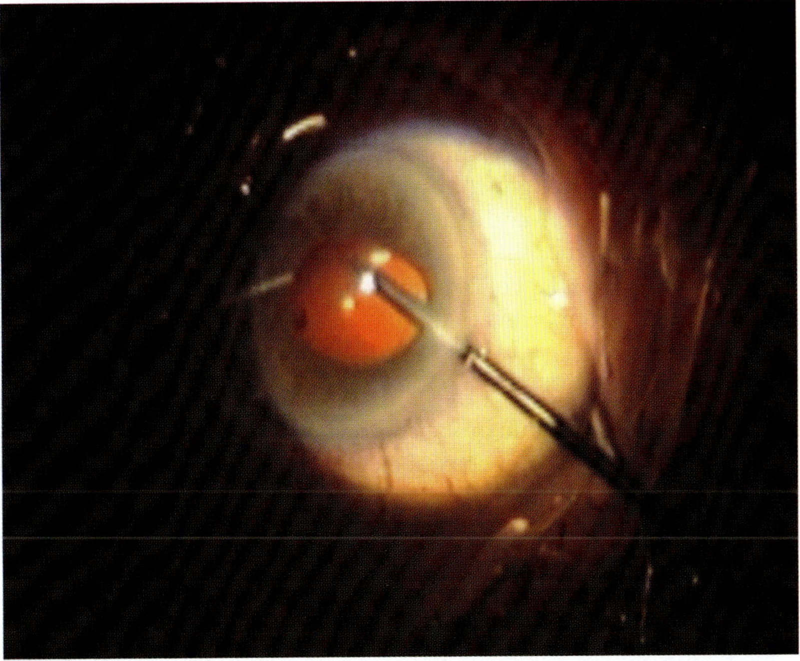

Fig. 3: Insertion of the high-frequency diathermic probe (Oertli) through the temporal corneal insertion

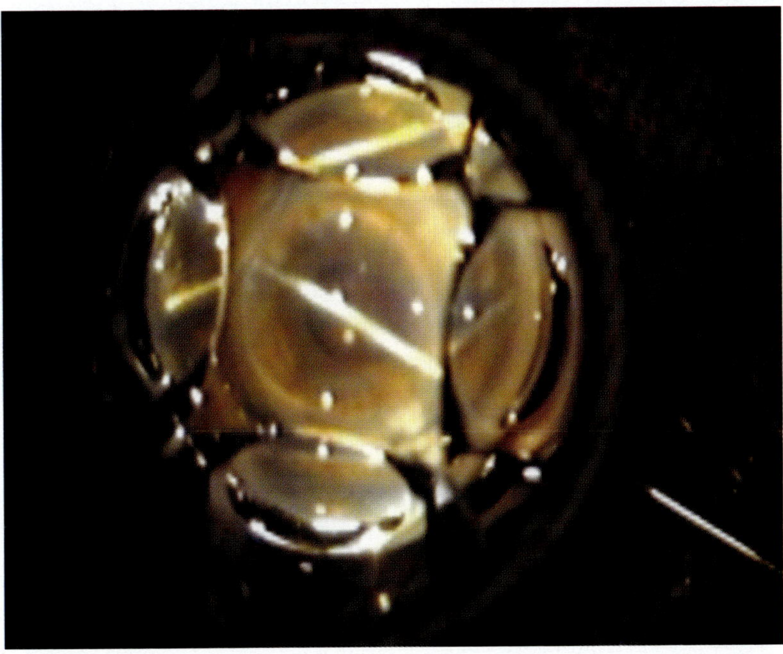

Fig. 4: Visual inspection of the target zone (opposite iridocorneal angle) by a 4-mirror gonioscopic lens

A complete ophthalmologic status check was carried out in each patient prior to surgery including: uncorrected and best corrected visual acuity, IOP applanation tonometry, biomicroscopy of anterior segment, funduscopy (in particular, stereoscopie evaluation of the optic nerve head) and computerized visual field testing (Octopus 101, program G2).

Complete ophthalmologic follow-up examinations were carried out postoperatively at day 1, 2, 3 and 4, after 1, 2 and 4 weeks, and 2, 3, 6, 12, 15, 18, 21, 24, 27, 30, 33 and 36 months.

In a pilot study with at least of 24 months follow-up, 5 patients with therapy-resistant juvenile glaucoma were treated.

High-frequency Diathermic Probe

The high-frequency diathermic probe consists of an inner platinum electrode which is isolated from the outer coaxial electrode. The platinum probe tip is 1 mm in length, 0.3 mm high and 0.6 mm width and is bent posteriorly at an angle of 15°. The external diameter of the probe measures 0.9 mm. Modulated 500 kHz current generates a temperature of approximate 130°C at the tip of the probe. The set-up provides high frequency power dissipation in close vicinity of the tip. As a result, heating of tissue is locally very limited and is applied as a rotationed ellipsoid.

Surgical Procedure

A clear cornea incision (1.2 mm wide) was placed in the temporal upper quadrant using a diamond knife. A second corneal incision was performed 120° apart from the first followed by injection of Healon GV. The high-frequency diathermic probe (Oertli) was inserted through the temporal corneal insertion. Visual inspection of the target zone (opposite iridocorneal angle) was observed by a 4-mirror gonioscopic lens. The high frequency tip penetrates up to 1 mm nasal into the sclera through the trabecular meshwork and Schlemm canal, forming a deep sclerotomy (i.e. "thalami") of 0.3 mm high and 0.6 mm width. This procedure was repeated 4 times within one quadrant. Healon GV was evacuated from the anterior chamber with bimanual irrigation/aspiration. Tobramycin/dexamethason eyedrops were then applied 3 × daily for 1 month and pilocarpin 2% eyedrops 3 × daily for 10 days.

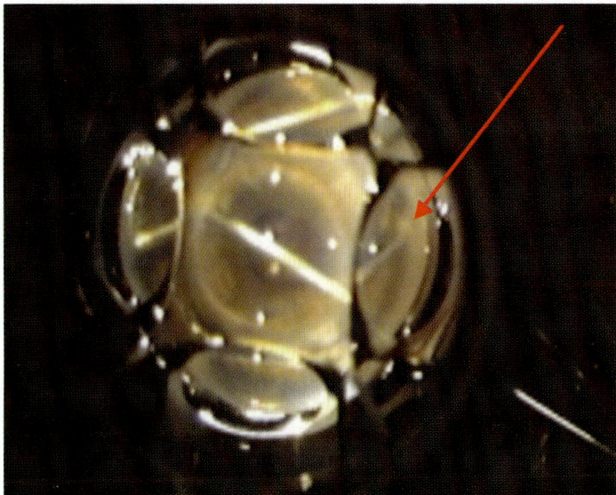

Fig. 5: Penetration of the high frequency tip

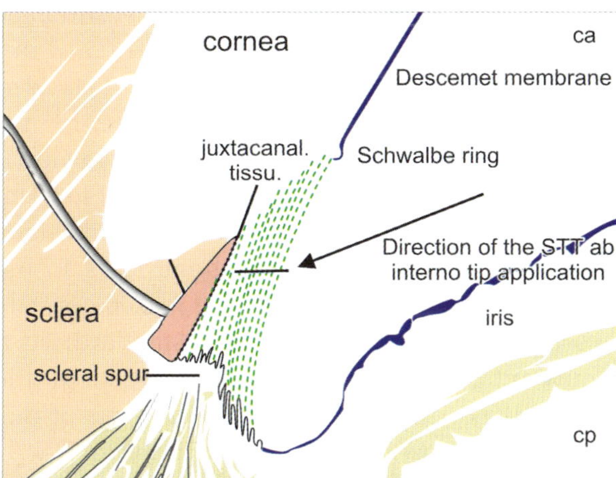

Fig. 6: Penetration up to 1 mm nasal into the sclera through the trabecular meshwork and Schlemm canal

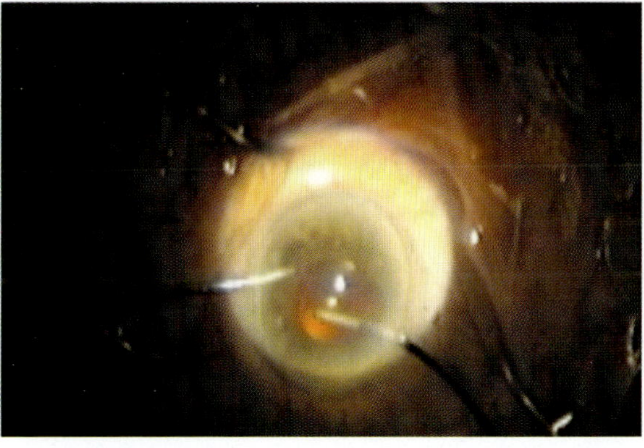

Fig. 7: Healon GV was evacuated from the anterior chamber with bimanual irrigation/aspiration

Evaluation of the Results

Statistical evaluation of results was calculated with SPSS Program Version 10. Two-tailed Student *t*-test was used for statistical evaluation of parametric data. The unit of significance was set at a critical p value of <0.05, including Bonferroni correlation for repetitive use of data sets.

RESULTS

Mean preoperative IOP in the study population of 53 patients with primary open-angle glaucoma was 25.6 ± 2.3 mm Hg (range 18 to 48 mm Hg). Average IOP was 17.6 ± 2.7 mm Hg (range 2 to 36 mm Hg) after a follow-up period of 1 day, 14.9 ± 2.4 mm Hg (range 2 to 30 mm Hg) after 2 days, 15.7 ± 2.4 mm Hg (range 4 to 28 mm Hg) after 3 days, 16.0 ± 2.6 mm Hg (range 4 to 36 mm Hg) after 4 days, 19.0 ± 2.6 mm Hg (range 12 to 39 mm Hg) after 7 days, 16.9 ± 2.5 mm Hg (range 9 to 44 mm Hg) after 1 month, 15.1 ± 1.8 mm Hg (range 11 to 20 mm Hg) after 3 months, 14.7 ± 1.7 mm Hg (range 11 to 20 mm Hg) after 6 months, 14.8 ± 1.7 mm Hg (range 10 to 20 mm Hg) after 9 months, 14.7 ± 1.7 mm Hg (range 10 to 20 mm Hg) after 12 months, 15.5 ± 1.7 mm Hg (range 11 to 20 mm Hg) after 15 months, 14.1 ± 1.6 mm Hg (range 11 to 20 mm Hg) after 18 months, 16.5 ± 1.7 mm Hg (range 12 to 22 mm Hg) after 21 months, 15.0 ± 1.6 mm Hg (range 11 to 20 mm Hg) after 24 months, 14.7 ± 1.7 mm Hg (range 11 to 20 mm Hg) after 27 months, 14.7 ± 1.7 mm Hg (range 10 to 20 mm Hg) after 30 months, 15.5 ± 1.7 mm Hg (range 11 to 20 mm Hg) after 33 months and 14.6 ± 1.7 mm Hg (range 10 to 20 mm Hg) after 36 months a result which, at $p<0.005$, is statistically highly significant. Pressure reduction at any time of standardised follow up was statistically significant compared to preoperative data at a level of $\alpha<0.03$ (Bonferroni corrected). For all patients the follow-up was 36 months.

At month 36, 54.7% of patients had an IOP<15 mm Hg, 77.4% had an IOP<18 mm Hg and 83% had an IOP<21 mm Hg. After 36 months, 86.8% achieved >20% reduction in IOPs and 77% of treated patients achieved >30% reductions of the IOP. The complete success rate, defined as an IOP lower than 21 mm Hg

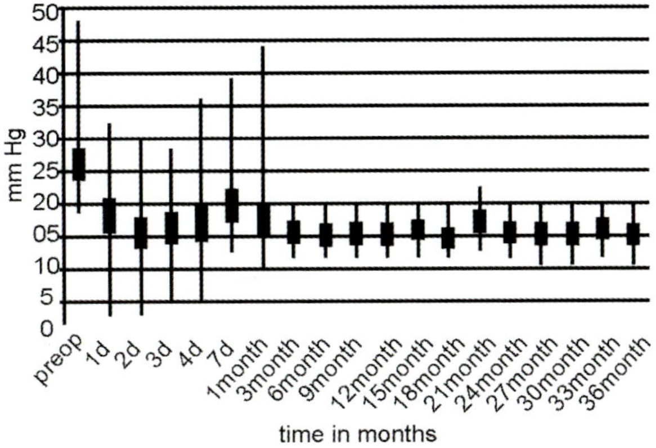

Fig. 8: Average level of intraocular pressure (IOP) after sclerothalamotomy (STT) ab interno surgery for all 53 cases at the time of scheduled examination

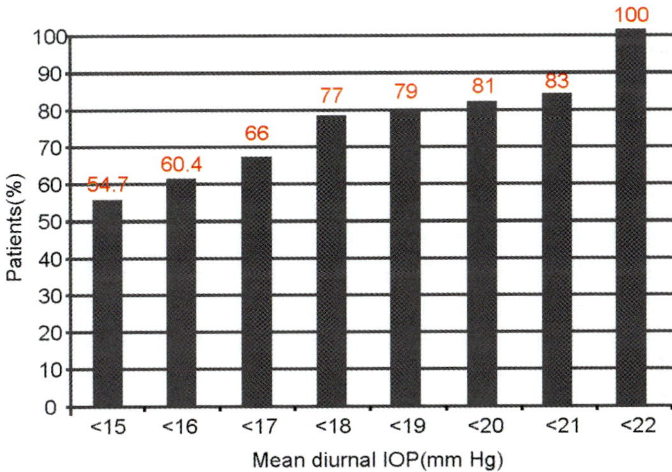

Fig. 9: Percentages of patients reaching specified intraocular pressure (IOP) levels

without medication, was 83% at 36 months. Qualified success rate, defined as an IOP lower than 21 mm Hg with medication, was 100% at 36 months.

The average preoperative administration of pressure-reducing eye agents was 2.6 ± 1.0. Following surgery, this value was decreased to 0.45 ± 0.72 after 1 month, 0.38 ± 0.60 after 3 months 0.38 ± 0.69 after 6 months, 0.19 ± 0.52 after 12 months, 0.21 ± 0.53 after 24 months and 0.50 ± 0.90 after 36 months. After 36 months, it was necessary to administer IOP reducing medication in only 9 eyes, a figure which corresponds to 17% of all cases.

Average visual acuity after treatment was 0.69 ± 0.31 (range 0.05 to 1.0). In 6 eyes (11.3%) moderate cataract development after surgery which was without influence of visual acuity. Another 3 eyes (5.7%) developed cataract with decreased visual acuity of one Snellen's line.

There is no significant difference regarding the cup/disc ratio at baseline with 0.65±0.18 and at 36 months with 0.66±0.19 ($p = 0.11$).

There is no significant changes comparing the visual field at baseline with mean defect MD 9.45±2.32, loss variance LV 30.0±5.11 and at 36 months with MD 9.29 ± 2.59, LV 31.4 ± 5.66 ($p = 0.78$ for MD, $p = 0.96$ for LV).

Temporary IOP elevation higher than 21 mm Hg was observed in 12 of 53 eyes (22.6%). These patients responded well to pressure-reducing treatment with one agent and medication could gradually be withdrawn in all of these patients. A single case of hypotension (1.9%) that lasted for 3 days after surgery was observed. Hyphema was present in 6 cases (11.4%) which disappeared within the first 2 weeks after surgery. One eye (1.9%) exhibited transient fibrin formation at pupillary level. Fibrin was cleared within one day after frequent application of topical dexamethason.

In a pilot study 5 patients with therapy-resistant juvenile glaucoma were treated. We observed an IOP reduction from 41 ± 6.4 mm Hg prior to surgery to 12 ± 2.6 mm Hg after surgery, a result that has remained stable without any additional pressure-reducing therapy for 24 months.

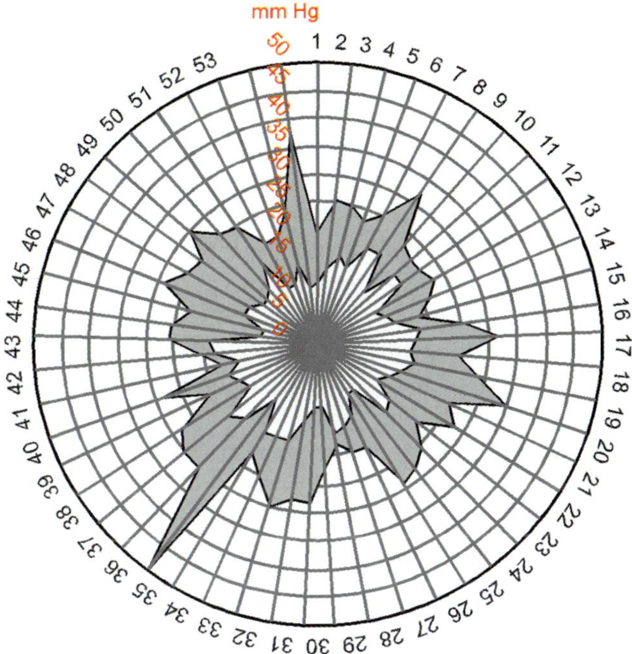

Fig. 10: Preoperative and postoperative level of IOP 36 months of follow-up

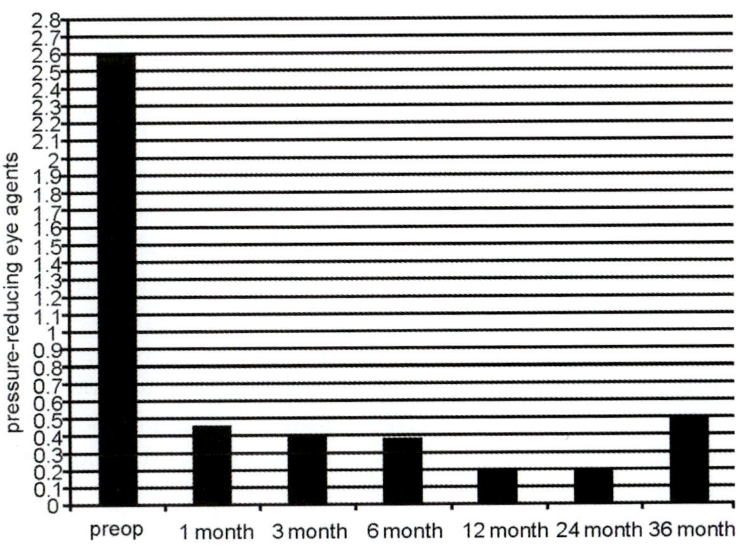

Fig. 11: Administration of pressure-reducing eye agents during 36 months

DISCUSSION

This study reports long-term results of a new surgical technique for treating open angle glaucoma. The STT ab interno method intends the creation of a direct channel between the anterior chamber and the Schlemm canal. Persistence of the sclerotomy can be investigated with a 3-mirror Lens (Goldmann 903). The STT ab interno tip creates a deep sclerotomy with subsequent access of aqueous to the scleral layer. Both aspects may facilitate a bypass effect of aqueous outflow. In light of the fact that about 85% of the aqueous humor drains (in physiological terms) trans-trabecularly, we suspect an additional route for aqueous humour absorption in the case of elevated IOP. There is evidence in literature that such bypass effects may be present after surgical intervention which do not lead to the formation of filtering blebs. In a previous study, it was ascertained that eyes without filter bleb exhibited very stable long-term IOP regulation postoperatively. In addition to the bypassing of trabecular outflow resistance caused by STT ab interno treatment, outflow resistance may be further reduced by scleral thinning at the base of the thalamus. In addition to that aqueous humor could perhaps be absorbed by the ciliary body. After early postoperative reduction, the average IOP continued to decline gradually over a period of 6 months before reaching a relatively a constant level . It can be speculated that newly formed blood vessel and lymph vessel close to the surgical site, may contribute to the decrease of IOP level during follow-up.

In literature the success rate range for trabeculectomy ranges between 57% and 96% for deep sclerectomy without collagen device between 57% and 74%, and for deep sclerectomy with collagen device between 58% and 90 %. The STT ab interno technique with a complete success rate of 90.6% is comparable with other so far published surgery methods.

Advantages of the STT ab interno method, compared with trabeculectomy and perforating and non-perforating deep sclerectomy seem to be a rate of postoperative complications and a constant level of reduced IOP. Hypotension, a frequent finding in trabeculectomy, perforating deep sclerectomy and non-perforating deep sclerectomy, is a relatively rare postoperative complication. The most frequent early complications in trabeculectomy are hyphema (24.6%), shallow anterior chamber (23.9%), hypotony (24.3%), wound leak (17.8%) and choroidale detachment (14.1%). The most frequent late complications are cataract (20.2%), visual loss (18.8%), iris incarceration (5.1%) and encapsulated bleb (3.4%). After STT ab interno cataract development was seen in 17% with only 5.7% loss of one line of visual acuity after 36 months. Compared with other techniques STT ab interno seems to be a relatively save surgical technique.

Transient IOP elevation after STT ab interno may occur in the first 6 weeks and can be effectively brought under control with the use of a topical medication. In most cases, IOP-reducing therapy could be gradually withdrawn after 3

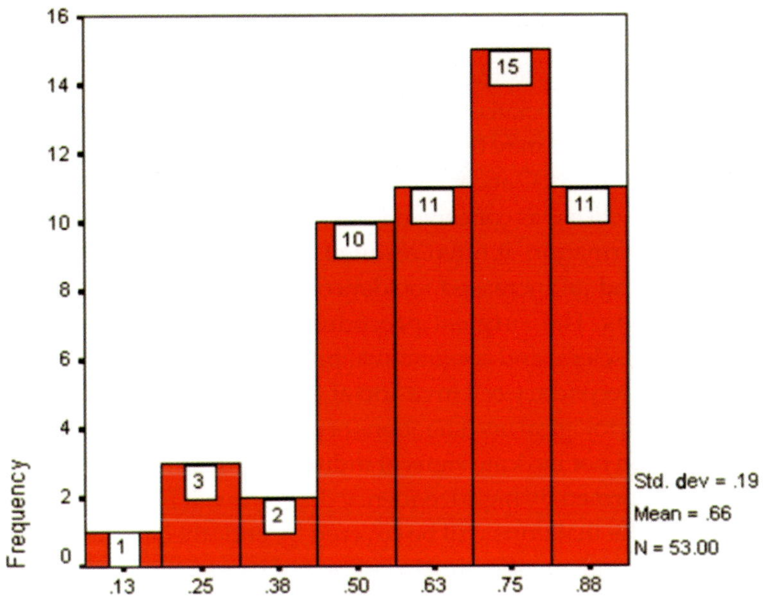

Fig. 12A: Cup/disc ratio at baseline

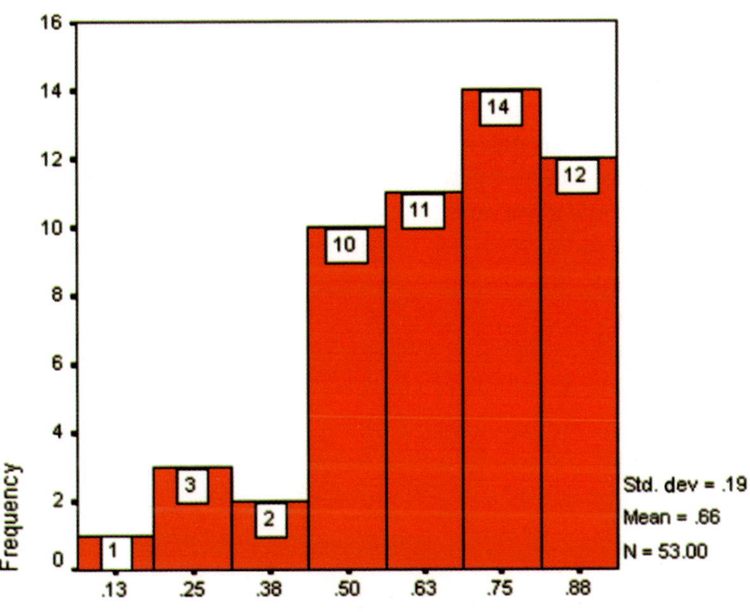

Fig. 12B: Cup/disc ratio at 36 months

weeks post surgery. It was necessary to continue pressure-reducing therapy in 5 of 53 eyes, in all this cases medication was effective in controlling IOP.

Problems of scarring to the Tenon's capsule, fibroblast proliferation and secondary occlusion associated with trabeculectomy which are induced by the surgical procedure itself may the reason behind the practice of antimetabolites applications (Mitomycin C at concentration of 0.2–0.4 mg/ml for 1-5 minutes). Although this practice was conceived to modulate wound healing and thus to counteract scar formation, it often resulted in serious complications, such as scleral necrosis and an increased incidence of avascular filter bleb and their late complications. The surgical procedure applied in this study avoids stimulation of episcleral and conjunctival proliferations and may therefore be related with less secondary cell invasion at the filtrating bypass.

Preliminary histological investigations of postmortem human eyes following STT ab interno did not indicate signs of indirect necrosis in cell layers adjacent to the thalamus formed by high-frequency diathermy. It is yet unknown, if the inner surface of the thalamus will be covered by endothelial cells of corneal or trabecular origin, and whether the thalamus and its function will remain intact on a much longer time scale.

Advantages to STT ab interno include the comparative simplicity and quickness of the surgical procedure itself.

This study point out, that the performance of 4 thalami has so far proved sufficient, what corresponds to a resorption surface area of 2.4 mm^2. The number of 4 thalami was defined empirical. Regarding the results of this study the creation of 4 thalami seems to provide a sufficient long-term decrease of IOP as a low rate of postoperative complications. For a further potentiality of IOP decreasing effect we recommend to perform up to 6 thalami.

A randomized multicentre study will be conducted in the future to compare STT ab interno, trabeculectomy, and deep sclerectomy for the surgical treatment of primary open angle glaucoma.

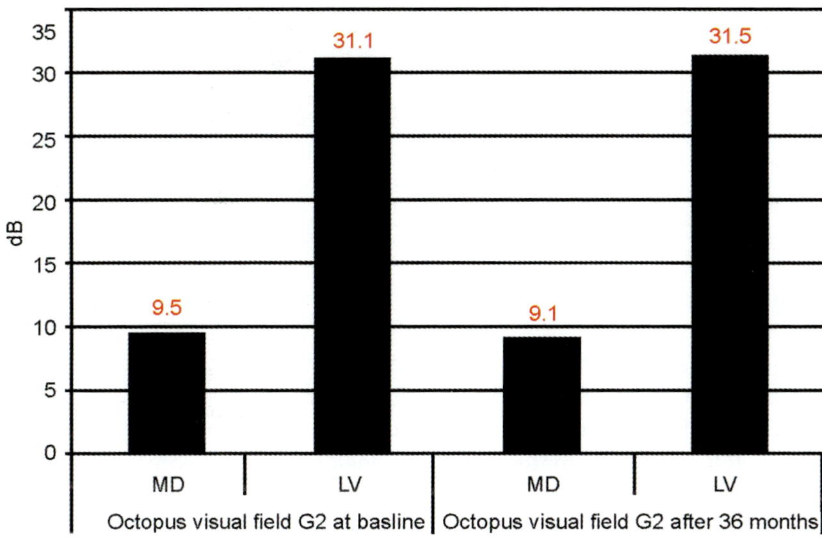

Fig. 13: Visual field analysis

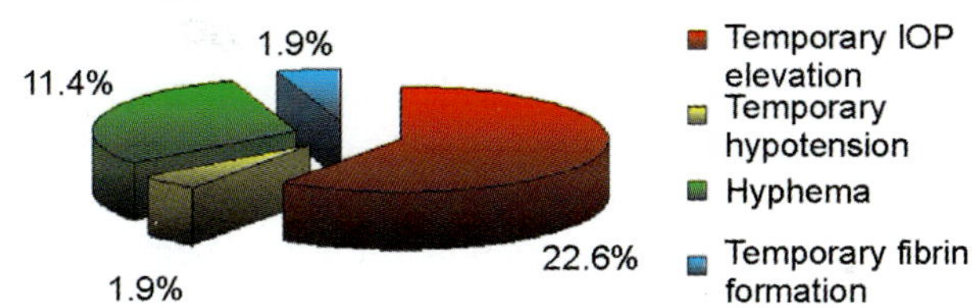

Fig. 14: Complications after sclerothalamotomy (STT) ab interno surgery

30

Sutureless Filtration Surgery in Glaucoma

RC Nagpal (India)

INTRODUCTION

WHO-NPCB (national program for control of blindness) survey in 1995 revealed that glaucoma accounts for blindness in 5.1 million persons (13.5% of the global blindness). In the United States glaucoma is the second leading cause of blindness. It has been estimated to be responsible for approximately 0.6 million new cases of blindness every year. In India with population of blind of 12 million, 0.8 % is due to glaucoma.

The management of glaucoma is directed towards reduction of intraocular pressure to a level that allows good perfusion of the optic nerve head so that it remains viable. It can be achieved medically, surgically or by a combination of both. In pre-surgical era, different medicaments have been used to lower intraocular pressure to a safer level, but surgical intervention became necessary when there was progressive glaucomatous damage despite maximum available medical therapy. Compliance to the medical treatment has always been a problem in the management of glaucoma in developing countries and a need was felt to find a really reliable successful, predictable, practicable surgical procedure to manage this complicated ocular disorder with minimal / negligible complications.

In earlier times, surgical procedures were full thickness fistulising procedures like Elliott's trephine and Schie's thermosclerostomy. These surgical procedures reduced intraocular pressure to safer levels but were associated with a host of complications. Cairns trabeculectomy (a partial thickness scleral flap filtering procedure introduced in 1967) was an attempt to optimize the surgical treatment of glaucoma. But cairns trabeculectomy and its later modifications had their own share of complications such as laceration of the scleral flap, excessive tissue trauma due to prolonged grasping of the scleral flap, foreign body reaction and local irritation because of problems with preparation of scleral flap and suture induced astigmatism.

Keeping in mind these complications, a study was published in 1996 by Lai and Lam in which they did trabeculectomy with iridectomy through a sutureless scleral tunnel. The newer technique has overcome many of the complications associated with classical trabeculectomy with sutures. This technique of sutureless trabeculectomy through scleral tunnel with peripheral iridectomy had also complications like hemorrhage, lamellar iridectomy injury to the lens and local iris atrophy as a result of iridectomy.

Keeping in view the aforesaid complications of classical trabeculectomy newer concept of sutureless filtration surgery through scleral tunnel has been

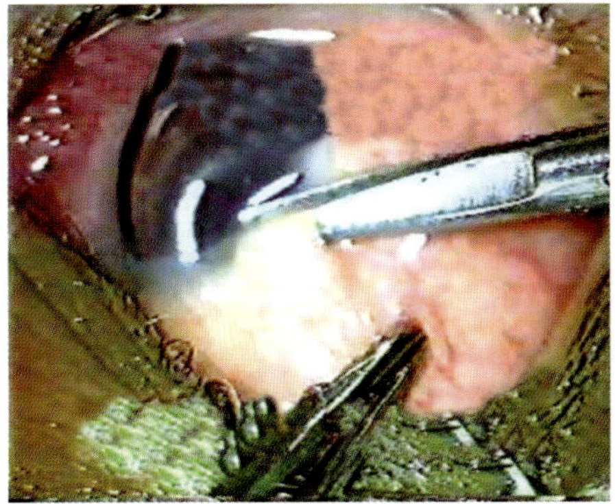

Fig. 1: Fornix-based conjunctival flap

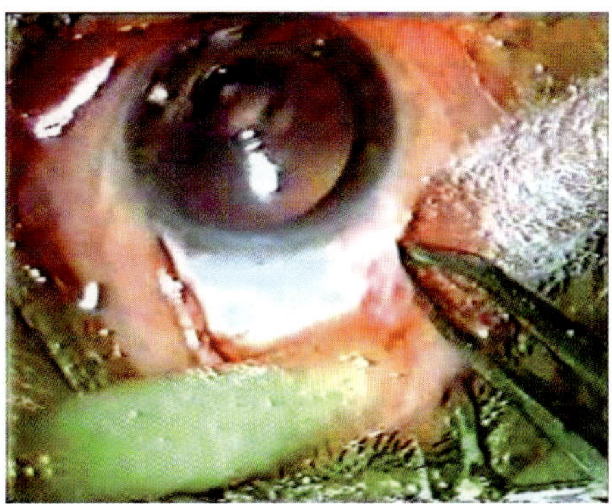

Fig. 2: Wet-field cautery

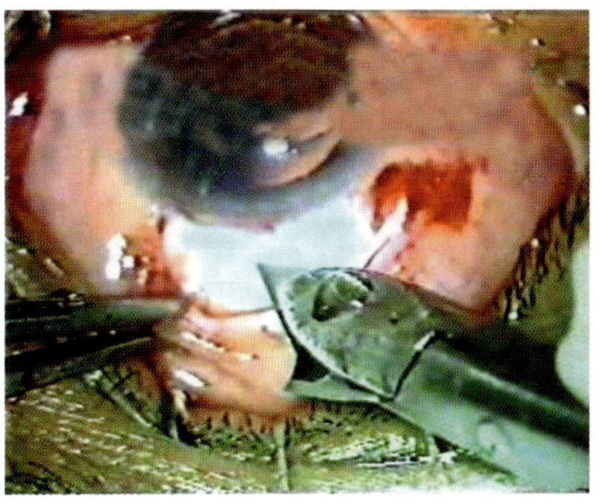

Fig. 3: Scleral incison and tunnel

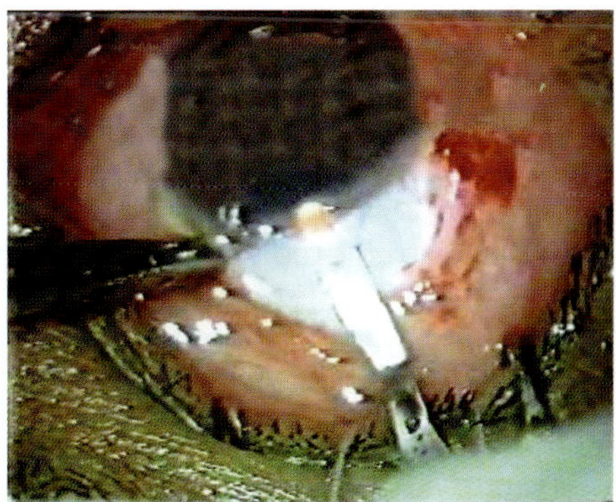

Fig. 4: Scleral tunnel

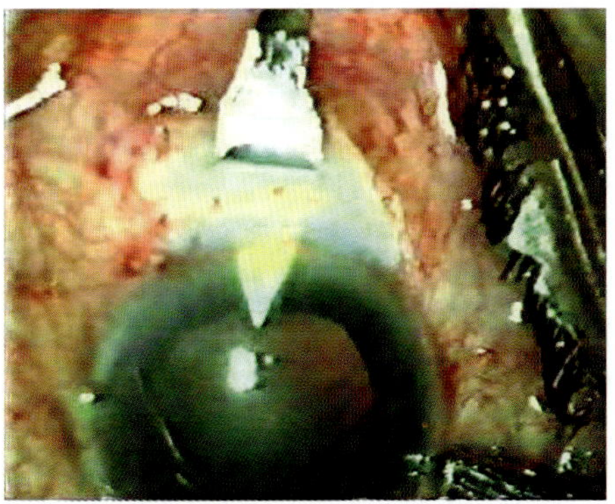

Fig. 5: AC entry with keratome

introduced after a successful, preliminary trial study in 50 patients of POAG and 50 patients of PNAG without and with peripheral iridectomy respectively at the Pt. BD Sharma, PGIMS, Rohtak over a period of 4 years.

Subjects Suitable for Sutureless Filtration Surgery

- Patients with medically uncontrolled POAG
- Patients with poor compliance to medical therapy
- Patients of PNAG with synechial angle closure more than 180 degree.

Preoperative Documentation

Visual acuity, slitlamp examination, funduscopy, applanation tonometry, gonioscopy, perimetry, keratometry and refraction.

SURGICAL PROCEDURE

Under all aseptic conditions and peribulbar block, fornix-based conjunctival flap raised from 10 to 2 o'clock position, bleeding episcleral vessels cauterized with wet-field cautery. A linear, partial thickness scleral groove 5 mm long was made 2 mm behind the surgical limbus with a razor blade piece knife. A scleral tunnel was made through a groove using a 2 mm crescent knife. The tunnel was extended into the clear cornea up to 1 mm in front of the limbus. The anterior chamber was entered with 3 mm keratome through the scleral tunnel already made. Anterior chamber was formed with 2% methyl cellulose. The trabecular tissue was punched out with Kelly descemet's membrane punch through the scleral tunnel. Iridectomy/no iridectomy was performed as per the case. The anterior chamber was irrigated with ringer lactate solution and viscoelastic was removed. The conjunctival flap was brought back to its original position by getting it anchored by means of wet-field cautery. 0.5 ml sub-conjunctival injection of gentamycin and decadron was given 180 degree away from the drainage site. Pad and bandage for 24 hours.

Photographic Illustrations of Surgical Steps

Postoperative Documentation

Visual acuity, slitlamp examination, funduscopy, perimetry, applanation tonometry, keratometry, and refraction at 1 month, 3 months and every 6 months till a period of 4 years.

Author's Personal Observations

Sutureless filtration surgery through scleral tunnel in POAG and PNAG has met with a high success rate regarding control of IOP (86% and 84% respectively) in contrast to conventional trabeculectomy (50%) with the added advantage of negligible postoperative surgical induced astigmatism (0.30 to 0.55 D) as compared to that reported with conventional trabeculectomy (1.0 to 2.5 D). The present technique of sutureless filtration surgery through scleral tunnel has obviated all those complications related to the use of sutures.

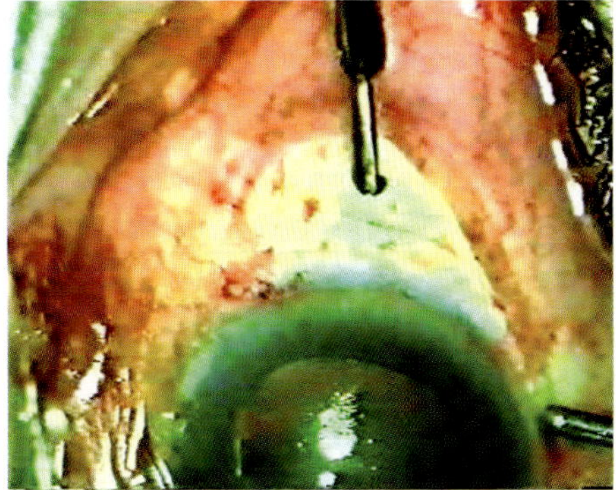

Fig. 6: Kellys Descemet's punch

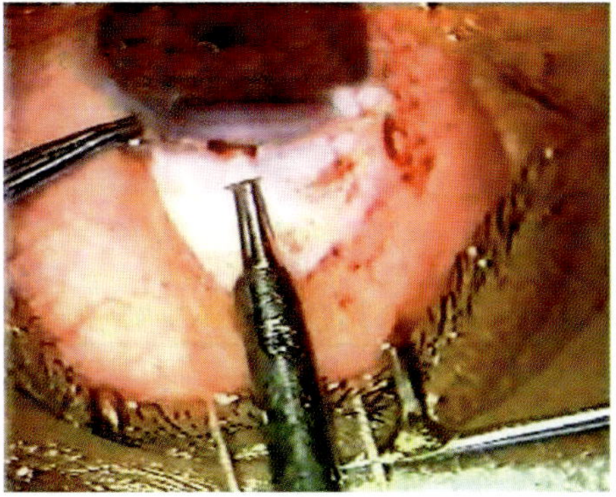

Fig. 7: Kellys punch in use

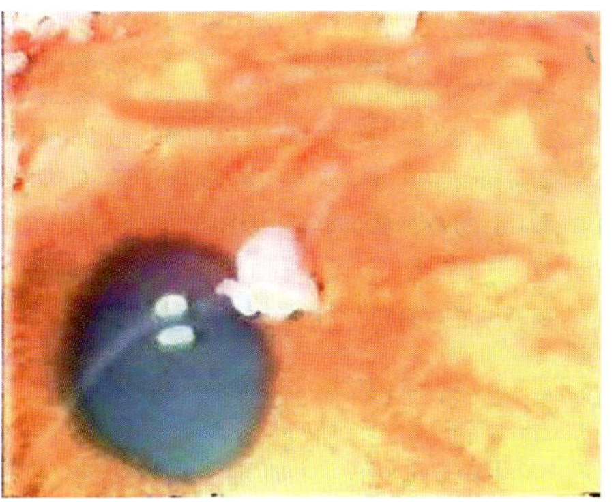

Fig. 8: Trabecular tissue removed

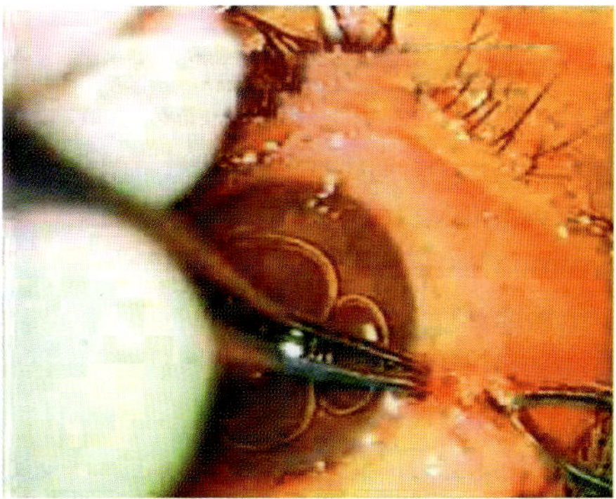

Fig. 9: Conjunctival flap in position with wet field cautery

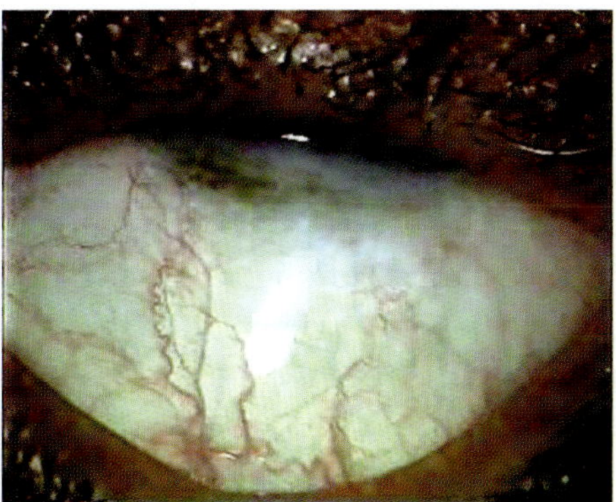

Fig. 10: Diffuse thin translucent filtering bleb

31

Viscocanalostomy

Roberto G Carassa (Italy)

INTRODUCTION

In the last years non-penetrating glaucoma surgery achieved great interest as a possible alternative to trabeculectomy. This class of procedures are mainly represented by *deep sclerectomy* and by *viscocanalostomy* (which was introduced by R. Stegmann in the early nineties), and are based on the original studies by Krasnov and by Zimmerman on "non-penetrating trabeculectomy". Similarly, both procedures are aimed at allowing drainage of the aqueous humor from the anterior chamber not through a patent scleral opening, but by slow percolation through the inner trabecular meshwork and/or descemet membrane (sclerodescemetic membrane). This avoids sudden IOP drops, hypotonies and flat chambers. The absence of anterior chamber opening and iridectomy limits the risk of cataract and infection. Compared to deep sclerectomy, viscocanalostomy is a step forward. In fact this procedure is aimed not only at taking the advantages of being non-penetrating, as deep sclerectomy, but, most important, in restoring the physiological outflow pathway, thus avoiding any external filtration. This would make the success of the procedure independent of conjunctival or episcleral scarring, leading cause of failure in trabeculectomy, with less indications for wound healing modulation. Moreover, the absence of the filtering bleb avoids related ocular discomfort, and the procedure can be carried out in any quadrant.

MECHANISM OF ACTION

Viscocanalostomy increases the aqueous outflow through different mechanism of action. It creates a by-pass by which aqueous humor can reach Schlemm's canal skipping the trabecular meshwork, which is the site of the increased outflow resistance in open angle glaucoma. This is obtained by producing a "chamber" inside the sclera which directly communicates both with Schlemm's canal and with the anterior chamber through the "sclerodescemetic membrane". The aqueous enters the "chamber" by percolating through the membrane, and leaves it via Schlemm's canal. A recent experimental study on monkeys also showed the evidence of micro-openings throughout the wall of Schlemm's canal over 360 degrees which may be invoved in the increased aqueous facility. Finally,

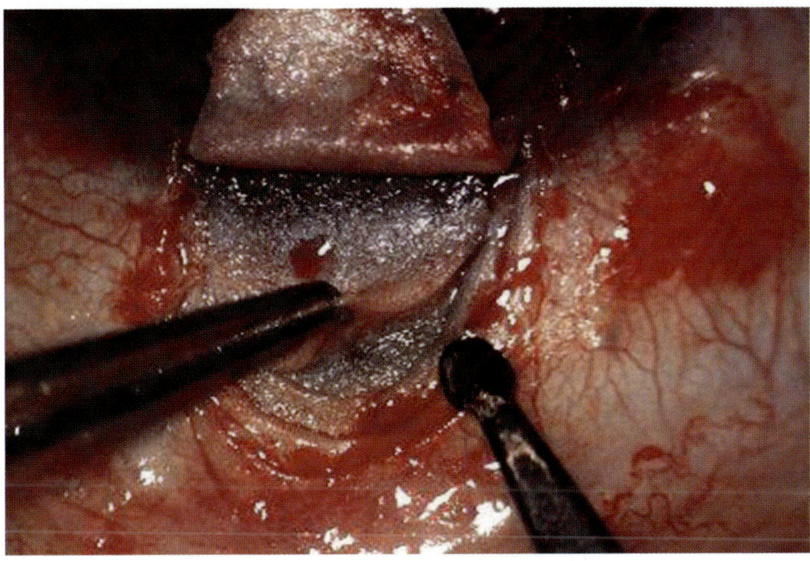

Fig. 1: Dissection of the internal flap

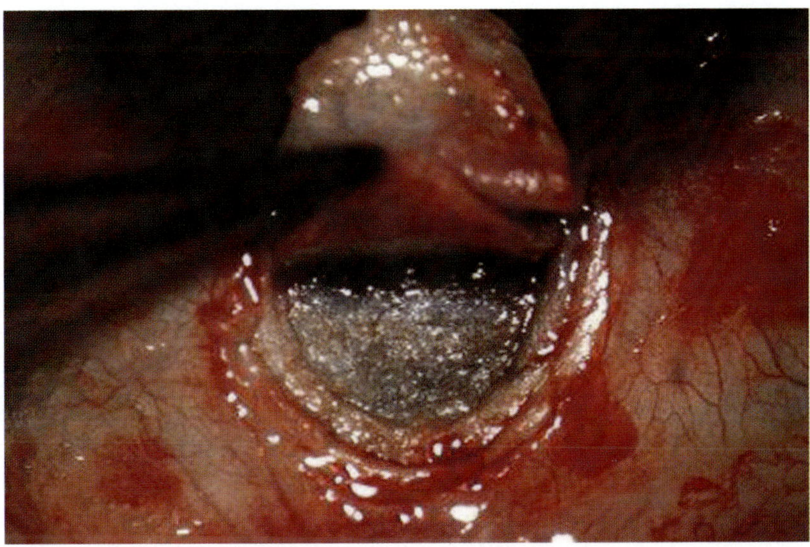

Fig. 2: Opening of Schlemm's canal

as in deep-sclerectomy, aqueous humor can also leave the intrascleral chamber through the subconjunctival space and through the supracoroidal space by uveoscleral absorption.

SURGICAL TECHNIQUE

In order to simplify the technique, a specific surgical set, composed by a 0.5 mm diamond knife, a 1 mm round steel bevel-up blade, and a 165 µm blunt needle to cannulate Schlemm's canal (Grieshaber, Switzerland) should be used.

Viscocanalostomy is performed under retrobulbar or peribulbar anesthesia and usually requires 25 to 40 minutes depending on bleeding control. In fact, in order to avoid damage to outflow channels (Schlemm's canal, aqueous veins, collector channels, etc.), wetfield cautery is used as little as possible, and bleeding is reduced by frequent irrigation of the surgical area with vasoconstrictive solutions as ornipressin. To provide optimal visualization of the surgical site, a bridle suture should be passed either on the superior rectus or in clear cornea.

The surgical technique can be divided in 9 steps:

1. **Conjunctival flap dissection**

Viscocanalostomy does not require any specific accuracy in the dissection of the conjunctival flap, and can be performed in any quadrant, although the upper and temporal ones are most commonly chosen. The surgical field is prepared by creating a fornix-based conjunctival flap, using as little wetfield cautery as possible.

2. **Outer scleral flap dissection**

A 5 × 5 m parabolic cut approximately 200 µm deep, is made using the diamond knife (the incision can be outlined using a calibrated diamond knife to assure a constant depth of cut). After reaching the correct plane of cut the flap is dissected anteriorly in clear cornea by advancing the incision with the bevel-up spatula which allows easier following of the plane.

3. **Inner scleral flap dissection**

A 4 × 4 mm parabolic cut parallel to the outer incision is made beneath the outer flap. The choroidal plane must be almost reached, and this is revealed by the observation of a dark reflex at the bottom of the cut. Using the specific beaveled spatula a precise dissection is advanced until Schlemm's canal is reached and deroofed leaving two patent openings on the lateral edges of the cut. In order to maintain the same plane of dissection and provide sharp lateral edges, progressive deepening of the lateral cuts is often needed.

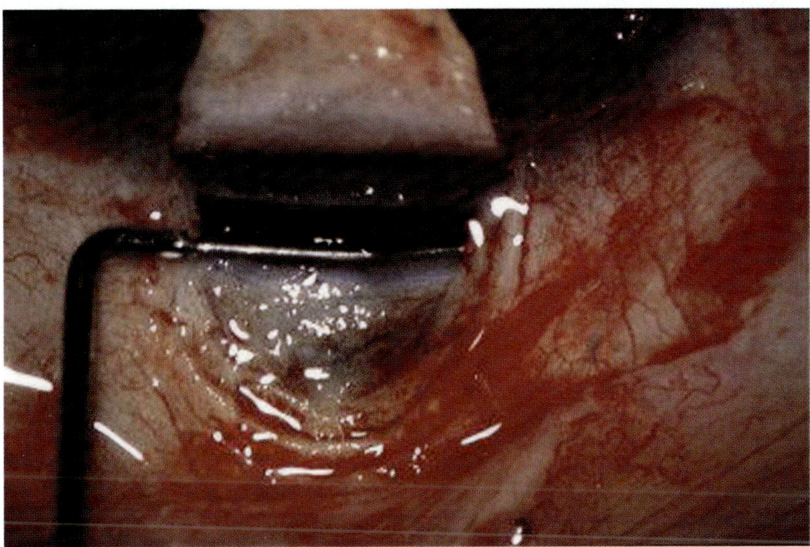

Fig. 3: Injection of high molecular weight sodium hyaluronate into Schlemm's canal

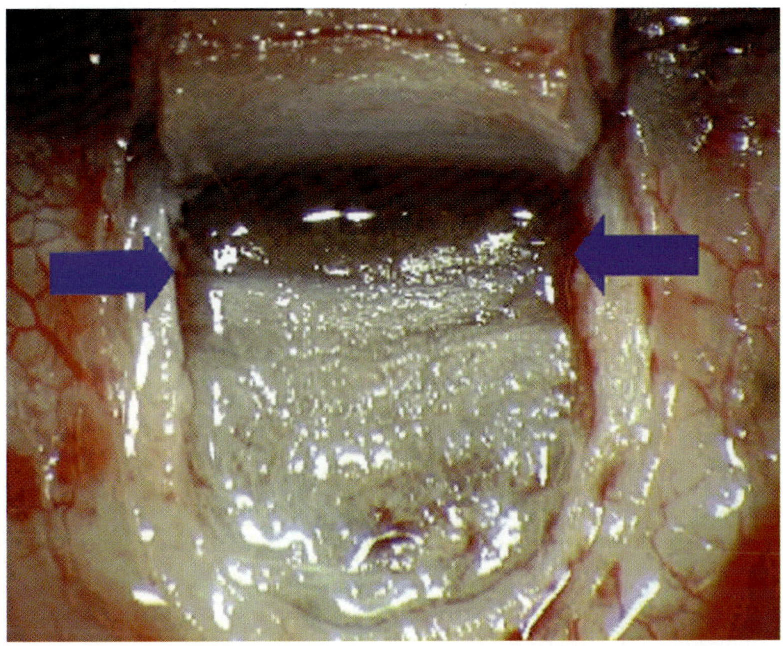

Fig. 4: Showing Sclerodescemetic membrane and the 2 openings of Schlemm's canal (Arrows)

4. **Paracentesis**

A paracentesis should be always made in order to decrease intraocular pressure, to make incannulation of Schlemm's canal easier and to reduce bulging of Descemet's membrane during its cleavage from the corneal stroma, which is at high-risk of tear formation. To avoid external pressure on the eye, the traction on the bridle suture should also be removed.

5. **Cannulation of Schlemm's canal**

Using the specific 165-μm cannula, high molecular weight sodium hyaluronate is slowly injected into Schlemm's canal by cannulating the two ostia at the lateral edges of the inner flap. To avoid damage to the canal endothelium, the insertion of the cannula should not exceed 1–1.5 mm from the ostia. The injection of viscoelastic substance allows progressive atraumatic dilatation of Schlemm's canal up to 1-2 clock hours from the ostia. Moreover, its hemostatic properties avoid bleeding and fibrin clot formation, thus limiting healing processes and scarring of Schlemm's canal openings. The slow injection should be repeated 6-7 times on each side.

6. **Creation of Descemet's window**

The alternative route by which aqueous humor bypasses the trabecular meshwork and reaches Schlemm's canal is a "window" created right anterior to the canal, and represented by the anterior portion of the trabecular meshwork and by the intact Descemet's membrane. The window is realized by gently pulling the inner scleral flap upwards and delicately depressing the floor of the canal and Descemet's membrane with the tip of a cotton swab. By delicately repeating the procedure, the membrane is progressively cleaved from the scleral flap. The flap itself is then advanced in clear cornea for approximately 1 mm by a careful deepening of the lateral cuts with the round bevel-up spatula.

7. **Inner scleral flap excision**

The inner scleral flap is then excided using very sharp Vannas' scissors in order to avoid damage to Descemet's membrane.

8. **Outer scleral flap suture**

In order to seal the intrascleral "chamber", the outer scleral flap should be tightly sutured by placing 6 or 7, 10-0 nylon stitches. The step created by the different size of the two flaps allows a better and tight apposition of the external flap. Finally, in order to minimize bleeding and prevents collapsing and scarring of the intrascleral chamber, high molecular weight sodium hyaluronate is injected underneath the flap.

9. **Closure of the conjunctiva**

The procedure ends by repositioning the conjunctiva with two lateral stitches, and by giving a subconjunctival injection of steroids-antibiotics.

INDICATIONS

Viscocanalostomy has specific indications and contraindications. It cannot be effective when the angle is closed or neovascularized, or when Schlemm's canal is likely to be damaged. This is the case of previously operated eyes where an extensive cautery of the perilimbar area was made. Due to its final results the procedure is indicated in primary open angle glaucoma when target IOP is not very low (as indicated by the Guidelines for Glaucoma of the European Glaucoma Society). The advantage of the absence (or very reduced) external filtration make the technique safe and particularly indicated in eyes with chronic blepharitis, in lens contact wearer, or when the surgery has to be perform in the lateral or inferior quadrants. Viscocanalostomy was shown effective also in uveitic glaucomas with well controlled inflammation.

RESULTS

Viscocanalostomy seems effective in lowering IOP with a good safety profile. It has low complications, an easy postoperative management and is inducing significant less eye discomfort than trabeculectomy, as could be expected considering the absence of the filtering bleb in the majority of the cases.

When compared with trabeculectomy many of the studies lack to find significant differences between the procedures; nevertheless final IOPs seem higher after viscocanalostomy when compared with trabeculectomy.

A direct comparison between different studies is difficult because criteria for success, length of follow-up and techniques are different.

These can be grouped in retrospective, prospective and randomized controlled trials.

Retrospective Studies

Stegmann and co-workers reported results of viscocanalostomy in 214 eyes of 157 African patients with open-angle glaucoma and a mean preoperative IOP of 47.4 ± 13.0 mm Hg. After an average follow-up of 35 months, mean IOP was 16.9 ± 8.0 mm Hg; 83% of eyes achieved an IOP less than 22 mm Hg off all glaucoma medications.

Two recent studies showed viscocanalostomy a successful procedure in glaucoma secondary to uveitis. Miserocchi et al found a complete and qualified success rate of 54.5% and 90.9% respectively, after 46 months of follow-up. Final IOP was 18.1±/11.6 mm Hg. Auer et al after performed NPGDS (including viscocanalostomy) on 14 eyes: complete and qualified success rate were 45.4% and 90.4% at 12 months. Final IOP was 12.1±- 4.0.

Prospective Studies

Carassa et al reported a series of 23 VCs performed in 23 patients. In four eyes, the procedure was converted to trabeculectomy. Of the 16 eyes with IOP less than 21 mm Hg, mean IOP was 11.6 ± 4.4 mm Hg.

Sunaric-Mégevand et al evaluated the procedure in 67 eyes of 67 consecutive patients with chronic open angle glaucoma. Complete success was an IOP = < 20 mm Hg with 30% or greater IOP reduction without ongoing medical or additional surgical treatment. Qualified success was an IOP = < 20 mm Hg with further treatment or an IOP reduction less than 30% from preoperative level. The overall success rate was 88% at 1 year, 90% at 2 years and 88% at 3 years. The complete success rate was 68% at 1 year, 60% at 2 years and 59% at 3 years. No serious complications were reported in this series.

Luke et al when comparing viscocanalostomy with and without a SKGel implant showed a success rate (IOP < 22 mm Hg without medications) of 40% in both groups at 12 months, with a very low complication rate.

Shaarawy et al in a 5 year, follow-up study, showed a final IOP of 13.9 mm Hg and a complete success rate with IOP < 21 mm Hg in 60% of the eyes. Goniopuncture was performed in 37% of the cases.

Randomized Controlled Studies

Jonescu-Cuipers et al in 2001, showed at 6 months, a complete success rate (IOP < 20 mm Hg) of 0% after viscocanalostomy and 50% after trabeculectomy on 20 eyes. The same group in 2002, showed an IOP < 22 mm Hg without medications in 30% with VC and 56.7 after trabeculectomy group at 1 year on 60 patients. Viscocanalostomy showed significant less complications compared with trabeculectomy.

O'Brart et al. showed a 1 year success rate (IOP < 21 mmHg on no medications) of 60% after viscocanalostomy and of 91% after trabeculectomy.

In a 24 months controlled randomized trial comparing viscocanalostomy with trabeculectomy, Carassa et al. reported similar final IOP levels of 14.1 ± 4.7 mm Hg after viscocanalostomy and 16.3 ± 5.1 mm Hg after trabeculectomy. No significant difference was found between the 2 procedure as for IOP < 21 mm Hg (76% versus 80%) or < 16 (56% versus 72%) on no medications.

A recent study by Yalvac et al on 50 eyes followed for 36 months found similar results. At 3 years, the mean IOP was 17.8 ± 4.6 mm Hg in the viscocanalostomy group and 16.0 mm Hg ± 7.07 in the trabeculectomy group (P = .694). Complete success (IOP 6 to 21 mm Hg without medication) was achieved in 35.3% after viscocanalostomy and 55.1% after trabeculectomy (P > .05). Postoperative hypotony and cataract formation occurred more frequently in the trabeculectomy than in the viscocanalostomy group (P = .002).

O'Brart et al in a 20 months RCT comparing viscocanalostomy with trabeculectomy with adjunctive use of antimetabolites on 50 eyes, found a significantly lower complete success rate (IOP < 21 mm Hg) after viscocanalostomy (34%) than after trabeculectomy (68%). Early transient complications such as anterior chamber shallowing and encysted blebs were more common in the trabeculectomy group ($p < 0.05$). Late postoperative cataract formation was similar between the two groups.

CONCLUSIONS

Viscocanalostomy seems a promising surgery for lowering IOP in glaucomatous eyes. It has several potential advantages over trabeculectomy, the major being the absence of external filtration and thus the independence of conjunctival and episcleral scarring. When considering final IOPs between 16 and 21 mmHg, the rate of failure overtime is similar between the two procedures. The procedure is affected by few and minor complications, it requires an easy postoperative management and induces significant less eye discomfort than trabeculectomy. Viscocanalostomy is nevertheless technically demanding and requires a long learning curve.

Results from basic researches aimed at defining the exact mechanism of action will certainly provide improvements in the surgical technique and more appropriate indications.

32

Open Angle Filter Surgery for Glaucoma Deep Sclerocanalostomy (DSC): New Technique

Jerome Bovet (Switzerland)

HISTORY

The goal of all surgery for glaucoma is to lower the ocular pressure in order to reduce postoperative risk as much as possible.

Surgical techniques using perforation have several postoperative disadvantages.

A certain number produce complications such as hyphema, flat anterior chamber, choroid detachment, cataract, and endophthalmitis,

Non-penetrative surgical techniques do not have the postoperative complications of the first, penetrative, surgery, but they are more difficult to carry out. An exact knowledge of the micro-anatomy of the region is important and a learning curve necessary.

The main drawbacks with these new techniques are that they are less effective with weak hypertensions, and, importantly, they increase the number of times the operation needs to be performed due to poor healing and flap collapse.

1909 Elliott's trepanation

1960 Burian's trabeculectomy, Sugar 1961

1968 Cairn's trabeculectomy for open angle glaucoma

1962 Krasnov's sinusotomy: this technique aims to remove the external wall of the Schlemm Canal

1984 Zimmermann: Non-penetrating trabeculectomy

1984 Fiodorov and Koslov suggest the term 'non-penetrating deep sclerectomy' (NPDS)

1990 Koslov improves his technique by adding a collagen implant into the base of the flap. At the same time, many others tried different types of implants to increase the duration of the drainage life of the aqueous humour.

1991 Arenas: *Archila Trabeculotomy ab externo*. Areans uses the same technique but employs the help of a trepan to open the Schlemm Canal

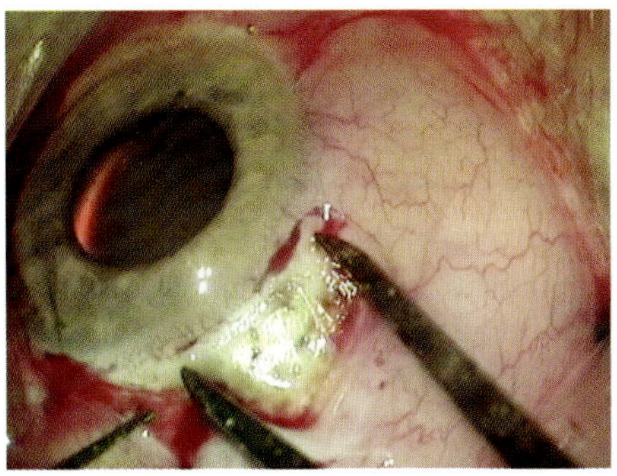

Fig 1: Measure the width being of less importance than the length

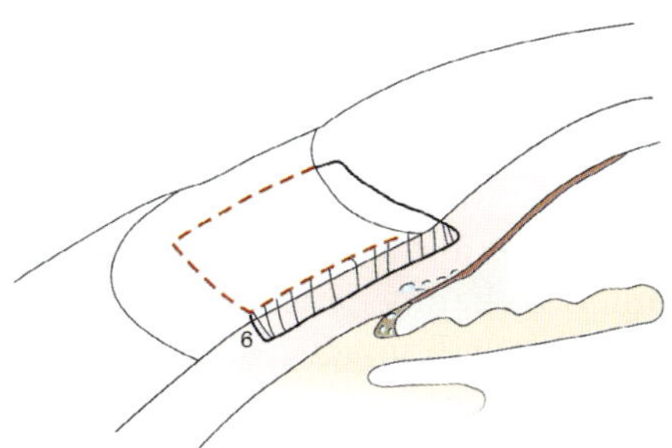

Fig 1A: The path of dissection and flap's localization are chosen to spare the penetrating vessels Conjunctival Flap at the limbus L shape

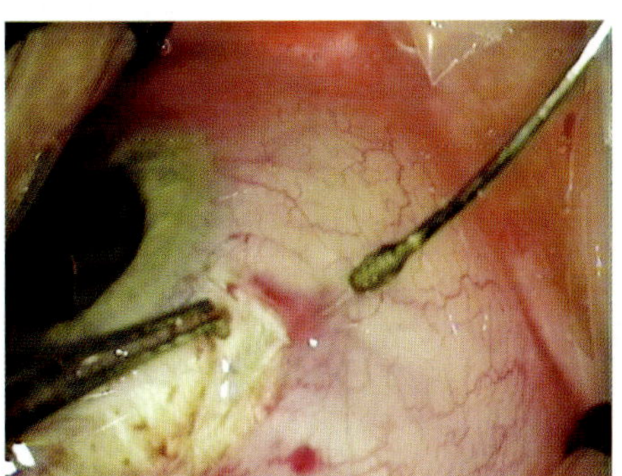

Fig 2: Dissecting the first flap

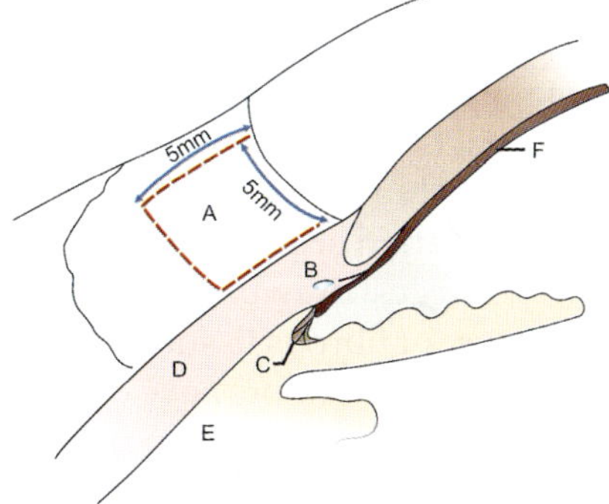

Fig 2A: A First scleral Flap 6 × 4mm × 300 micron
B Schlemm's canal
C Scleral spur
D Sclera
F Descemet membrane

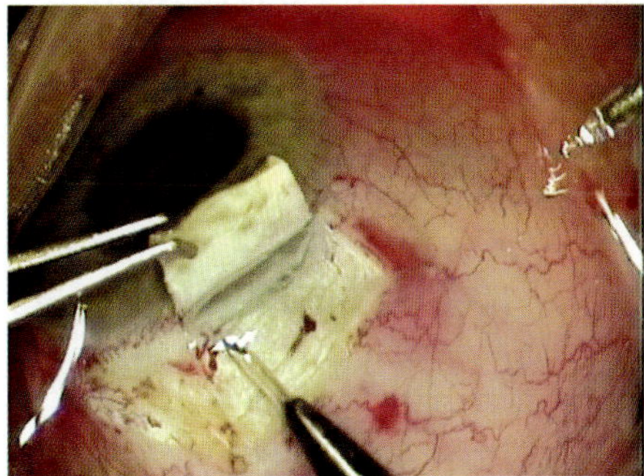

Fig 3: First flap's dissection to the stromal lamellae

1999 Stegman: *Viscocanalostomy* The author proposes a dissection and an injection of viscous fluid into the Schlemm Canal.

ANATOMO-PHYSIOLOGY

Goldman demonstrated by using manometric experiments, the main point of resistance to the drainage of the aqueous humour was situated between the anterior chamber and the Schlemm Canal. Nowadays, it is generally accepted that 75% of drainage resistance is situated at the level of the endothelium of the Sclemm Canal and of the trabeculum network.

New Techniques

The new techniques of filtering non-perforating are all connected with dissection or injection of the Schlemm Canal.

Krasnov(15) proposes the sinusotomy removing the endothelium of the Schlemm Canal using microdissection:

The principle of deep sclerectomy is to dissect the internal wall of the Schlemm Canal where the greatest resistance to drainage of the aqueous humour is situated, thus allowing a physiological filtration, since the external wall is kept intact.

The technique of using high viscosity to widen the Sclemm Canal, allows better filtration of aqueous humour.

The biggest drawback of these techniques, above all deep sclerectomy, is the formation of fibrous tissue on the sclerotic flap.

Numerous authors have described a multitude of implants that would keep the space of the second flap free.

We submit a new surgical technique which allows a synthesis of the three main surgical techniques for non-penetrative filter surgery. This reduces the risks of each, whilst increasing the long-term chances of success.

Surgical technique in outpatient surgery.
Local anesthetic.

This anesthetic technique has been described in the previous chapter.

Let us remember that this local anesthetic allows - thanks to the patient's ability to participate - exposure of the operative field for dissection and its best, and variable angles of work.

Choices for Dissection

The path of dissection and flap's localization are chosen to spare the penetrating vessels and to search for the zone that is the most avascular

The draining vessels are on the surface, as shown by Stegmann.

The choice of the best place for the flap to spare the penetrating vessels to find the most avascular zone, one must not forget that the draining vessels are on the surface, as shown by Stegmann in his film.

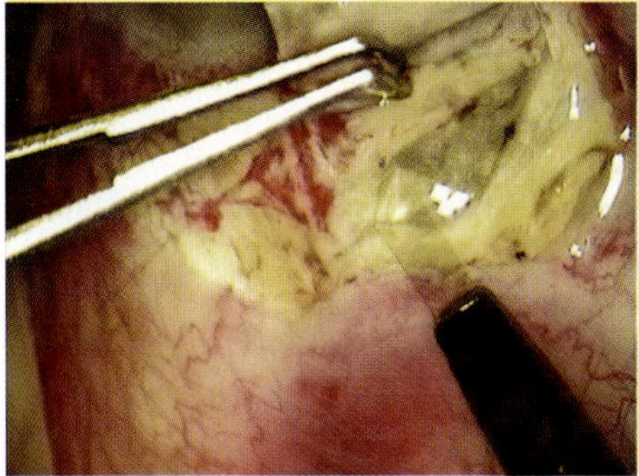

Fig 4: Second Flap's dissection

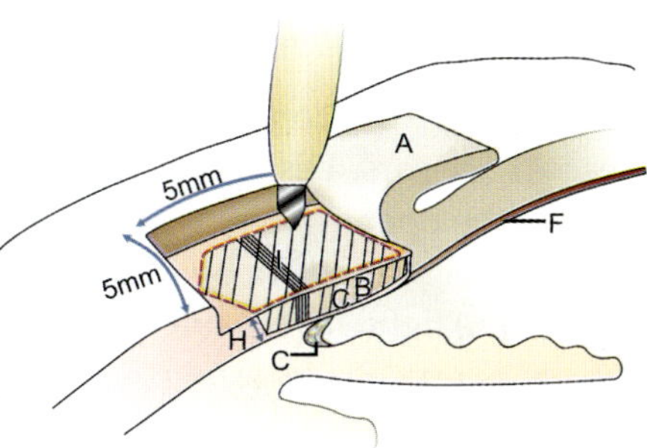

Fig 4A: Second triangular flap of all the depth of the sclera

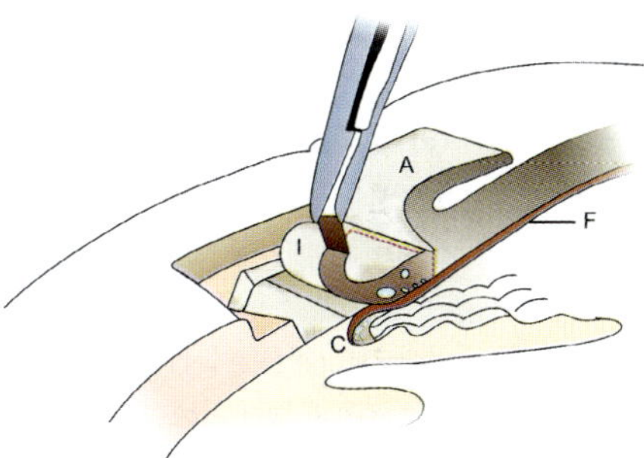

Fig 5: Second flap as to be deep enough. This allows getting exactly at the scleral spur, at the beginning of Descemet's membrane

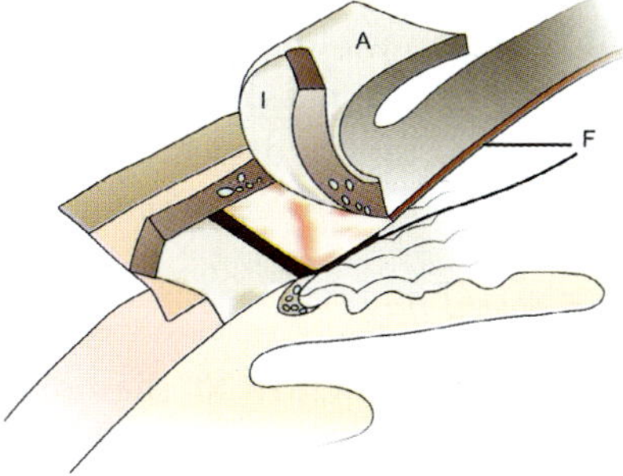

Fig 6: A slight bleeding can be seen at the cut in the drainage vein of the Schlemm canal

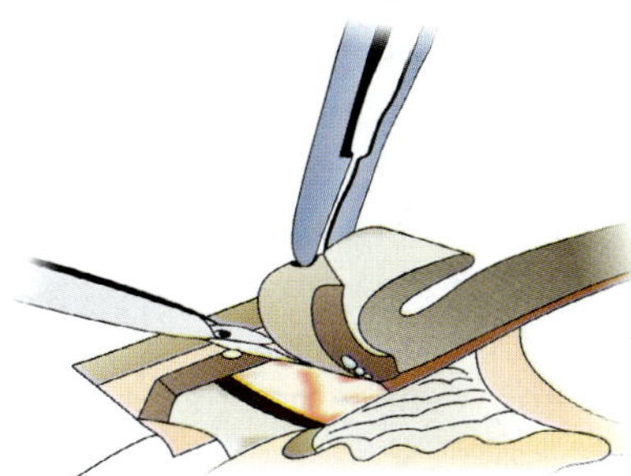

Fig 7: Removal of the second flap with the diamond or the Vannas scissor

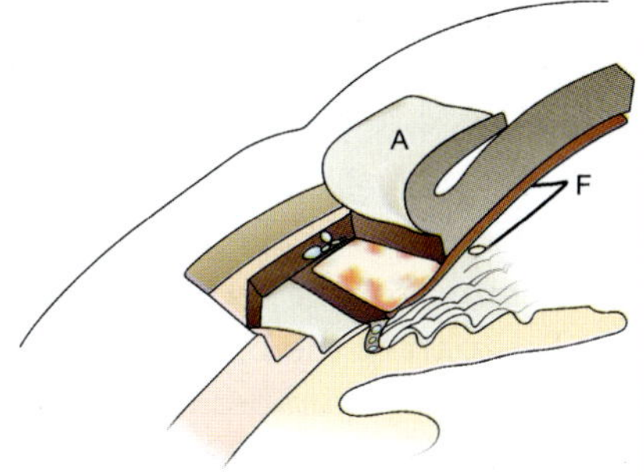

Fig 8: Schlemm canal dissection

Conjunctival shutter with limb

Stages are as follows

Dissection of the conjunctival shutter with limb, not less than 10 mm, with Vescoat scissors. Dissection in an L shape allowing the conjunctival flap to relax in the opening.

Exposing the sclera by dissecting Tenon's capsule with care

Use the lightest possible electro coagulation in order to spare the draining vessels as much as possible.

1st Scleral Flap

Incision of the scleral flap.

- 6 mm × 4 mm, the width being of less importance than the length
- depth of 300 microns, cut with a 30° diamond (Meyco Switzerland) or with a diamond for KR (Meyco, Switzerland) up to the lames corneostromales

It is important to make a flap which is thick enough not to tear when one arrives in the corneal stroma

It is important to dissect the lames corneennes, starting from the limb, the cut allowing more room when making the incision of the second flap

2nd Scleral flap

5 mm dissection, with a 30° diamond (Meyco, Switzerland), of the length of the second triangular flap of all the depth of the sclera leaving some lamelles sclerales in order to just reveal the choroidien tissue. This allows getting exactly at the scleral spur, at the beginning of Descemet's membrane.

Dissection, holding on to the second flap, au tampon triangulaire pour repousser le stroma. Thus, we free Descemet's membrane. Those who practice deep lamellar keratoplasty ("keratoplastie lamellaire") operations will have no difficulty in finding the plane of dissection.

Separation of the Descemet from the stromal tissue is quite easy, so long as one is in the right plane.

The 1.5 mm incision in Descemet's membrane is made in order that the Schlemm canal is not covered at the time of the cutting of the flap.

On this level, each side, in the scleral tissue, a slight bleeding can be seen at the cut in the drainage vein of the Schlemm canal.

Removal of the second flap with the diamond.or the vannas scissor.

This part of the operation is delicate and has to be done with great care. Because, on a number of occasions, when using Vannas or other scissors, Descemet's membrane has been torn.

Cut up the scleral flap in half: one half is soaked for 5 minutes in 0.04% mytomycin, then rinsed.

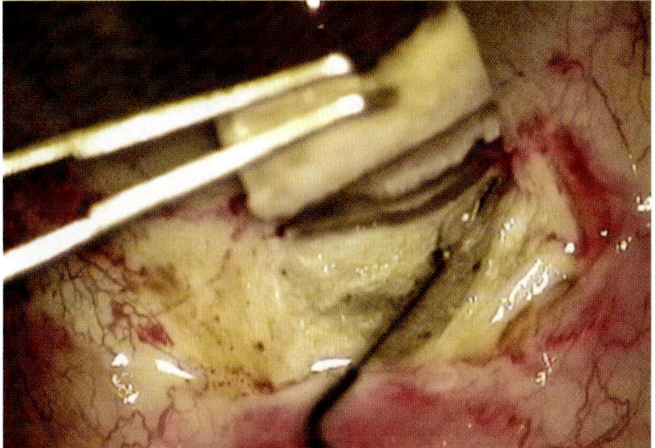

Fig 9: Canalostomy

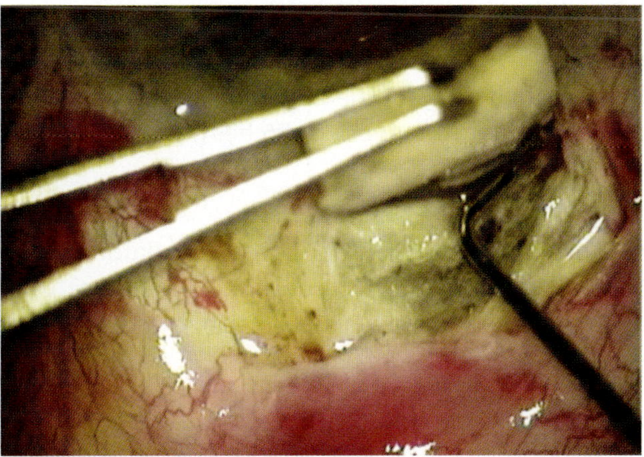

Fig 10: Introduction of an extra fine Grieshaber cannula

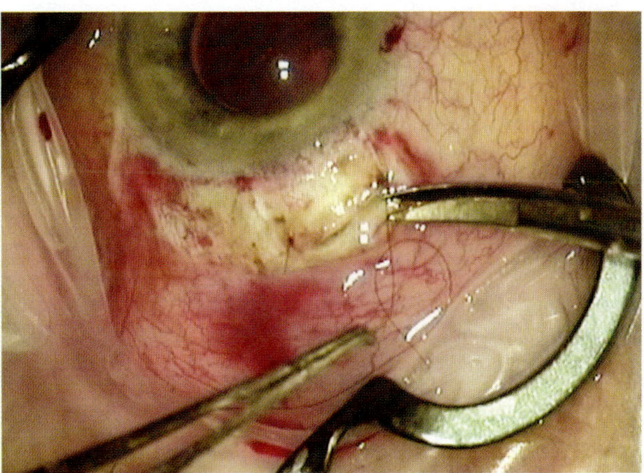

Fig 11: Closing the first flap with inverted stitches

Schlemm Canal Dissection

Using Bonn forceps with microteeth, a 5 mm dissection of the interior wall of the Sclemm canal is made, allowing us to see some seepage of the aqueous humour.

Canalostomy

The Schlemm canal vein gives the location of the Sclemm canal. Introduction of an extra fine Grieshaber cannula on both sides of the sclera of the Sclemm canal until some resistance is felt. Slow injection of high viscosity viscous fluid (Healon, G V *AMO*) whilst removing the microcatheter.

Implant/Mitomycin C

Put in place, in the bed of the second flap, the previously prepared implant, the implant having been, beforehand, soaked in mitomycine and rinsed before being used.

Close the first flap with inverted stitches using nylon 10.0, at each corner of the flap pulling the stitches tight.

Close the conjunctive with 3 inverted stitches using 9.0 reabsorbable thread.

Postoperative treatment

As this operation is extra-ocular, done with ambulatory surgery and local anesthetic, there is no need to cover the eye with a dressing.

Patients are treated using eyedrops of cortisone and antibiotics.

The dose is 1 drop 3x a day for 3 weeks.

Postoperative checkups

The postoperative follow-up must be rigorous,

The patient is checked, one hour after the operation, before leaving the clinic, after 1 day, 1 week, and 1 month.

Usually, all eye hypotensor treatments are stopped, even if it's necessary for them to be re-introduced at a later date.

The filtration bubble that is found when trabectomy is used, does not exist using this technique. As a result, the patient has to be checked controlling the ocular tension in both the eyes. If possible, the measure has to taken each time at the same hour, in order to avoid obtaining distorted results because of the curve of the nychthemeral ocular pressure.

Patients who are cortisone respondant need particularly special attention.

Continuous check-ups to control postoperative pressure are necessary in cases of glaucoma.

It is extremely important to check the pre- and postoperative pressures in the two eyes at the same times.

Preoperative Complications

The most frequent complication is rupture of the Descemet membrane when dissecting the second scleral flap: the rupture happens after the scleral spur and, especially, after the removal ? with diamond or Vannas scissors.

If this happens, it will be necessary to convert the deep sclerectomy into trabeculectomy without viscocanalostomy, whilst not forgetting to make an iridectomy.

When the canalostomy is done, the viscous fluid can leak into the anterior chamber. In the hours following the operation, this will cause a rapid increase in the intraocular pressure. The operation will have to be reviewed, by carrying out a paracentesis, emptying the viscous fluid and rinsing the anterior chamber.

The other possible complication is the perforation of the choroid, which has no postoperative importance.

Postoperative Complications

The most frequent complication from using this technique is increased post-operative pressure, more or less long-term, due to the collapse or closing up/ healing of the scleral flap on the bed of the operation. This is the reason why many authors have proposed different types of implants which very in the rapidity of their reabsorbtion.

Our technique uses an autograft from the sclera, soaked in mitomycin C which inhibits all fibrocyte proliferation. This produces the best results in the long-term and the lowest costs. When, after this operation, pressure increases occur rarely, they can still happen after 3-4 years.

If there is a recurrnce, nowadays we favour repeating the procedure in a more favourable quadrant. We have never had to repeat this operation more than twice.

We have stopped doing trabeculopasty au yag for patients who have increased pressure after three weeks, this technique not having brought the expected results.

We do no longer convert our deep sclerocanalostomy into a trabeculectomy, because the complications were too important.

33

Milling Trabeculoplasty: A New Technique for Non-penetrating Glaucoma Surgery

José L Rodríguez-Prats, Jorge L Alió, Ahmed Galal (Spain)

INTRODUCTION

Trabeculectomy has been the operation of choice for glaucoma since its introduction in 1961 and as a full-thickness operation it had its complications. Guarded filtration procedures were developed to reduce these risks such as hypotony, and infections. In the standard trabeculectomy, as reported by Cairns, the trabecular block is excised anterior to the scleral spur or alternatively from the posterior side as proposed by Watson. The success rate of trabeculectomy is influenced by several factors including patient's characteristics, type of glaucoma and wound healing processes. Other important factors that might reduce the success of this surgery include tissue scarring, anterior segment neovascularization, active uveitis, aphakia, previous ocular surgery and chronic conjunctival inflammation.

Over the past 10 years new modalities in glaucoma surgery have been introduced as possible alternatives to Trabeculectomy. Krasnov and Zimmerman have identified those procedures into deep scleretomy and viscocanalostomy. The non-penetrating glaucoma surgeries aim to allow drainage of the aqueous humour by slow percolation through the inner trabecular meshwork and/or Descemet membrane (trabeculo-descemetic membrane) rather than through a patent scleral opening, as in standard trabeculectomy. This avoids sudden reductions in IOP, hypotony and flat chambers. Performing such a non-penetrating glaucoma surgeries has great advantages are the absence of anterior chamber opening and iridectomy, the facts that limit the risk of cataract and infection. In the past 10 years new non-penetrating modalities in glaucoma surgery were introduced as possible alternatives to Trabeculectomy. Krasnov and Zimmerman have proposed these procedures as deep sclerotomy and viscocanalostomy. The non-penetrating glaucoma surgeries aim to allow drainage of the aqueous humour by slow percolation through the inner trabecular meshwork and/or trabeculo-descemetic membrane rather than a patent trabeculo-scleral opening, as in standard trabeculectomy. This avoids sudden reductions in IOP, hypotony and flat chambers. Non-penetrating

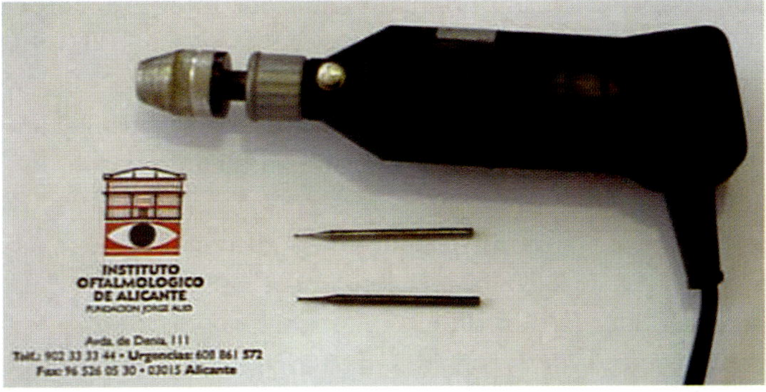

Fig 1: Milling drill with the tips used in the surgery of milling

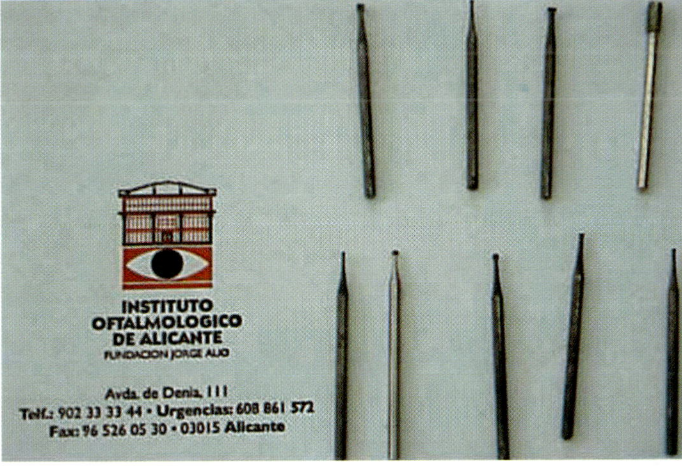

Fig 2: The drill held with the tip unassembled just before the surgery

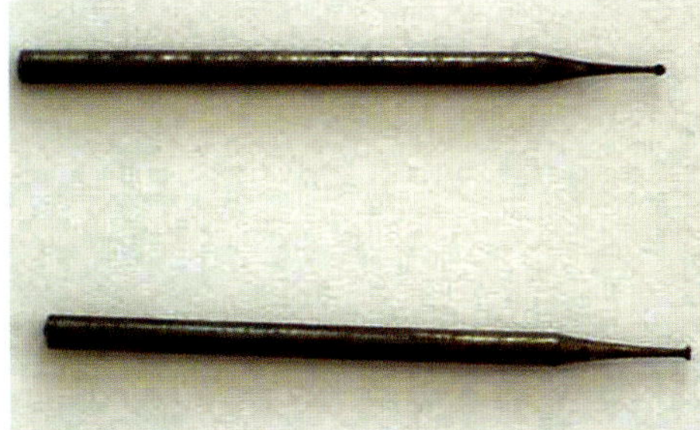

Fig 3: Milling set of metallic tips. The set includes tips for cutting, other for refining

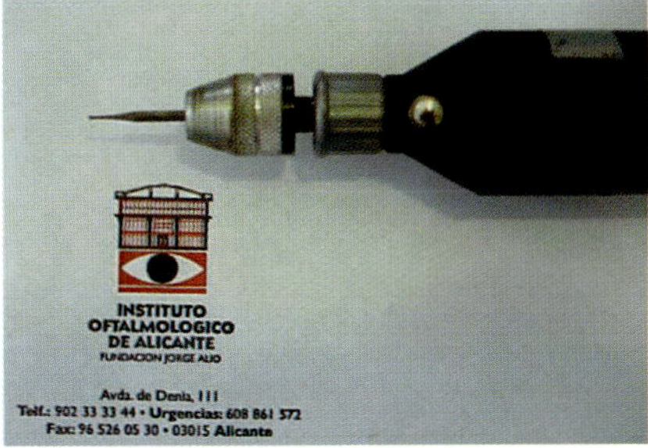

Fig 4: The notched hemispherical metallic tips to polish but not cut the remaining scleral thickness

glaucoma procedures have important potential advantages mainly the absence of anterior chamber opening and iridectomy, the fact that limits the risk of cataract and infection.

One of the important targets while performing trabeculectomy or non-penetrating glaucoma surgeries is to minimize the stimulation of fibroblast proliferation that might reduce the success rate of the procedure. The cutting, spreading, and tearing of tissue should be kept to a minimum. In addition, the surgeon should strive to keep the incisions linear, rather than multilaminate, to maintain as small and localized incisional scars as possible.

Milling trabeculoplasty is considered a variation of deep sclerectomy with more refining. The technique of milling trabeculoplasty provides the opportunity to perform a non-penetrating glaucoma surgery with greater attention for the dissection of the deep scleral flap or the deroofing of the Schlemm´s canal with the addition advantage that is being much faster.

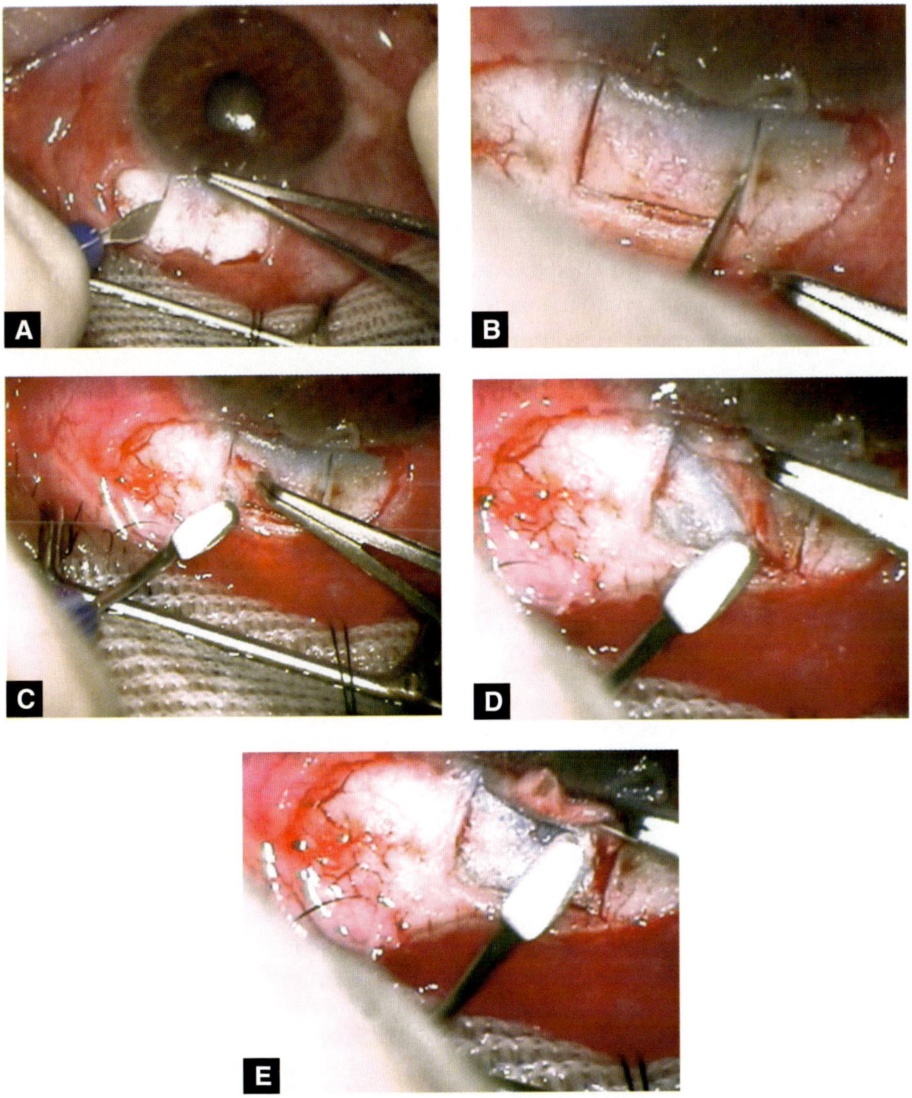

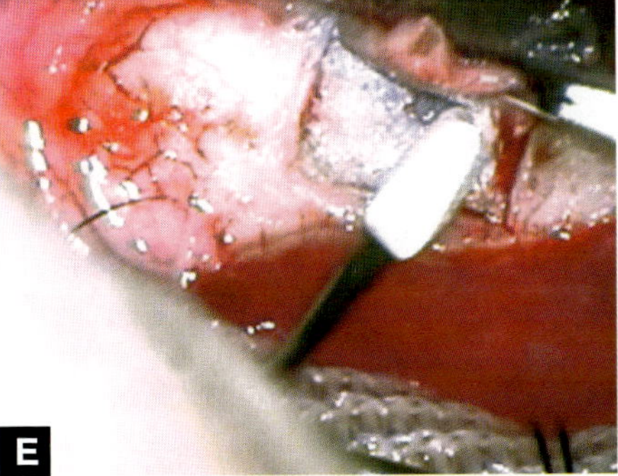

Fig 5: (A) Fashioning of the scleral flap size and site
(B) The scleral incision as being completed
(C) Beginning of the lamellar dissection
(D) Lamellar dissection of the scleral flap
(E) Completion of the lamellar dissection

INDICATIONS

Eyes with primary open angle glaucoma are the best candidates for the milling surgery. However, all indications of deep sclerectomy are cases of milling procedure.

PATIENT PREPARATION

Preoperative examination: Before surgery, each patient had manifest refraction, slit lamp biomicroscopy with measurement of IOP by using Goldman tonometry, gonioscopy and computerized perimetry.

Preoperative medications: Medications included Ciprofloxacin 0.3% eye drops 3 times/ day for a week. The topical antiglaucoma therapy was stopped 3 days before the surgery.

Anesthesia: Peribulbar anesthesia in the form of combination of 8 ml of 0.75% Bupivacaine and 2% Lidocaine was injected. Intravenous sedation was used when necessary. A light compression with the Honnan balloon was applied 15 minutes prior to surgery for 5 minutes to insure diffusion of the anesthetic agent.

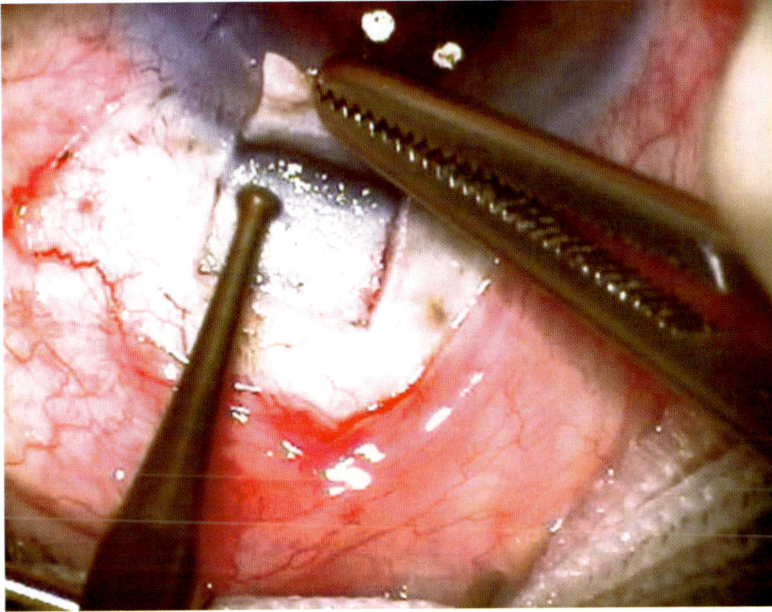

Fig 6: The scleral bed refined and grazed using the milling motorized drill in dry field through the remaining scleral thickness in a linear pattern to leave a thin layer of sclera below and a width of 3.5 mm.

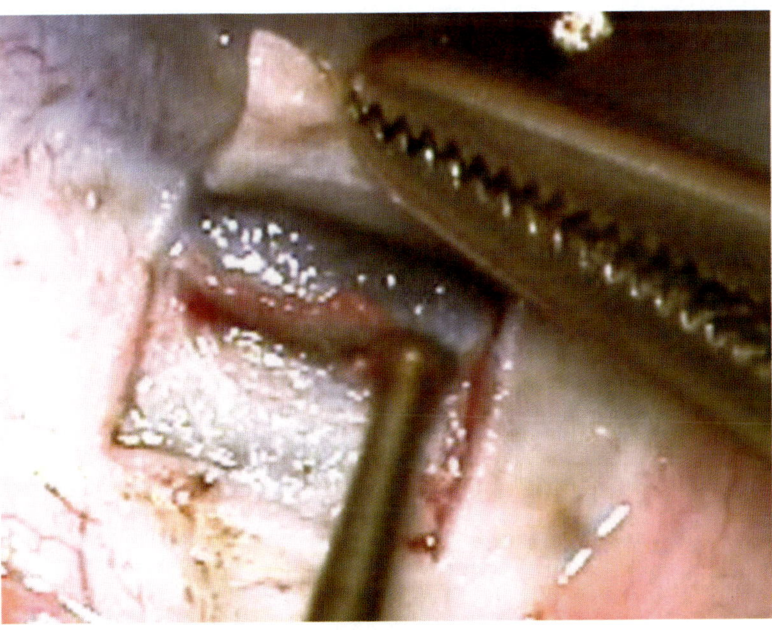

Fig 7: The refining is carried anteriorly and down until the roof of Schlemm´s canal can barely be visible

Milling surgical procedure

Instruments: Milling drill (Katena Inc, Denville, NJ USA) is the main instrument necessary to perform this procedure. The mode of action of the drill is similar to that used to burr the nasal bone in dacryocystorhinostomy (DCR) surgery or that used to polish the bed after removing corneal foreign bodies. The drill used in our milling procedure is handheld 150-mg weight equipment and made of autoclaveble material. Following the concept of refined tissue removal would decrease the rate of post-operative fibrosis, a high frequency and velocity motorized drill tip could be able to polish (no cutting method) the remaining scleral thickness with minimal tearing and smaller more localized scars at the end of the procedure.

The high speed Milling drill (6000 RPM) allows easy, quick and more controlled refining of the remaining scleral thickness by using sharp- metallic tip first to refine the sclera and later on as the tissue became thinner another notched hemispherical metallic tip was used to polish and not cut the remaining scleral thickness. A new tip covered with diamond powder is also needed for more delicate maneuvers as removing debris making the technique ideal to have an extremely smooth bed. In both Groups the procedure started as the initial steps of deep sclerotomy then the specific steps of milling surgery were continued. In Group II, the milling procedure is carried out until Schlemm's canal is identified. Thereafter, phaco is performed (through a separate clear corneal incision) and after the IOL was implanted, the milling procedure was finished.

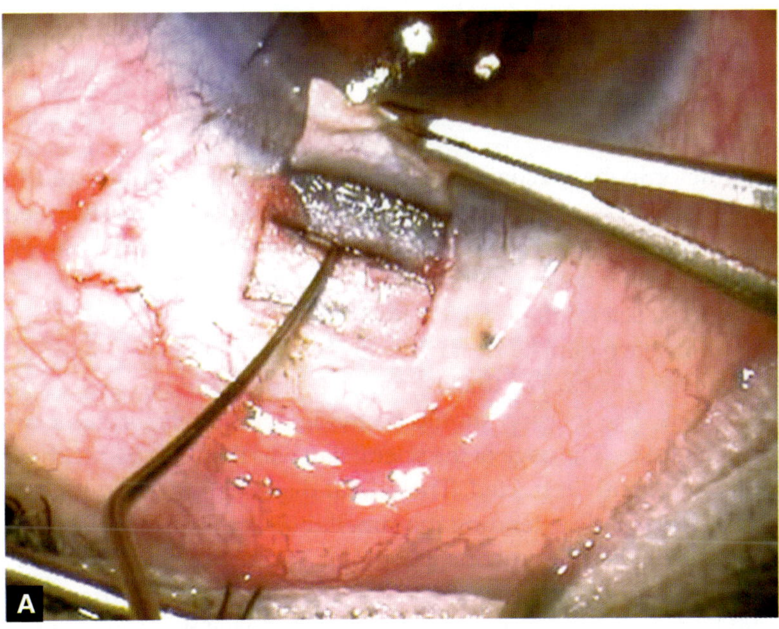

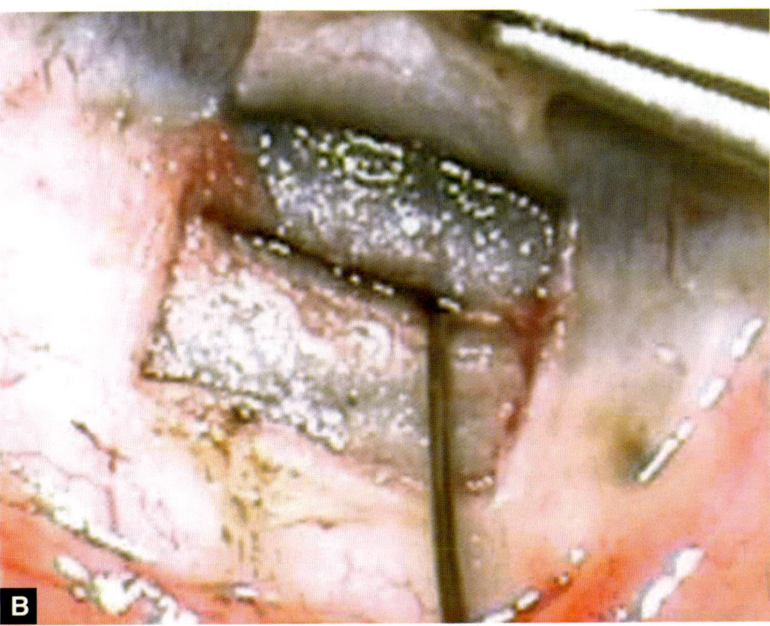

Figs 8A and B: A hook is passed though the opening of the canal to insure adequate level of dissection and milling

Surgical Steps

1. The eyelids are sterilized with ophthalmic Betadine solution (Purdue Frederick, Norwalk, CT), and after the sterile drape was placed, a lid speculum was inserted.
2. An 8-mm fornix-based conjunctival flap is prepared superiorly and Tenon's capsule was retracted. Bipolar cautery is then applied sparingly to cauterize individual limbal vessels one by one to achieve homeostasis preserving as much as possible the episcleral vessel.
3. A superficial scleral flap of 4 × 4 mm hinged at the limbus was designed using ultra sharp mini blade such as the No. 7511 Beaver, extending 1-mm into the clear cornea. The thickness of the flap should be between 200 and 250 microns. The incision should be made definitively, without multiple tentative strokes. The edge of the scleral flap was then grasped with Hoskins forceps and gently retracted. The scleral dissection is carried out using a crescent-style blade extending the lamellar dissection anterior tell the blue limbal zone then more anteriorly until 1 or 2 mm of a clear cornea is reached and the iris details can be seen through the deep layers of corneal tissue.
4. Under high magnification, a rectangular dry area of the scleral bed about 3 × 3 mm inside the superficially created flap is selected to start milling and the milling motorized drill was applied without pressure allowing to drill and refine the remaining scleral thickness in a linear pattern to leave a thin layer of sclera underneath. The site of milling should be applied at the surgical limbus in order to expose the canal of Schlemm. The refining is carried anteriorly and downwards until the blue-gray color of the choroid should appear through the residual scleral fibers. When reaching the appropriate depth, the canal openings are identified by passing a hook though them.

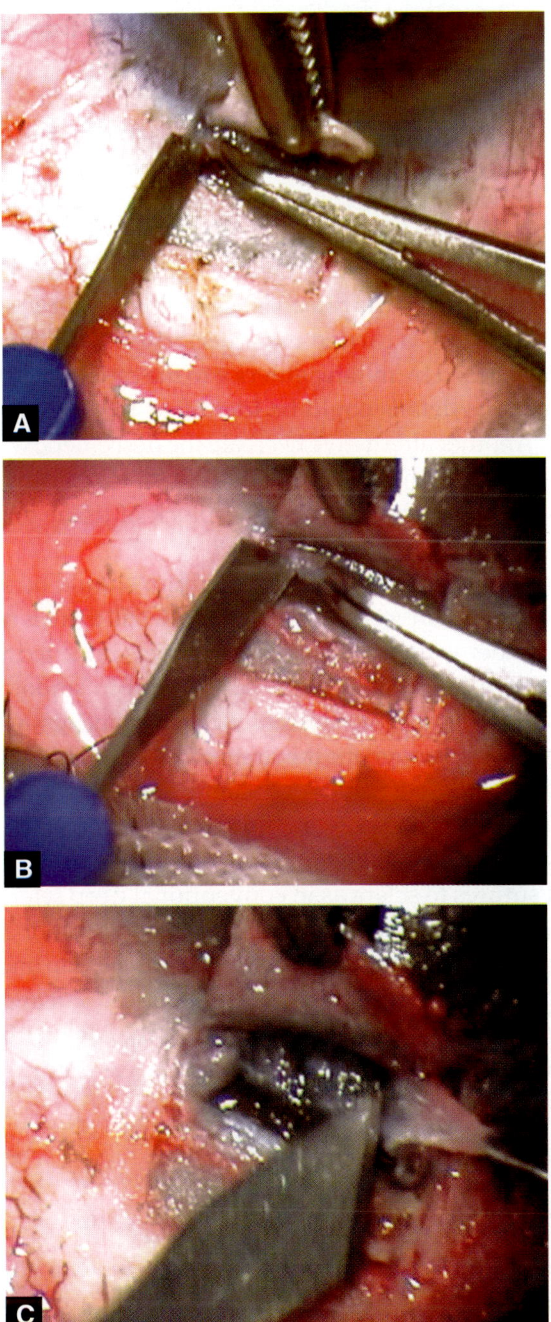

Fig. 9: Deroofing of Schlemm's canal is done:

(A) 2 incisions are created at both sides starting from the opened Schlemm's canal and anteriorly tell reaching the clear corneal under the flap

(B) The site of incision is checked again and repeated on the other side

(C) The roof of the canal is removed using the surgical knife

5. The process of "Unroofing" of the canal is automatically done using the motorized milling drill but care should be taken not to apply any pressure (maintaining the high velocity) and leave the drill to refine the tissues. After being unroofed, the inner wall of Schlemm's canal appears as a dark line, just anterior to the scleral spur. The milling is continued anteriorly towards the cornea to remove the sclero-corneal trabecular meshwork (T.M), which typically exhibits a granular texture. If phacoemulsification is combined with the procedure, the superficial corneal flap is reposted and a clear corneal incision is prepared then the phaco is performed. After the phaco has been completed the milling is carried out anteriorly and 1-2 mm of Descemet´s membrane is exposed by milling anterior to the canal till clear corneal tissue is reached and iris details could be identified though the remaining thin sheet of T.M. Another alternative to create the descemetic window is using a mini-blade starting with down-up incision at one of the two opening of the canal then with a shaving movement a block of tissue is excised moving towards the other opening of the canal.
6. At this stage of the procedure, aqueous humor should be seen percolating through the trabeculo-descemetic membrane. If still there is reduced outflow, stripping the inner wall of Schlemm´s canal was done to increase aqueous outflow and then further milling is carried out to smoothen the surface. Ultimately, only the trabeculo-descemetic membrane remains intact. Visible filtration of aqueous through the thin trabeculo-descemetic membrane should be obtained. Dilatation of Schlemm´s canal could be also done by inserting a cannula into the canal for 0.5 or 1 mm.
7. In case of glaucoma implant the implant should inserted at this level of the surgery and sutures to sclera as in conventional deep sclerectomy.
8. The flap is gently laid in its normal anatomic position. Two 10-0 nylon stitches were placed at both edges of the superficial flap and tied fairly (not very tight and not very loose). The suture ends were cut and the knots were parried to prevent the suture tips from eroding the conjunctiva. After closing the scleral flap repositioning of the conjunctiva was then done with 2 lateral 10/0 nylon stitches.

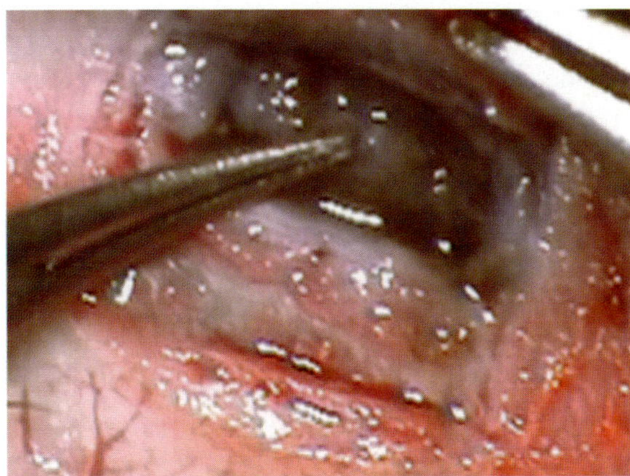

Fig. 10: Stripping of the floor of the canal is done if insufficient filtration is found

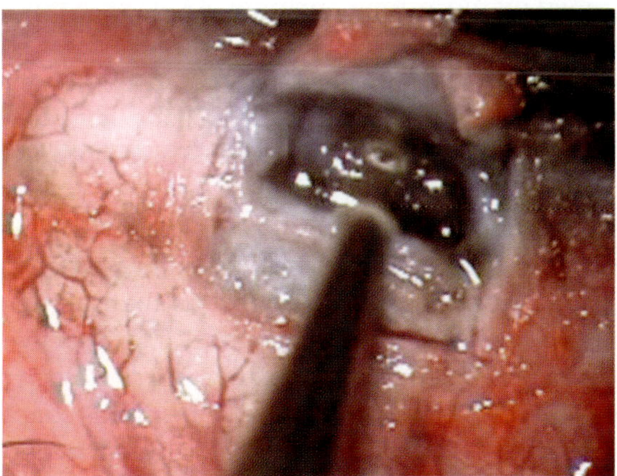

Fig. 11: Refining the descemet window is done using the drill and the milling is done applying no pressure

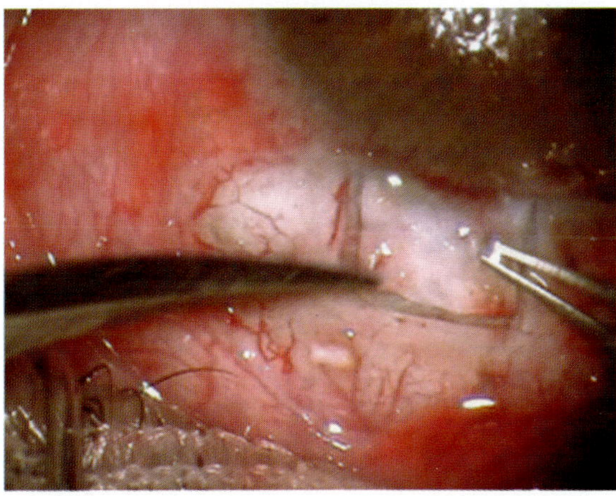

Fig. 12: The scleral flap is reposted at the end of the surgery

Postoperative Follow Up

Treatment: Antibiotic-steroidal combination; Tobradex® (Lab Alcon Cusi, Inc. Barcelona. Spain) eye drops were instilled postoperatively 4 times daily for 1 week and slowly withdrawn over one month period. No viscoelastics was injected into the Schlemm canal, and the procedure was completed without the use of collagen device or mitomycin C at any stage of the surgery in our series.

Follow up: Patients were scheduled for follow-up visits at 1 day, 1 week then 1, 3 and 6 months after surgery. The postoperative evaluation included the IOP, presence of functioning bleb, gonioscopy, visual acuity status and possible surgical and postoperative complications.

RESULTS

The study performed by the authors included 41 eyes (41 patients). The mean age of the patients was 67.9 ± 10.9 (range 50 to 80) years. The preoperative diagnoses had confirmed that all eyes have medically uncontrolled primary open-angle glaucoma. The mean pre-operative cup/disc ratio was 0.7 ± 0.25. The mean angle grading as reported by gonioscopic findings was 3.6 ± 0.61 according to shaffer grading system.

The eyes were divided into 2 groups: group I (20 eyes) underwent milling procedure and group II (21 eyes) underwent combined procedure, milling and phacoemulsification procedures. In both groups the milling procedure was done without the use of collagen device or MMC. The other eye of each patient was operated by conventional deep sclerectomy and combined phaco and deep sclerectomy and their results are behind the scope of this chapter.

The past medical history of the patients included hypertension in 36% patients, and one patient had history of diabetes mellitus. Among the eyes included in the study, 23.7% had history of cataract extraction and IOL implantation, 7.2% had history of previous glaucoma surgery (deep sclerectomy). Preoperative history of anti-glaucoma therapy is shown in Figures 16A and B.

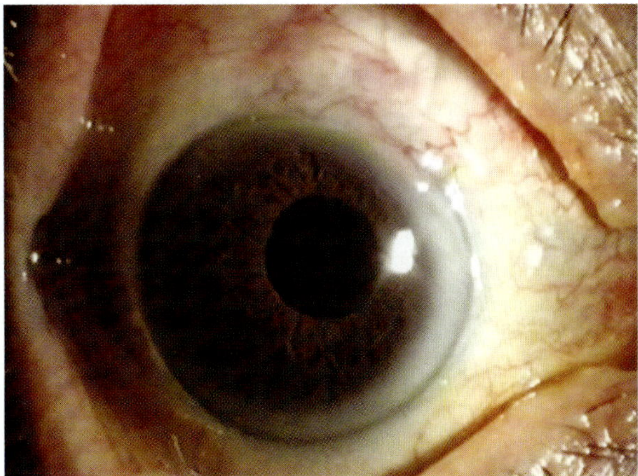

Fig. 13: Slit-lamp photo of the postoperative bleb obtained at 6-months in group I

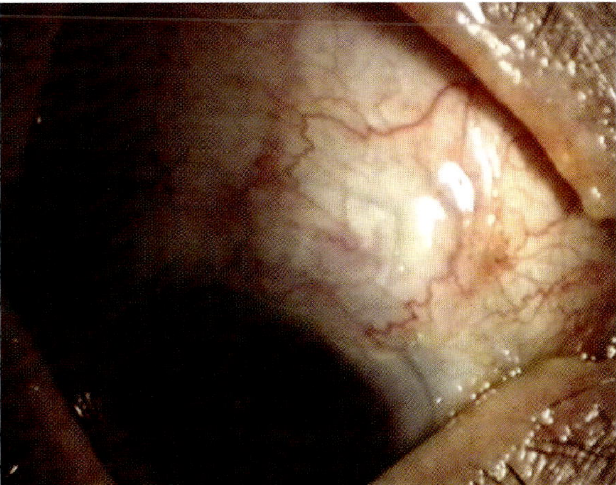

Fig. 14: Slit-lamp photo of the postoperative bleb obtained at 6-months in group II (Phaco-milling)

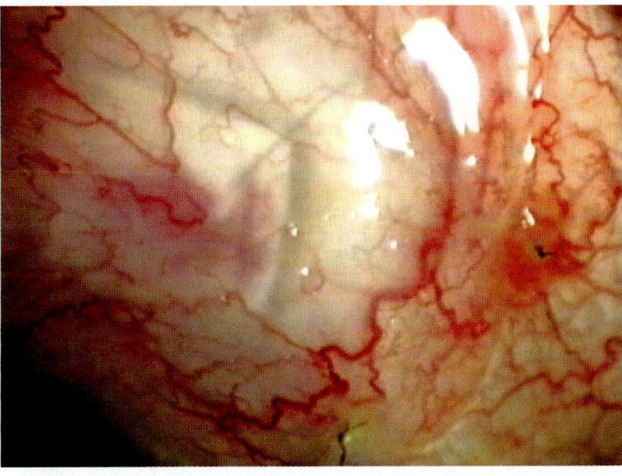

Fig.15: The diffuse filtering bleb as appeared at the end of the 6th month in group II

Group I (Milling procedure)

Visual results and refractive results of this group: refer to Table 1. Intraocular pressure (IOP) and its results during the study are shown in Table 2. Figure 17 shows the IOP results of both groups during the follow up period of the study.

Table 1: Shows the results of group I, milling trabeculoplasty

Group 1: Milling trabeculoplasty		*N*	*Mean ± SD*	*Standard error*	*Range* *Maximum*	*Minimum*
Pre-op refraction	BCVA	20	0.828 ± 0.279	0.0624	1	0.05
	Sphere		0.025 ± 0.648	0.145	1.5	–1.5
	Cylinder		–0.675 ± 1.067	0.239	0	–4
	SE		–0.313 ± 0.512	0.115	0.5	–1.5
	Defocus equivalent		0.725 ± 0.786	0.176	2.500	0.000
Post-op refraction at 1M	BCVA	20	0.792 ± 0.258	0.0578	1	0.05
	Sphere		–0.025 ± 0.858	0.192	1.25	–2
	Cylinder		–0.0875 ± 2.507	0.561	10	–3
	SE		–0.069 ± 1.302	0.291	4.5	–2.25
	Defocus equivalent		0.713 ± 0.762	0.170	2.500	0.000
Post-op refraction at 6M	BCVA	20	0.835 ± 0.262	0.0587	1	0.05
	Sphere		0.1 ± 0.357	0.0799	1	–0.5
	Cylinder		–0.713 ± 0.964	0.216	0	–4
	SE		–0.257 ± 0.336	0.0752	0.13	–1
	Defocus equivalent		0.625 ± 0.750	0.168	3.000	0.000

Table 2: Shows the results of group II, milling trabeculoplasty plus phacoemulsification at the same session

Group I1: Milling + Phaco		*N*	*Mean ± SD*	*Standard error*	*Range* *Maximum*	*Minimum*
Preop refraction	BCVA	21	0.298 ± 0.217	0.0473	0.8	0.01
	Sphere		–2.821 ± 5.946	1.298	2.5	–16
	Cylinder		–1.012 ± 1.1	0.24	0.5	–3.25
	SE		–3.328 ± 6.17	1.346	1.25	–17.5
	Defocus equivalent		4.024 ± 6.339	1.383	19.000	0.000
Postop refraction at 1M	BCVA	21	0.571 ± 0.313	0.0682	1	0.01
	Sphere		–0.464 ± 1.004	0.219	1.5	–2.5
	Cylinder		–1.179 ± 1.151	0.251	0	–4.5
	SE		–1.055 ± 1.247	0.272	0.5	–4.75
	Defocus equivalent		1.714 ± 1.603	0.350	7.000	0.000
Postop refraction at 6M	BCVA	21	0.636 ± 0.304	0.0663	1	0.05
	Sphere		–0.238 ± 0.835	0.182	1.5	–1.5
	Cylinder		–1.19 ± 0.898	0.196	0	–3
	SE		-0.835 ± 0.867	0.189	0.5	–3
	Defocus equivalent		1.524 ± 1.006	0.220	4.500	0.000

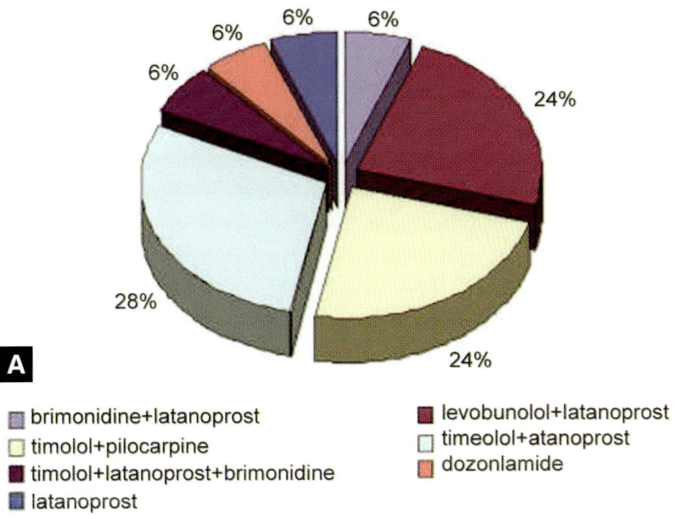

Combined eye drops used pre-op in Group I: Milling

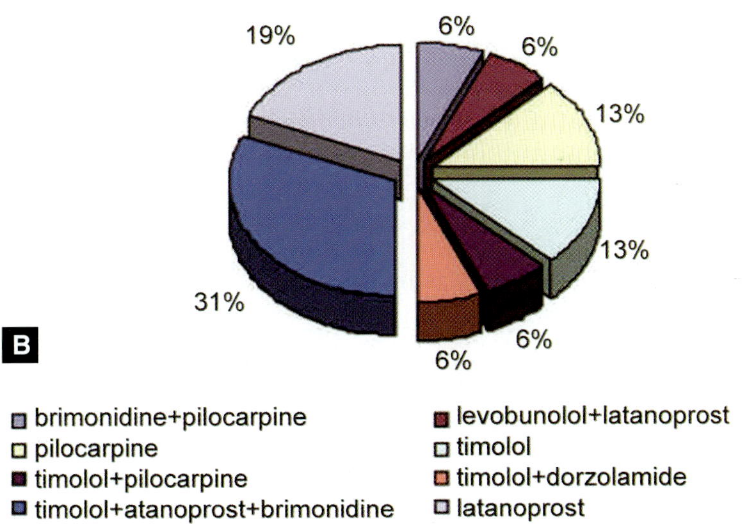

Combined eye drops used pre-op in Group II: Milling + Phaco

Figs16A and B: Graph showing the percent of pre-op combination of anti-glaucoma treatment in A) Group I and B) Group II

Group II (Milling procedure combined with phaco)

Visual results and refractive results of this group: refer to Table 3. Intraocular pressure (IOP) and its results during the study are shown in Table 4. Figure 17 shows the IOP results of both groups during the follow up period of the study.

Table 3: Shows the results of IOP in group I, milling trabeculoplasty

Variable	*N*	*Mean ± SD*	*Standard error*	*Range*	
				Maximum	*Minimum*
Initial IOP	20	23.9 ± 7.166	1.602	50	16
Basal IOP	20	32.640 ± 7.151	1.599	50.0	22.0
Objective IOP	20	20.650 ± 3.99	0.894	26.60	14.4
IOP at 1m	20	12.65 ± 4.945	1.106	22	2
Reduction IOP at 1m	20	−7.994± 5.853	1.309	6.50	−15.95
% Reduction IOP at 1m	20	47.205 ± 15.039	3.282	88.89	19.23
IOP at 1m	20	14.45 ± 3.379	0.756	24	10
Reduction IOP at 6 m	20	−6.200± 4.148	0.928	1.5	−14.6
% Reduction IOP at 6 m	20	36.821 ± 17.252	3.765	64	−5.26

Table 4: Shows the results of IOP in group II, milling trabeculoplasty plus phacoemulsification at the same session

Variable	*N*	*Mean ± SD*	*Standard error*	*Range*	
				Maximum	*Minimum*
Initial IOP	21	22.952 ± 7.619	1.663	42	10
Basal IOP	21	33.310 ± 14.487	3.161	65.1	13.0
Objective IOP	21	23.319± 10.154	2.216	25.2	6
IOP at 1m	21	15.762 ± 5.761	1.257	38	10
Reduction IOP at 1m	21	−7.546± 9.047	1.974	6.9	−27.9
% Reduction IOP at 1m	21	25.906 ± 28.22	6.017	56.67	−60
IOP at 1m	21	15.19 ± 3.473	0.758	23	10
Reduction IOP at 6 m	21	−8.11± 8.607	1.878	6.9	−24.8
% Reduction IOP at 6 m	21	27.91 ± 26.897	5.734	56	−60

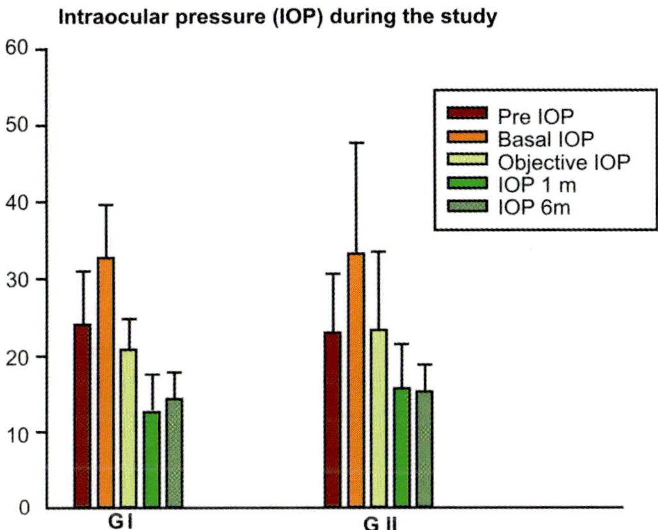

Fig.17: Graph showing the IOP changes during the follow up period in both groups

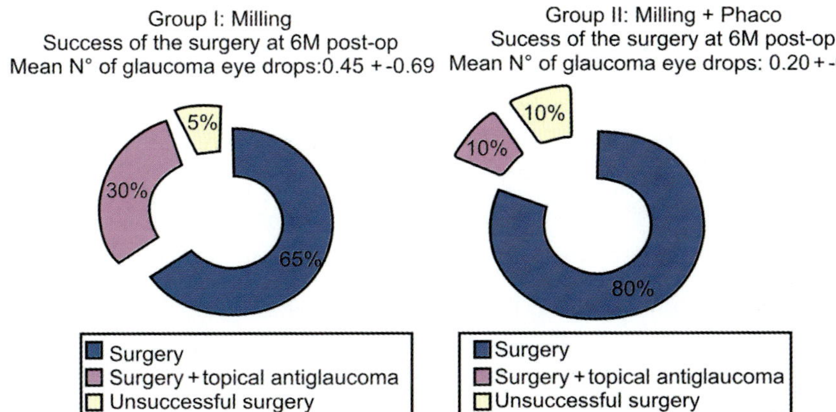

Fig.18: Graph showing the percent of success of milling surgery and milling-phaco after 65 months, the percent of eyes that had to use topical treatment and eyes that had to go back to treatment as the target pressure was not reached

DISCUSSION

Non-penetrating glaucoma surgeries including viscocanalostomy and deep sclerectomy are difficult to perform, need a high learning curve and time consuming. In both non-penetrating glaucoma surgeries and milling surgery, both the postoperative recovery and follow up are faster and the level of IOP reduction achieved is satisfactory when compared with the results of trabeculectomy.

Milling trabeculoplasty in this prospective, pilot study on 41 eyes has showing good results as it led to a 30-40% reduction of IOP in both groups operated with the technique. The percent of success of surgery at the 6th month without the use of collagen device or MMC was 60% for group I and 80% for group II. The rate of postop bleb fibrosis and the use of postop anti-glaucoma therapy was found to be similar to that found with deep sclerectomy.

The followings are the potential advantages of the Milling trabecuoloplasty over the non-penetrating glaucoma surgeries:

1. Facilitate the surgical procedure of non-penetrating technique as the refining is carried anteriorly and down until the roof of schlemm´s canal can barely be visible. Unlike deep non-penetrating sclerectomy, this technique does not require any specific accuracy in the dissection of the deep sclera.
2. To reduce the wound healing as a determinate factor for the IOP outcome as the diamond powder tip is available for more delicate maneuvers like removing debris, making the technique ideal and leaving an extremely smooth bed.
3. Offers less complications than deep sclerectomy and it prevents the "double-cut" sclera and hazards.
4. The economic coast of the drill.
5. Saves time as this technique has an easier approach to the trabeculo-descemetic membrane.
6. No need for the use of high expensive surgical set.

CONCLUSION

Milling trabeculoplasty is an evolving technique for easy scalpel-free non-penetrating glaucoma surgery. The milling surgery seems to be a promising technique for surgical management of POAG glaucoma. Milling trabeculoplasty is a fast, safe, effective technique to perform non-penetrating glaucoma surgery with low coast and simple instruments. Milling trabeculoplasty is a potential alternative to deep sclerectomy providing comparable results to conventional deep sclerectomy mainly the low level of IOP together with minimal intra and postoperative complications.

34

G-probe as Primary Glaucoma Procedure in Cases of Coexisting POAG and Cataract

Cyres K Mehta, Keiki R Mehta (India)

INTRODUCTION

Here we introduce a new concept in the **primary** therapy of glaucoma where a G-probe of an Iris Medical Diode laser is used to treat glaucoma along with phacoemulsification on a primary basis i.e. a first glaucoma procedure of choice!

Materials and Methods

During the course of a year at the Mehta International Eye Institute, Mumbai, 50 patients had combined phacoemulsification and G-probe performed in the same sitting for coexisting cataract and glaucoma. Only those patients with IOP>21 on maximum tolerated medication were chosen. A peribulbar block was given and the G -probe was applied for 24 applications circumferentially(1 for each clock hr) over the ciliary body at 2W for 2 seconds. Then clear corneal phaco was performed and an injectable intraocular lens implanted in all cases. The IOP was measured on day 1 week 1 and months 1, 3 and 6. All surgery was carried out by the same surgeon (CM) using the Alcon Infinity unit , Iris Medical Diode laser and G-probe. Pressures were measured with Topcon-CT80 air puff tonometer.

Results

At the end of one day all patients had pressure less than 10 mm Hg. At week one, 3 patients had pressures greater than 21. At month 1, the number of patients(IOP > 21) had increased to 6.

At month one these 6 underwent the same procedure again(G-probe). At month 6 all patients except one has pressures less than 21 mmHg on no additional medication.

Conclusion

Combined G-probe phaco with IOL implantation has proved to be safe consistent and reproducibly easy to perform. It's a very effective way to control glaucoma without any incisional surgery.

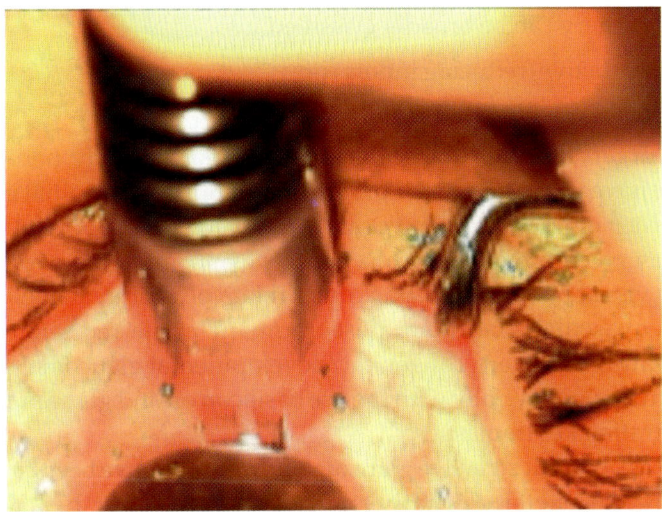

Fig. 1: Applications for 22 clock hour

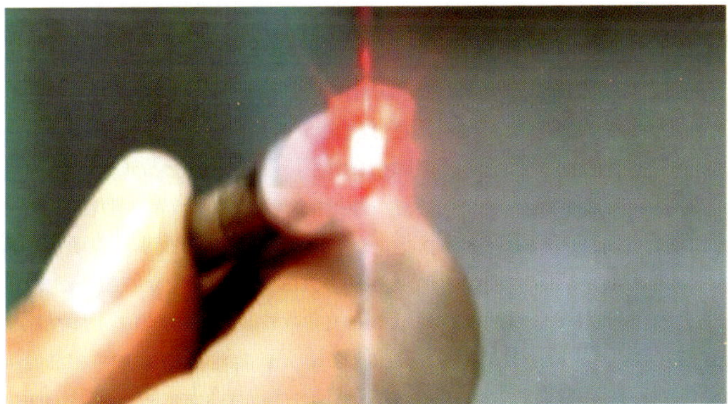

Fig. 2: Aiming beam of G probe

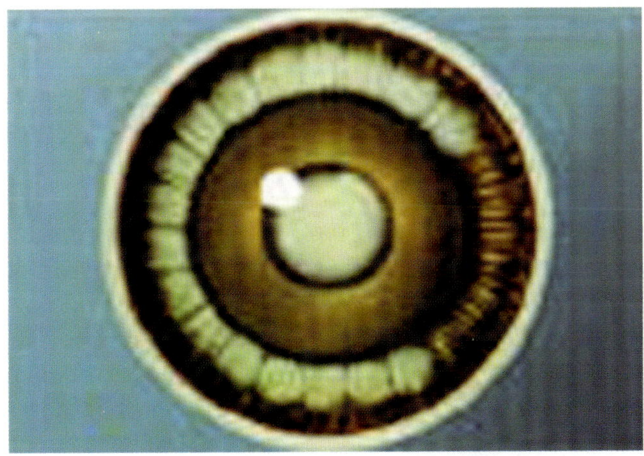

Fig. 3: Apple miyake view of spots

Glaucoma surgery can be broadly classified into

1. Cyclodestructive (reducing inflow) or
2. Filtering (increasing outflow).

Filtration surgery, typically trabeculectomy and more recently, non-penetrating techniques have usually been the procedure of choice as an initial intervention because of their efficacy and relative safety and predictability . Ciliary destruction has been reserved for more refractory cases of glaucoma and in eyes which have little or no visual potential. Refractory or relatively "untreatable" glaucomas include neovascular glaucoma, post-traumatic angle recession glaucoma, aphakic glaucoma severe congenital/developmental glaucoma, post-retinal surgery glaucoma especially with the use of silicon oil and glaucoma associated with penetrating keratoplasties.

In the past, cyclodestructive glaucoma procedures have been carried out by either surgical excision, diathermy, cryotherapy, or by laser. Laser cyclophotocoagulation has now become the principal method for what has been termed as "turning down the tap. " Beckman and Sugar pioneered the use of trans-scleral cyclophotocoagulation (TCP) thirty odd years ago. In the beginning they tried the procedure with a Ruby laser but they found that the (Nd:YAG) laser was more effective in penetrating the sclera and optimizing energy absorption by the ciliary epithelium. The delivery of laser energy through the sclera may be performed by either the non-contact or contact method. In the non-contact approach, a slit lamp is employed to apply laser energy through the conjunctival/scleral eye wall. The focus of energy delivery is 1–1. 5 mm behind the limbus , through a contact lens so that maximal effect is at the level of the ciliary body. The total number of laser applications are usually about 32 (eight per quadrant), avoiding the 3 and 9 o'clock positions in order to preserve the long posterior ciliary arteries.

More recently, contact cyclophotocoagulation has gained favour as a preferred modality. Using the Nd:YAG laser (Surgical Laser Technologies (SLT), a hand held sapphire tipped probe is placed on the conjunctiva and sclera, 1–2 mm behind the limbus. Depending on the requirement, 28 spots are applied, also avoiding the 3 and 9 o'clock positions. Energy levels are titrated to avoid an audible "pop" which signifies an overtreatment and explosion of the ciliary body tissue.

The semiconductor diode laser (Iris Oculight SLx, Iris Medical Inc, Mountain View, CA, USA) emits at 810 nm wavelength and is better absorbed by melanin than the Nd:YAG. The spade shaped tip of the hand piece (known as the "G-probe") protrudes 0.7 mm deeper than the contact surface. There is better absorption of this wavelength by the pigmented tissues of the ciliary body than the 1064 nm Nd:YAG laser. Also a lower incidence of the complications seen with other cyclodestructive techniques—namely, phthisis, hypotony, uveitis, pain, and loss of visual acuity are reported in the literature . The most widely

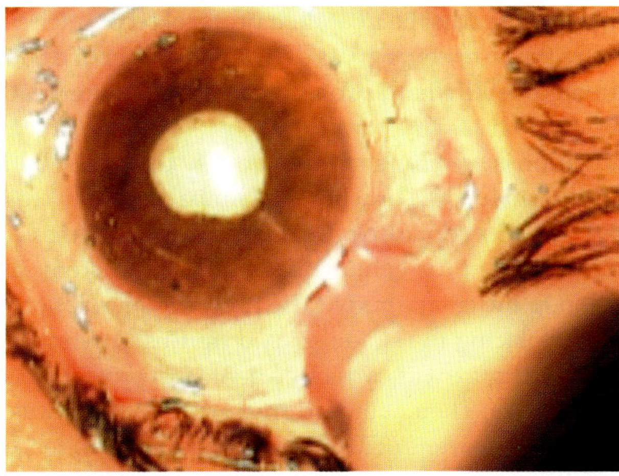

Fig. 4: Applying the G-probe laser energy

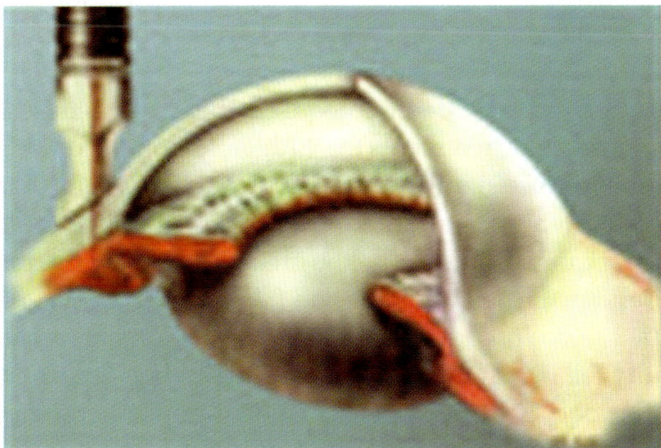

Fig. 5: Cross section view of laser

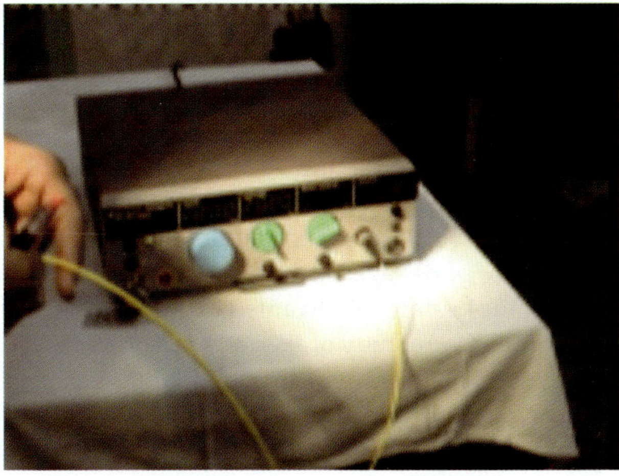

Fig. 5: Iris medical base unit with PR

adopted treatment strategy is the treatment protocol recommended by Spencer and Vernon. Here the laser energy was delivered through the 600 μm diameter quartz fiber oriented within the G-probe handpiece to centre treatment 1. 2 mm behind the limbus.

Transillumination is recommended to identify the ciliary body position in eyes with congenital glaucoma or where the limbal anatomy was distorted by previous surgery. The fiberoptic tip protrudes 0. 7 mm from the G-probe contact surface in order to indent the conjunctiva and sclera thereby improving the laser transmission to the ciliary body. The posterior angulation of the fiber is ensured by simply placing the spade shaped tip flush with the limbus in the manner shown in the figure was correctly oriented to protect the lens of phakic eyes from laser damage. Their standard treatment protocol was used at each "session" to treat three quarters (270 degrees)of the circumference of the ciliary body. This usually resulted in 14 . An energy of 2. 0 W was used for 2. 0 seconds, resulting in a power delivery of 4. 0 J per application (56 J per session for 14 applications). This was not altered even if "pops" were heard during treatment. In the first treatment session the temporal 90 degrees was left untreated. A different 90 degrees was left untreated if further treatment sessions proved necessary. On subsequent treatments the 90 degrees untreated varied depending on the appearance of the sclera and conjunctiva at the limbus that is, if an area of scleromalacia from previous surgery was present this area could be avoided. In Spencer and Vernons(S&V) study, the mean IOP before treatment was 33. 0 mm Hg (10. 7) and by the last visit this had fallen to 16. 7 mm Hg at 6 months It is apparent that the cyclodiode gives a mean reduction of at least 33% in IOP . The visual acuity fell in half the patients by 1 line, when utilising the Iris diode laser with the G-probe. In their experience , when "pops" were heard continually with a consistent energy level they did not have any eyes with marked inflammation post-laser. They did not find a particular association between race and hearing "pops".

Different Protocols and Treatment Strategies are Found in the Literature

Kosoko *et al* , delivered between 17 and 19 applications to 270 degrees of the ciliary body for a 2. 0 second period and commencing at 1. 75 W increasing to 2. 0 W, if no "pops" or "snaps" were heard. The theory behind reducing the energy so as not to hear "pops" at each application is that these are indicative of tissue disruption, thus leading to unwanted extra inflammation. No eyes in Kosoko and others' multicentre study of 27 eyes had a previous cyclodestructive procedure and only two eyes had repeat treatment (after 9 and 13 months). About 60% of eyes were controlled (IOP < 22 mm Hg) which is less than the figure of 81% from the S&V study.

In a study carried out by Philip Bloom , they allowed more than one treatment session but 18% of their eyes had cyclodestructive procedures before cyclodiode

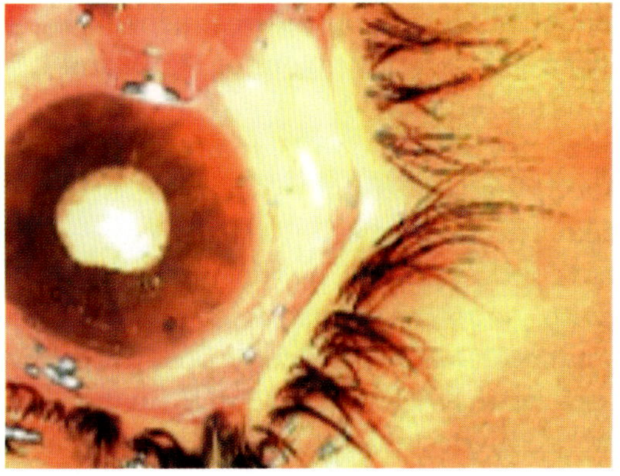

Fig. 7: Note the pressure of mature T

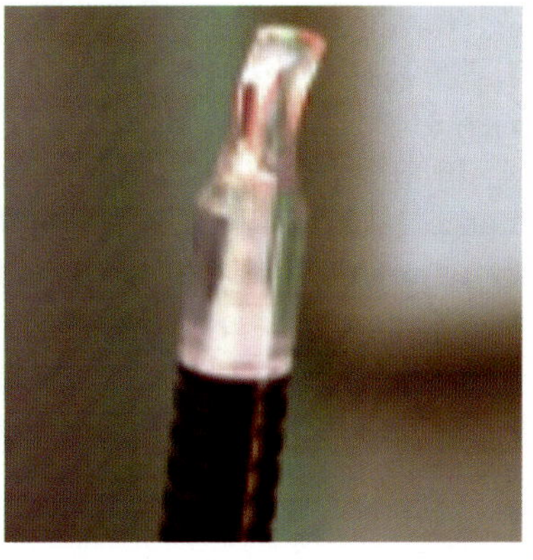

Fig. 8: Spade shaped footplate

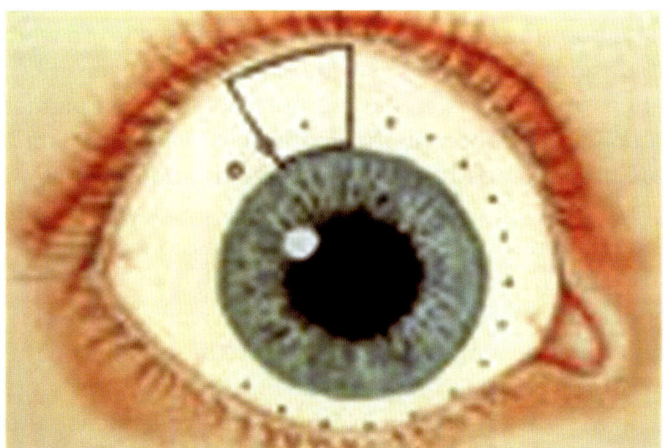

Fig. 9: Proper placement of spots

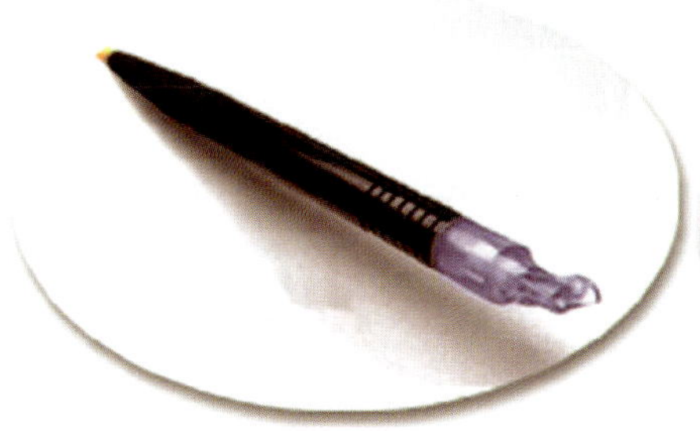

Fig. 10: The G probe

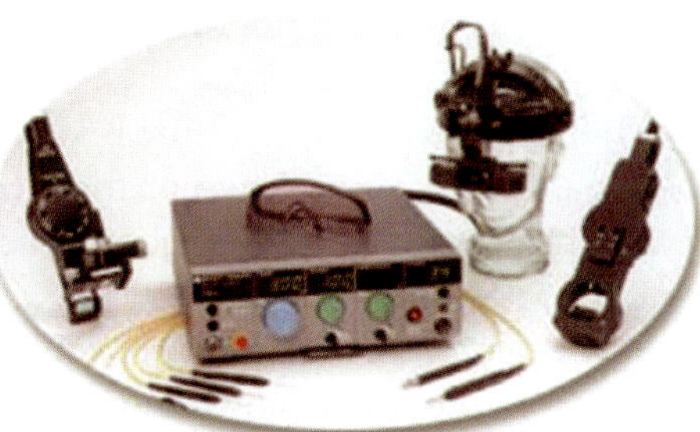

Fig. 11: The Iris Medical d10 Nm

and the mean follow up was only 10 months. In addition, the treatment protocol varied considerably between eyes, from 20 to 40 applications of 1. 5 W and 1. 5 seconds "titrated against risk of phthisis".

Brancato *et al* 20 had a higher retreatment rate of 65% than Spencer and Vernons, 45%. This is probably due to patient group differences as 10/48 patients in Brancato's series had "pediatric glaucoma".

Different types of glaucoma behaved differently. The rubeotic eyes, those with silicone oil glaucoma, those with glaucoma related to corneal disease (including post-keratoplasty glaucoma), and those with chronic post-traumatic glaucoma had the greatest percentage drop in IOP (56. 7% to 65. 6%) in the S&V study. These groups, however, had the highest pretreatment pressures and therefore would have required a larger drop to achieve the target pressure.

In our practice the following procedure is followed.

The eye to be operated, undergoes G-probe applications, over 360 degrees with the probe in the proper orientation, we use 2 watt power and 2 second exposure time. We aim for a "pop-less" endpoint. To simplify, I put 2 or 3 applications . If popping occurs, the energy is decreased in 0. 5 watt increments till popping subsides, usually at 1. 5 watts or sometimes even at 1 watt. Twenty two applications are administered with care taken to avoid pigmented lesions on the conjunctiva , common pigmented Indian eyes. Also 3 and 9 , o' clock meridians are best avoided to avoid pain, uveitis and ischemia which occurs with damage to the long ciliary nerves and vessels. The applications are put with firm indentation so as to maximize transmission of energy through the sclera and also as indentation leaves a mark which helps to position and space the next application. Once the applications are over, the eye is washed with betadine solution and cataract surgery is carried out either with a standard 2. 8 mm clear corneal phaco technique involving direct backcracking after tipping the nucleus up in hydrodissection in a procedure called lens salute phaco, or by employing a Microphaco technique and the same chopping maneuver with a Cyres Scythe chopping tip on the MST Duet inflow system.

In my (CM) experience, of combining phacoemulsification wth G-probe as a primary procedure for coexisting cataract and primary open angle glaucoma the dreaded complication , phthisis has never occurred, probably as these were "virgin" eyes and had not undergone any surgical intervention for glaucoma previously.

Phthisis bulbi in the literature review occurs in less than 1%of cases. Typically these patients have had two or three trabeculectomies and a healthy dose of cryotherapy as well. The G-probe application adds the final straw on the camels back so to speak.

Phthisis has never been reported in a case where no previous intervention (surgery or cryo) has been attempted in "virgin" eyes.

No patient had significant pain apart from a feeling of heaviness of the head.

Postoperatively the patient is typically on topical dexa or beta methasone eye drops and Moxifloxacin eye drops. Oral diclofenac sodium tablets 50 mg twice a day is all that is needed for any pain control for three to four days. Oral steroid is administered in a dosage of 16 mg triamcinolone tablets for 4 days.

There was no extra uveitis seen in these patients and no appreciable cells or flare, apart from that expected in a simple clear corneal phacoemulsification with a good quality viscoelastic.

This procedure in our hands has proved its safety and efficacy and deserves a try. When you consider, bleb failures, bleb leaks, bleb related endophthamlitis, overhanging blebs, bleb failure, persistent hypotony, maculopathy, etc. simply turning down the tap, may prove to be a more attractive alternative.

35

Very Deep Sclerectomy or How to Increase Uveoscleral Outflow

Kaweh Mansouri, André Mermoud (Switzerland)

INTRODUCTION

Standard non-penetrating glaucoma surgery (NPGS) currently consists of different methods, the most popular of which are deep sclerectomy and viscocanalostomy. The goal of NPGS is to create a surgical procedure as efficient as trabeculectomy but with less complications. The main idea of NPGS is to target the portion of the aqueous outflow pathway responsible for the main resistance to outflow, and to create filtration through the thin trabeculo-Descemet's membrane.

The uveoscleral pathway was described more than 30 years ago. It was also termed unconventional outflow route (as opposed to the conventional or trabecular meshwork outflow) and showed to be responsible for up to 50% of aqueous humour drainage in monkey eyes. The aqueous percolates through the tissue spaces of the ciliary muscle into the supraciliary and suprachoroidal spaces.

We have observed that by tightly suturing the scleral flap, bigger amounts of the percolating aqueous could be forced through the remaining sclera into the uveoscleral outflow. Deep sclerectomy with collagen implant (VDSCI) is a modification of deep sclerectomy that was devised with the goal of increasing aqueous outflow via the uveoscleral pathway. By dissecting part of the deep sclera, the drainage of aqueous humor into the suprachoroidal space should be enhanced. Aqueous in the supra choroidal space may hypothetically reach the uveoscleral outflow, and it could also induce a chronic ciliary body detachment thus reducing aqueous production.

At the same time, we aimed to reduce dependency on subconjunctival outflow to minimize the size of the filtering bleb and bleb-related discomfort and complications.

We furthermore aimed to gain further knowledge in the mechanisms of function of NPGS that are not yet properly understood.

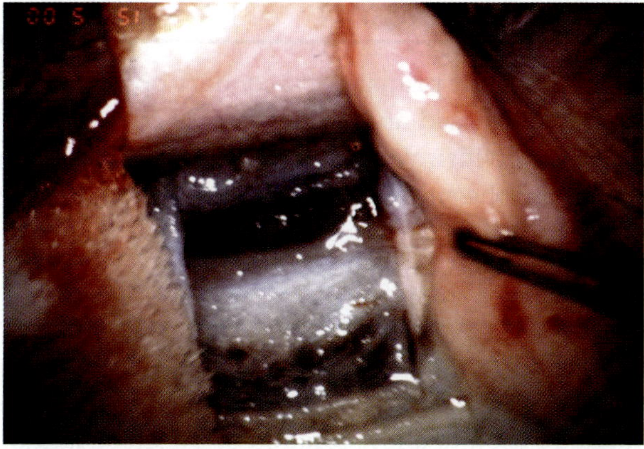

Fig. 1: Standard deep sclerectomy after dissection of the deep scleral flap

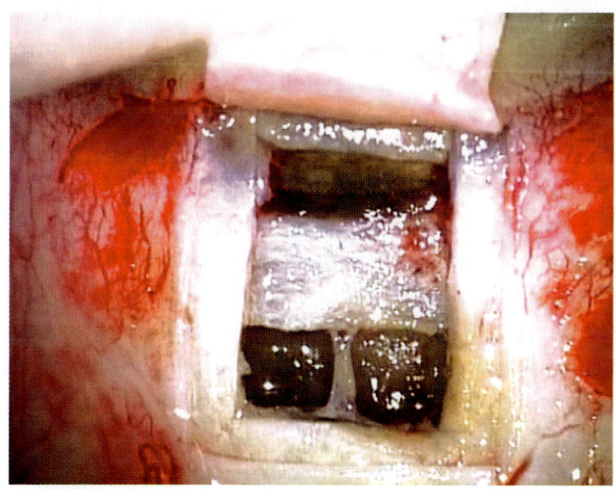

Fig. 2: Very deep sclerectomy after dissection of two 1.5 × 1.5 mm very deep scleral flaps. A scleral bridge is left to prevent choroidal prolapse, and the collagen implant is placed to re-inforce it for the early postoperative period

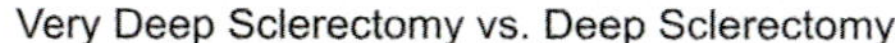

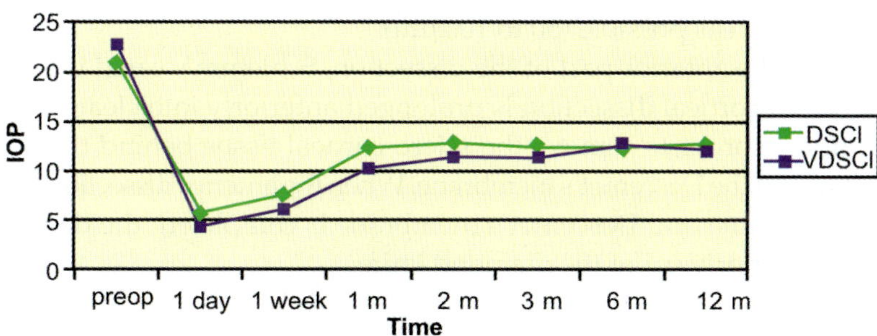

Fig. 3: IOP over time for VDSCI and DSCI groups. There was no significant difference at any point at time. Mean follow-up period was 6.5 months (maximum 12 months)

GENERALITIES

Indications for NPGS include primary or secondary open-angle glaucoma, and exclude neovascular and closed-angle glaucoma. The procedure is particularly well adapted for patients with myopia due to the slow and gradual postoperative pressure reduction and the smaller subconjunctival filtering bleb size which enhances the comfort of wearing a contact lens.

SURGICAL TECHNIQUE

Retrobulbar, peribulbar or topical anesthesia can be used at the discretion of the surgeon. With peribulbar or retrobulbar block, the smallest amount of anaesthetic should be used to allow rotation of the globe and thus give good exposure for the deep sclerectomy dissection. The initial steps for VDSCI are identical to those for standard DSCI, for which we give a short description here.

Conjunctiva and Tenon's capsule are opened on 8–10 mm either at the limbus or at the fornix. Some light wetfield cauterization should be performed on the sclera as necessary at this stage.

A superficial scleral flap measuring 5 × 5 mm and including 1/3 of the scleral thickness (about 300 μm) is first delineated using a metal blade and then dissected with a crescent ruby blade (Huco vision SA, St-Blaise, Switzerland). In order to be able to later dissect the corneal stroma down to Descemet's membrane, the scleral flap is dissected 1 to 1.5 mm into clear cornea. A sponge soaked in mitomycin-C, 0.02%, is used at this stage in patients at high risk of scarring (i.e., age below 60; melanoderm patients; previous history of conjunctival surgery; long standing history of glaucoma treatment; previous uveitis; or trauma).

Deep sclero-keratectomy is done by performing a second deep scleral flap (4 × 4 mm). The two lateral and the posterior deep scleral incisions are made using a 15-degree diamond blade. The deep flap is smaller than the superficial one leaving a margin of sclera on the three sides. This will allow a tighter closure of the superficial flap in cases of a preoperative perforation of the TDM. The deep scleral flap is then dissected horizontally. The remaining scleral layer should be as thin as possible (50 to 100 μm).

Reaching the anterior part of the dissection, Schlemm's canal is unroofed and the sclero-corneal dissection is prolonged anteriorly into clear cornea for 1 to 1.5 mm in order to remove the sclero-corneal tissue behind the anterior trabeculum and the Descemet's membrane. When the anterior dissection between the corneal stroma and Descemet's membrane is completed, the deep scleral flap is cut anteriorly using the diamond knife.

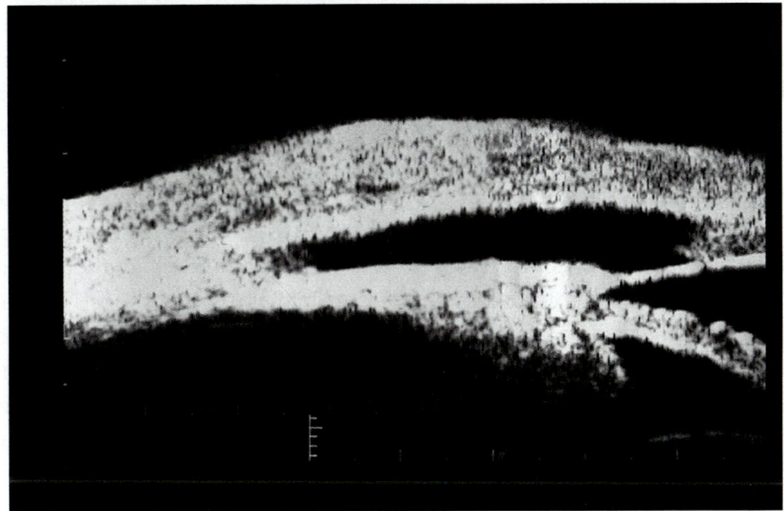

Fig. 4: UBM of a nice subconjunctival filtering bleb after DSCI

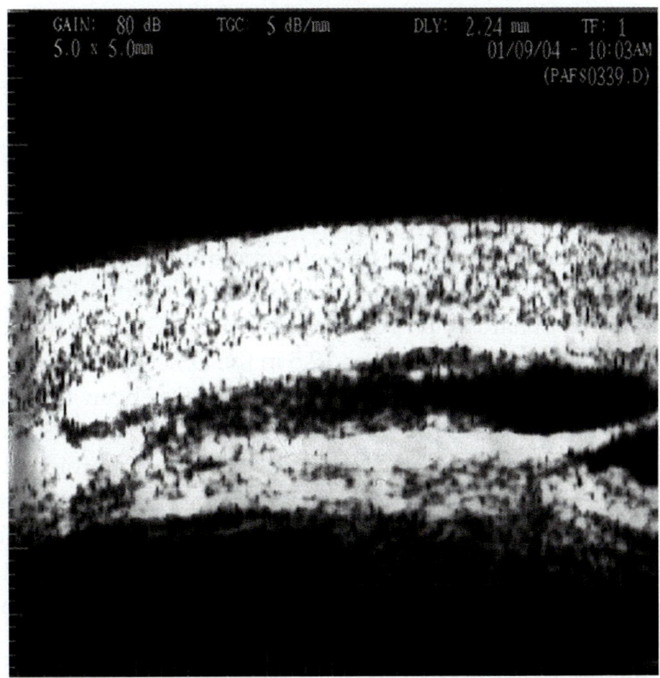

Fig. 5: UBM after VDSCI. Hypoechoic areas in the suprachoroidal space indicative of uveoscleral outflow can be seen

At this stage of surgery, the very deep scleral dissection is performed. In the posterior quadrant of the sclera, two very deep flaps (each 1.5 × 1.5 mm) of the remaining 5-10% of sclera are excised and the choroid is exposed. A thin bridge of deep scleral tissue is left between the two flaps in order to prevent a possible choroidal prolapse.

At that last stage of the procedure, there should be a diffuse percolation of aqueous through the remaining trabeculo-Descemet's membrane. The juxtacanalicular trabeculum and Schlemm's endothelium are then removed. To avoid a secondary collapse of the superficial flap over the TDM and the remaining scleral layer, a collagen implant is placed in the centre of the scleral bed over the remaining bridge of deep sclera and secured inside the scleral bed with a single 10/0 nylon suture. The superficial scleral flap is then repositioned into place, and closed with two loose 10/0 nylon sutures. Conjunctiva and Tenon's capsule are closed in two layers with a running 8/0 vicryl suture.

PRELIMINARY RESULTS

In a prospective randomised trial that involved 50 patients we looked at the intraocular pressure lowering effect and safety of the new method of very deep sclerectomy with collagen implant (VDSCI, 25 patients) and compared it to standard deep sclerectomy with collagen implant (DSCI, 25 patients). The two groups were well matched with respect to gender, age, race, and glaucoma type. Mean preoperative IOP was 21.5 mm Hg (±7.4) in the VDSCI and 22.7 mm Hg (± 4.4) in the DSCI group. After a mean follow-up of 6 months, the two procedures produced similar outcomes with respect to IOP, success rates, reduction of medication use, and safety. On the first postoperative day IOP fell to 4.4 in the VDSCI and 5.6 mmHg in the DSCI group, a positive prognostic sign for IOP control as shown by Shaarawy and co-workers. Mean IOP at six months' follow-up was 12.0 mm Hg in the VDSCI and 12.5 in the DSCI eyes.

The safety profile of the new procedure has also been favourable with significantly fewer patients requiring postoperative MMC (3 VDSCI vs. 10 DSCI eyes) and only two eyes in the VDSCI group developing a choroidal detachment versus none in the DSCI group. There were no significant postoperative complications in this series. No shallow or flat anterior chamber, no-bleb-related endophthalmitis, and no surgery-induced cataract was observed in either group. There was one case of a malignant glaucoma in a patient of African origin in the DSCI group.

Goniopuncture with the Nd:YAG laser was performed on 3 VDSCI-treated eyes and 5 DSCI-treated eyes.

High frequency ultrasound biomicroscopy (UBM), as developed by Pavlin and Foster, provides in vivo detailed anatomic evaluation of the anterior segment of the eye. Using ultrasound biomicroscopy, it was possible to observe greater

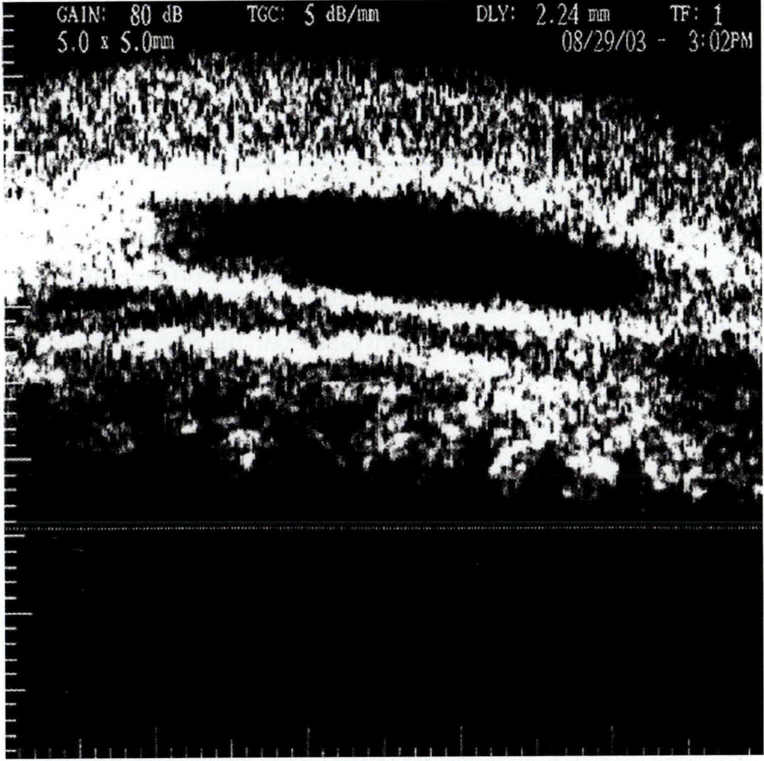

Fig. 6: UBM after VDSCI. Hypoechoic areas in the suprachoroidal space indicative of uveoscleral outflow can be seen

uveoscleral outflow in VDSCI eyes as measured by suprachoroidal effusion in 80% of VDSCI vs. 20% of DSCI patients. Mean subconjunctival bleb size was smaller in VDSCI eyes compared to DSCI eyes (9.1 vs. 29.6 mm^3)

POSTOPERATIVE MANAGEMENT

As in standard NPGS, the first postoperative weeks are crucial for the success of the new procedure. Experience has shown that the appropriate postoperative management can have the same magnitude of influence on the surgical outcome as surgery itself. The following regimen for postoperative check-up is recommended as a guideline: the patient is seen on the first postoperative day, where a complete ophthalmic examination is performed, with particular attention given to the appearance of the bleb and the depth of anterior chamber. After that, the patient is seen weekly for the first month, and then at month 2 , 3, 6, and, finally every 6 months with visual field examinations every year.

We use a topical regimen of corticosteroids and antibiotics in the immediate postoperative period. Tobradex© (Tobramycin and Dexamethasone) is administered beginning on the first postoperative day. Drops are given every 6 hours during waking hours for at least four weeks. In the next stage, patients are treated with a non-steroidal anti-inflammatory drug for two months.

CONCLUSION

In our first study with up to 12 months of follow-up, there is no statistically significant difference between very deep sclerectomy with a collagen implant and standard deep sclerectomy in terms of intraocular pressure, complete and qualified success rates, and reduction of number of medications. In VDSCI, UBM showed a statistically significant increase in amount of suprachoroidal effusion associated with a tendency towards smaller size of the subconjunctival bleb compared to DSCI. We therefore conclude that VDSCI might be a good alternative to standard penetrating surgery by decreasing the complications and discomfort related to the subconjunctival bleb. However, at this stage, longer follow-up is needed to assess the safety and efficacy of this new procedure.

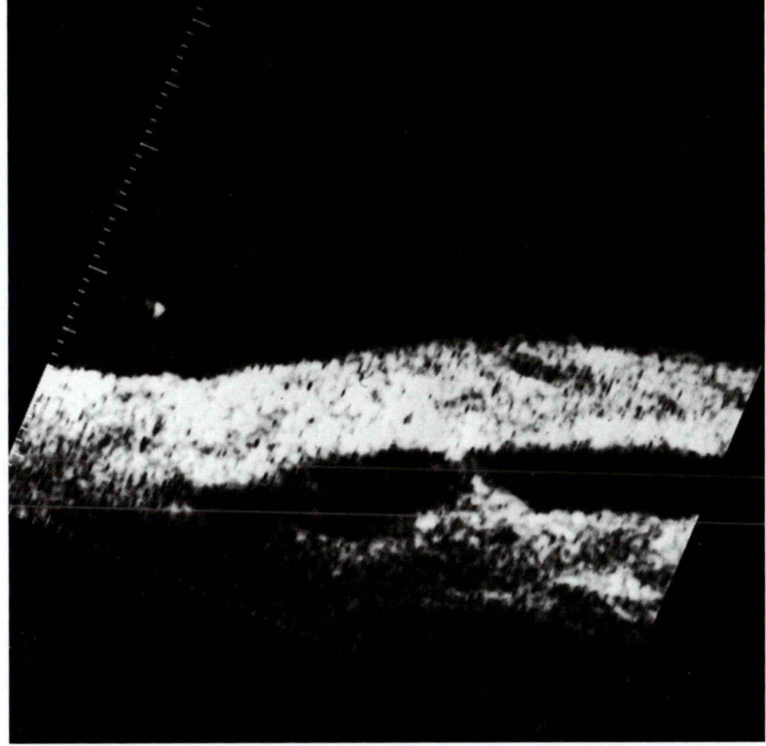

Fig. 7: UBM after VDSCI. The suture securing the collagen implant can be seen

36

Glaucoma Surgery with Fugo Plasma Blade

Daljit Singh, Kiranjit Singh (India)

Fugo blade is a unique electro-surgical device that ablates much like an excimer laser. The focused plasma energy developed at the surgical tip is absorbed by the tissues by resonance. The tissue macro-molecules become unstable, when they have additional energy. As a result they shatter. Clinically this is seen as an incision, a pit formation or a track formation. The tissue is actually removed in the path of the incision, without collateral thermal damage. This peculiarity of Fugo blade can be used in any kind of glaucoma surgery – a classical trabeculectomy or newer ways of making filtration tracks as described below.

TRANS-CILIARY FILTRATION (SINGH FILTRATION)

This technique allows the drainage of the posterior chamber to the sub-conjunctival space. The track passes through the ciliary body. The steps of operation are as follows. The conjunctiva is detached from the limbus for about 6 mm and is retracted to expose the sclera. A 600 micron Fugo blade tip is used to make a scleral pit, about 1 mm behind the posterior edge of surgical limbus, till it reaches the ciliary body. The ciliary body is also partially ablated by the same tip. The entry in to the posterior chamber is effected with a 100 micron or a 300 micron ablation tip. The tip is directed at an angle that takes it through the anterior part of the ciliary body in to the posterior chamber.

Post-operative recovery is quick. Transciliary filtration cases do not get flat anterior chamber. Choroidal detachment is rare. Neovascular glaucoma cases often develop blood leakage from the angle, but the blood stays as hyphema and is absorbed slowly.

After a century of anterior chamber filtration, posterior chamber filtration is a good idea. I have been doing this since year 2000.

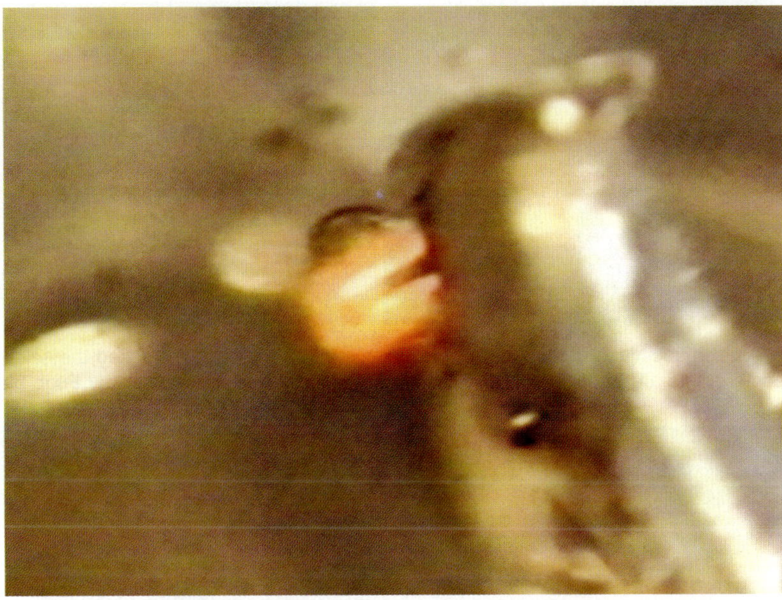

Fig. 1: The plasma energy of Fugo blade as visualized under a high power microscope. The central 100 micron steel filament is surrounded by yellow plasma cloud, which is in turn surrounded by orange coloured photon cloud. Only the plasma cloud has the cutting power

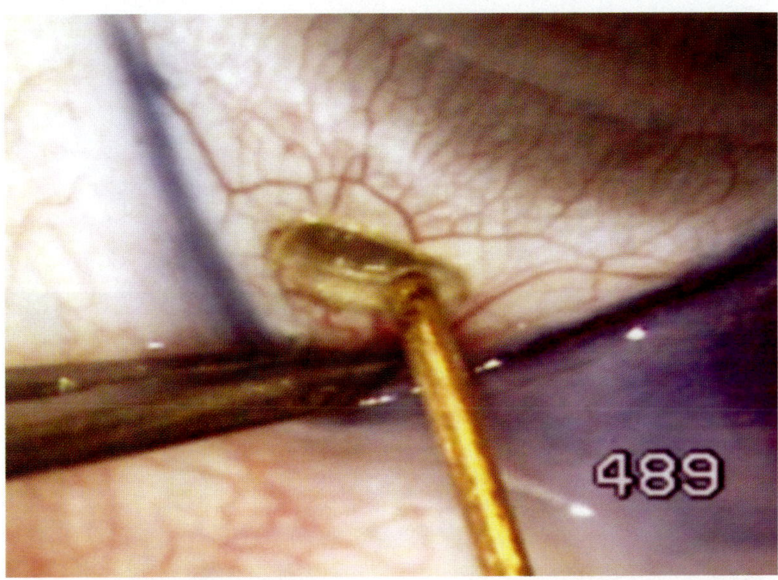

Fig. 2: Ablating the sclera to reach the ciliary body, to perform cyclodialysis. The sclera just disappears from the area that is touched by the Fugo blade

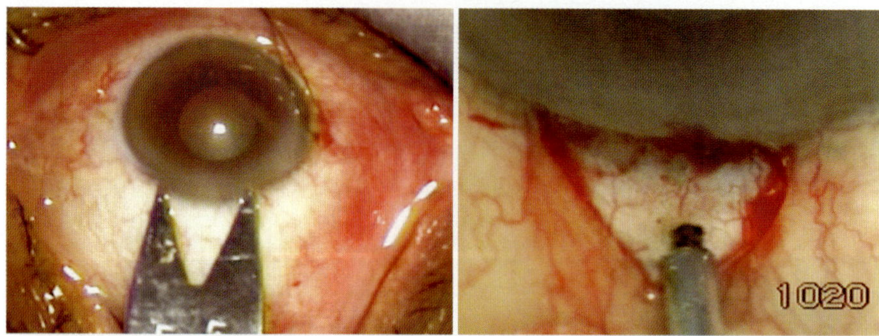

Fig. 3: The conjunctiva is detached from the limbus and retracted to exposed the sclera. The bleeding points are either allowed to close by themselves or are ablated by Fugo blade

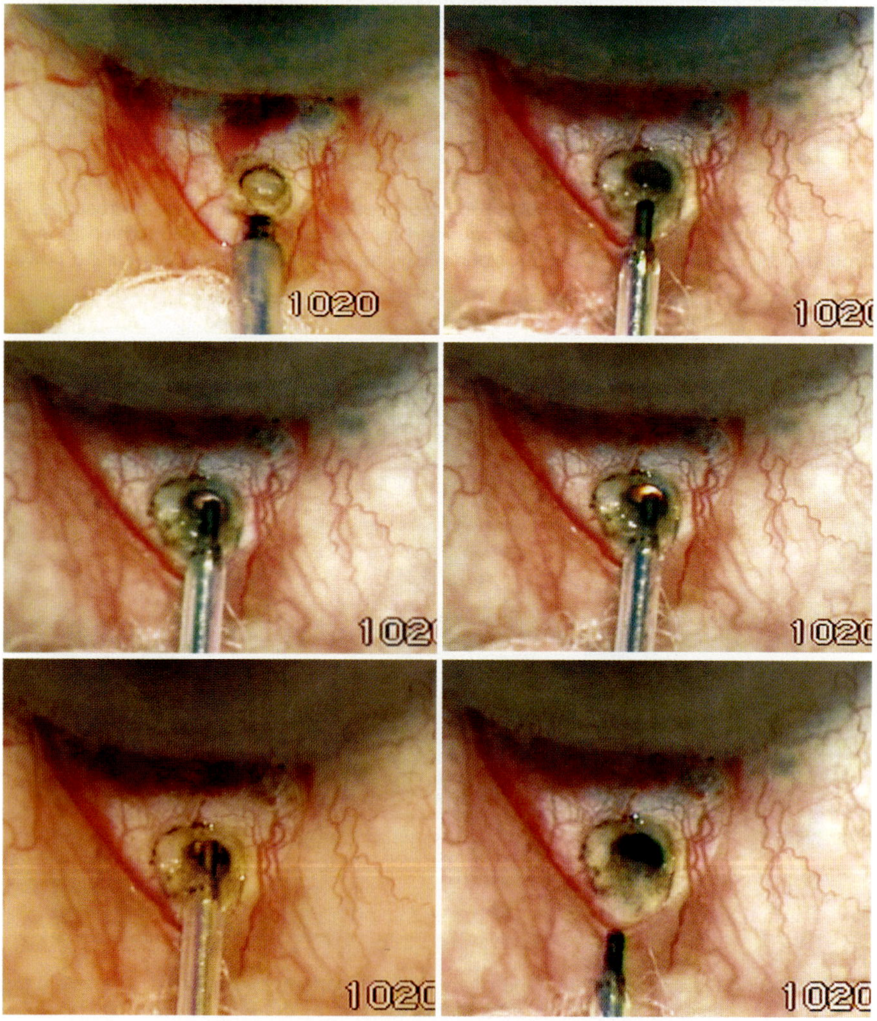

Fig. 4: The scleral pit is made 1 mm proximal to the surgical limbus till the ciliary body is reached. The ciliary body is ablated with a 300 micron Fugo blade tip till aqueous starts flowing

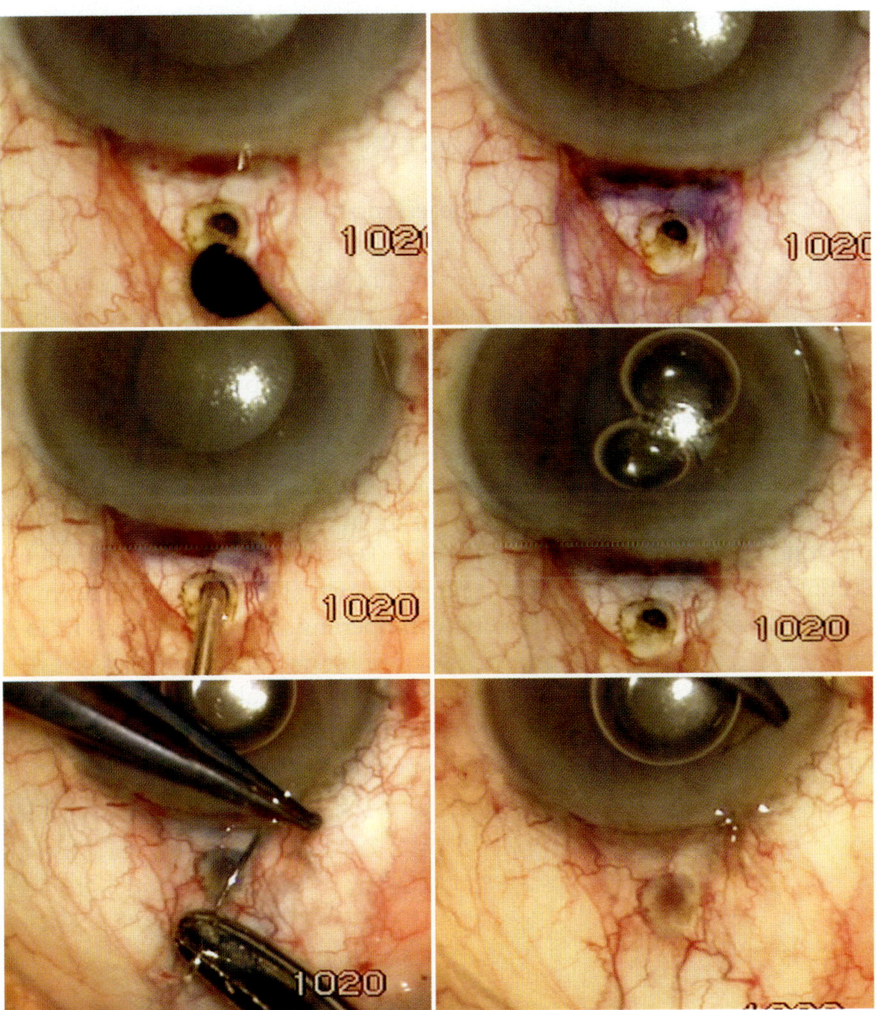

Fig.5: The flow of aqueous can be verified by a drop of trypan blue. When air is injected in the filtration track, it passes under the iris before appearing in the anterior chamber through the pupil. The conjunctiva is brought down and a suture is applied at the limbus

Trans-conjunctival Trans-ciliary Filtration (TC-TCF)

If the surgeon has confidence about the surface marking and the direction in which the ablation tip shall move, it is possible to make a trans-ciliary track without making a conjunctival flap. The example given below was a 94 year old patient, who also had parkinsonism.

Full local anesthesia was given. The jerking head was steadied by the grand sons. A non-cutting blunt diamond knife was used to mark a line, one mm behind the perceived posterior limit of the limbus. The same knife was used to push towards cornea a fold of conjunctiva, up to the marked line. The blunt diamond knife was pushed towards the sclera, so that the folded conjunctiva could not slip from under it. A 300 micron ablation tip was used to open the posterior chamber. It was placed in direct proximity of the diamond (non-conductive it is). The tip was directed in the direction of the posterior chamber, i.e. just posterior to the plane of the iris. The tip was activated and pushed. In no time the resistance free ablation took the tip in to the posterior chamber. The fluid followed, as the tip was withdrawn. The TCF track was confirmed by injecting air through the track. The conjunctiva was allowed to retract normally. A suture was applied to the conjunctival opening. The patient was fit to go home.

This technique is eminently suitable in cases of phakomorphic glaucoma, immediately prior to lens surgery. It is also very helpful in cases of acute glaucoma and many cases of malignant glaucoma.

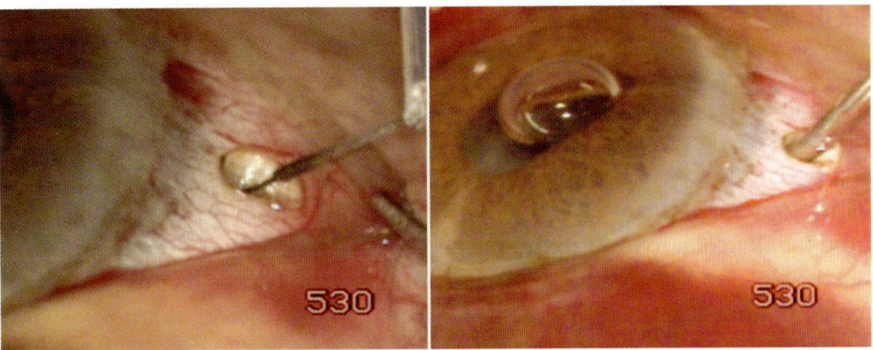

Fig. 6: A side view of the surgery of trans-ciliary filtration. Note the angle at which the ablation tip is directed towards the posterior chamber

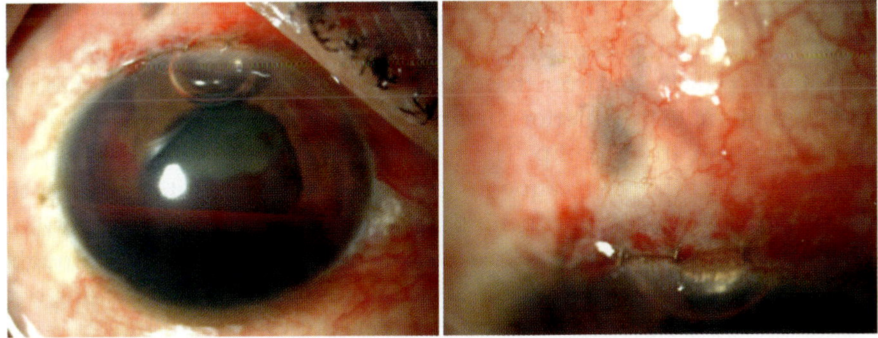

Fig. 7: Transciliary filtration in neovascular glaucoma. Hyphema started at the time of surgery and increased thereafter. Clear aqueous kept draining through TCF track, while it took about a fortnight for the blood to clear up

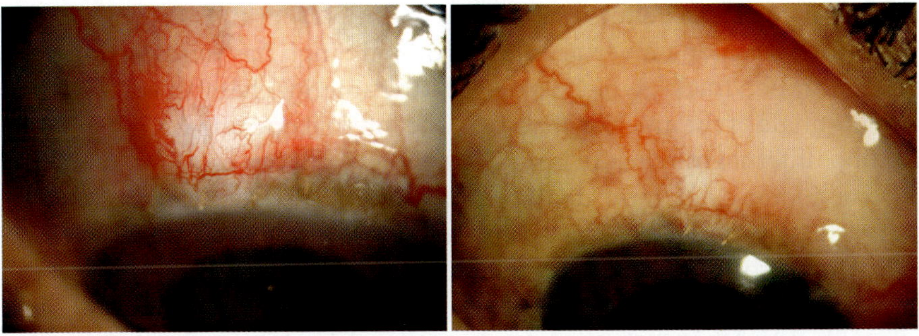

Fig. 8: A month later the same patient came for follow up. He had no pain and the eye was quiet. However, the IOP was 50 mm and tenon cyst formation was visible. The tenon cyst was opened and drained from a small conjunctival button-hole, about 6 mm away, through which 300 micron Fugo blade tip was introduced. In a fraction of a second the tenon cyst was drained with two 400 micron holes

Singh Microtrack Filtration

This is the simplest way to create a filtration track. Surface anesthesia is enough. The conjunctiva is held with a plain forceps about 3 mm from the limbus. It is pulled down over the cornea. The limbal area is visible through the transparent conjunctiva. It is for the surgeon to decide, at which point of the limbus he wishes to make a filtration track. A vertical entry at the posterior edge of the limbus shall take it to the anterior corneo-scleral trabeculae. I prefer to make the track as close to the conjunctival attachment to the cornea as possible, which means making the track in the clear cornea. A 100 micron ablation of 1 mm length is selected for the purpose. Since the forceps is metallic, it is important that the ablation fiber should not touch it. An better alternative is to push down the conjunctiva with a non-conductive dulled diamond or a sapphire blade, so that the ablation filament can actually touch the retracting device prior to track making.The time taken for making the filtration track is a tiny fraction of a second. The filament is kept steady with a light pressure on the target tissue. The moment it is activated from the foot switch, it passes through the conjunctiva and the limbus in to the anterior chamber. Fine bubbles are seen to arise in the anterior chamber from the tip. The foot switch is stopped instantly. As the ablation tip is withdrawn, aqueous ooze follows, which starts lifting the conjunctiva over the external opening. The conjunctiva retracts to its position. Air, miotic or viscoelastic can be injected in to the anterior chamber through a fine cannula. A bandage contact lens is placed, that helps in preventing over filtration and keep the anterior chamber under control.

Compared to TCF cases, the anterior chamber microfiltration cases need more careful follow up and management. The pupil needs to be contracted to keep the iris away from the internal opening of the filtration track. Cases with deep anterior chamber do better. A pre-filtration laser PI helps to some extent. A larger manual PI is better.

Instead of making a vertical track, Kiranjit Singh has innovated a "Clear cornea filtration track", which opens in to the anterior chamber some distance from the angle of the anterior chamber. The internal opening is visible under a slit lamp. Internal iris closure is readily visible and it can be released either by a strong miotic, by extreme dilatation or by a single shot of Nd:Yag laser. His approach is to let the iris block the internal opening for a few days, during which period some resistance develops in the subconjunctival tissues. Releasing the iris after a period of 2-3 weeks seems to give better and more lasting results. Internally blocked track can also be opened by injecting air or sodium hyaluronate through a small corneal incision.

Microtrack filtration is a minimally traumatic filtration procedure. It is easy to do and redo. It can take care of failed cases by other techniques. It can take care of dire emergencies, like trauma. Acute or chronic uveitis and corneal ulcer cases with very high unmanageable rise in intraocular pressure, need help in this kind of emergency.

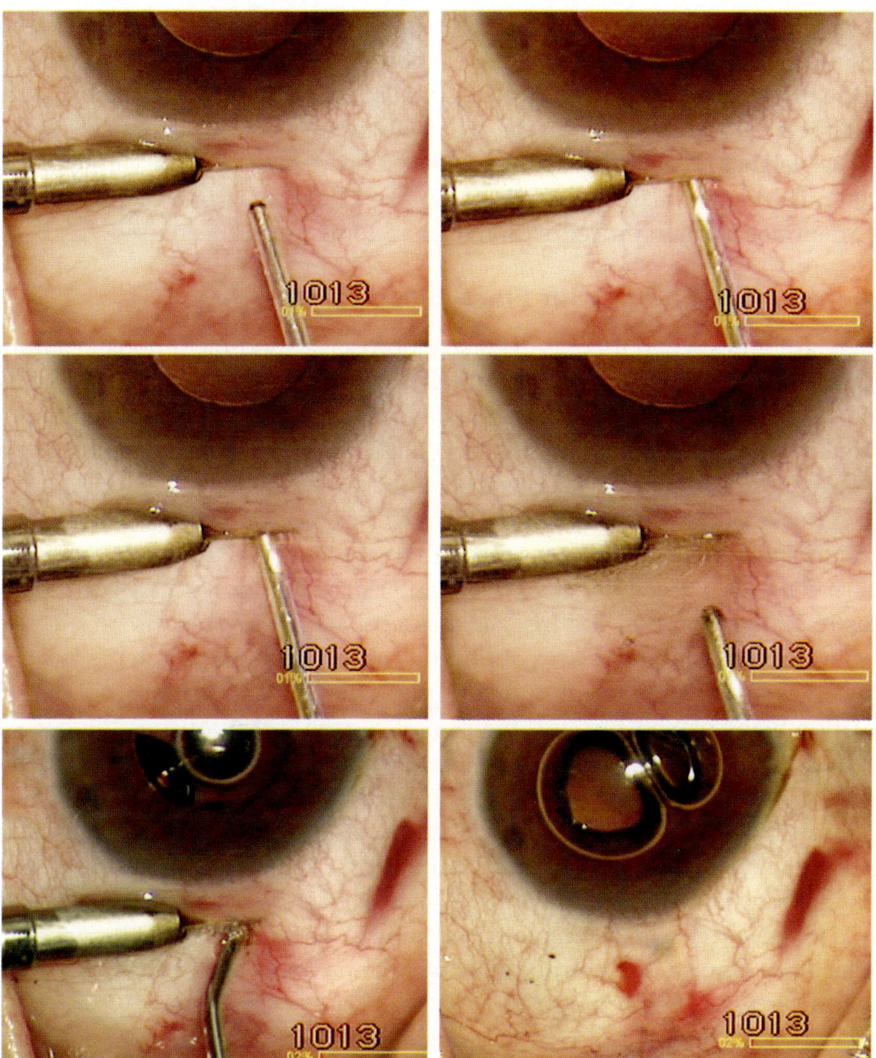

Fig. 9: Transconjunctival TCF, is done by pushing the conjunctiva to a point 1 mm behind the surgical limbus, with a blunt diamond knife (it is non-conductive). 300 micron ablation tip is passed in to the posterior chamber. The injected air appears from under the iris in to the anterior chamber

One interesting variation of MTF is making a filtration track, through a conjunctival opening made close to the limbus. The track making is then entirely in the pre-tenon potential subconjunctival space. The bleb formation is such that it seems to be over the surface of the tenon capsule, in stead of being inside it. The bleb has no visible border and it is widely spread over the surface of the sclera. The bleb is healthy and is quite unlike a large avascular bleb often seen in a routine filtration procedure in which mitomycin has been used.

Ab-interno Filtration with Fugo Blade

There are times when there is extensive fibrosis around the limbus, resulting from a variety of causes including anti-glaucoma operations. A very small sector with virgin conjunctiva might be available for an additional attempt at filtration surgery. If the anterior chamber is deep, it may be reasonable to attempt an ab-interno filtration surgery. The steps of surgery are as follows:

A pocket incision is made in the clear cornea at such a point, from where a straight Fugo blade tip can pass through the limbus, and the tenon capsule to reach the subconjunctival space. The anterior chamber is filled with visco-elastic material so that the iris get pressed back. A big bleb is raised with lignocaine in the intended area of filtration. The idea is that when the ablation tip comes out, it should not puncture the conjunctiva.A straight 100 micron ablation tip is passed through the pocket section, till it touches the corneal endothelium anterior to the corneo-scleral trabeculae. It is then activated and pushed through the limbal tissues, to reach the already raised bleb area. The surgery is over. The aqueous drainage starts the moment the ablation tip is withdrawn from the track. Air and sodium hyaluronate are injected to reform the anterior chamber. A peripheral iridectomy in line with the filtration track is good to prevent closure of the internal opening of the track. Fugo blade peripheral iridectomy may be done through the very same pocket incision, or with Yag laser, a few hours before surgery.

The role of lymphatics in health and after glaucoma surgery:

The lymphatics is a totally neglected subject, even by glaucoma surgeons. We have studied lymphatics in health under a slit lamp microscope, and by injecting trypan blue in surgical settings. In our 8 years long study, we have ample proofs to show that there is a network of channels in the cornea which is prominent around the canal of Schlemm. This network communicates with the conjunctival lymphatics at the limbus and further to wider channels around the limbus and beyond. The conjunctival network is a part of a three dimensional lymphatic system that unites it with the lymphatics in tenon capsule and the episclera. There are channels in the sclera too that communicate with the suprachoroidal space, the channels around the canal of Schlemm and with the episcleral channels.

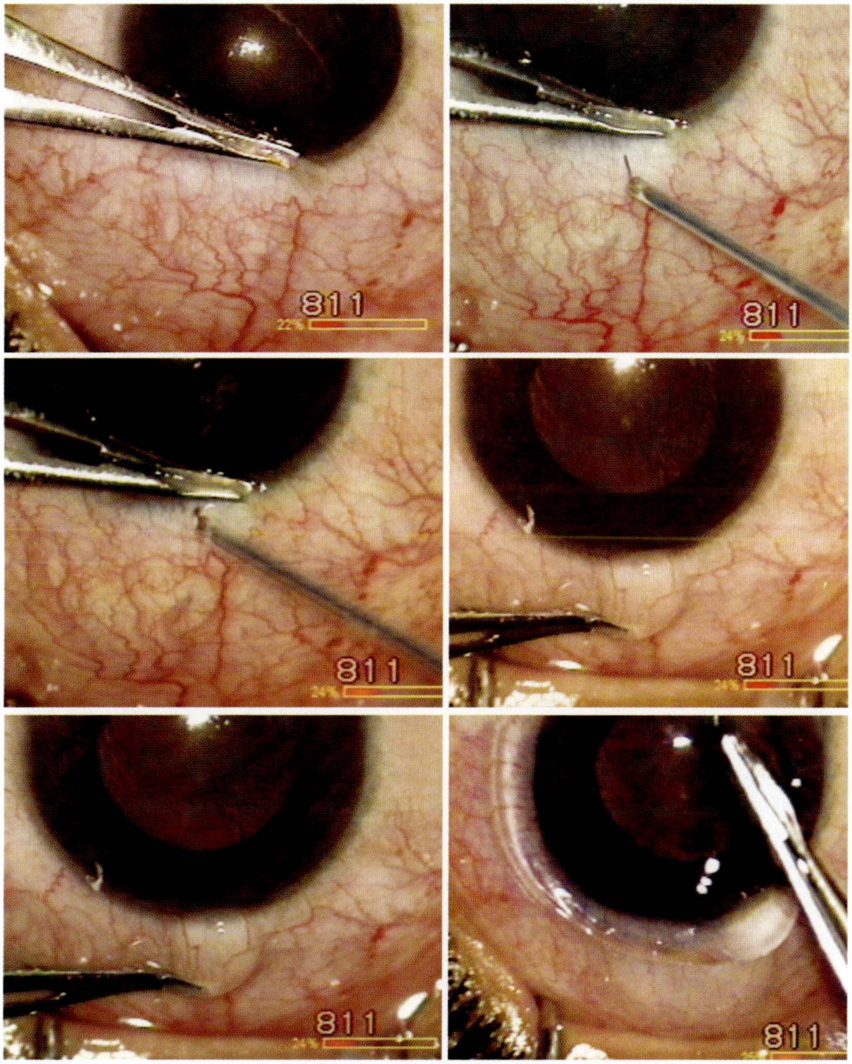

Fig.10: The conjunctiva is pulled over the cornea and a 100 micron Fugo blade tip is used to create a trans-conjunctival filtering track. A bandage lens is applied at the end of surgery. This is my first case that was done in 2004

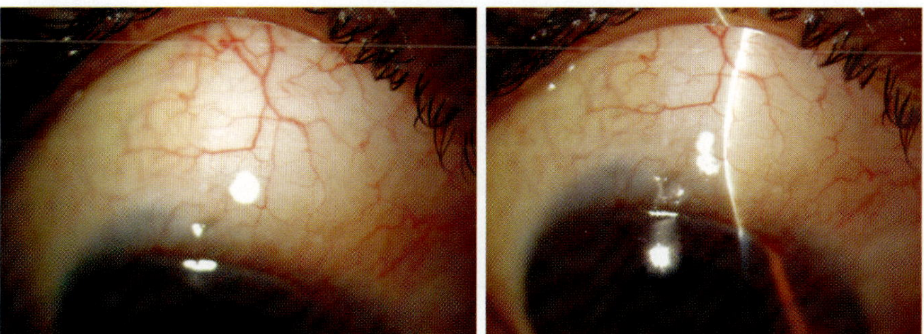

Fig. 11: Extensive borderless bleb in a microtrack filtration that was carried out in the pre-tenon potential (opened forcibly with a blunt cannula) subconjunctival space.The aqueous seems to cover the surface of the tenon capsule

What is the function of the lymphatics? Like elsewhere in the body, they drain interstitial fluid. And what could be the major fluid source in ocular area? The aqueous. It is well known that more than 40 % of aqueous drainage is through uveo-scleral route and the rest through canal of Schlemm and aqueous veins. Even the aqueous veins are bound to leak somewhat and add to the interstitial fluid. If the lymphatics were non-existent there would be a perpetual oedema. In other words the lymphatics act as flood drains. This especially true after a filtration surgery. Presence of a bleb is a sign of bottleneck. Filtration in an already failed operation case is never done in the scarred area, but in a virgin area of conjunctiva. Lymphatics shall never be seen in the scarred area, as we have seen after trypan blue injection studied. Preservatives in anti-glaucoma drops, if medication is carried out for a long time, can damage the lymphatics. Thus increases the chances of failure of anti-glaucoma surgery. During surgery, any kind of cutting, cauterization and even application of anti-mitotics can damage lymphatics.

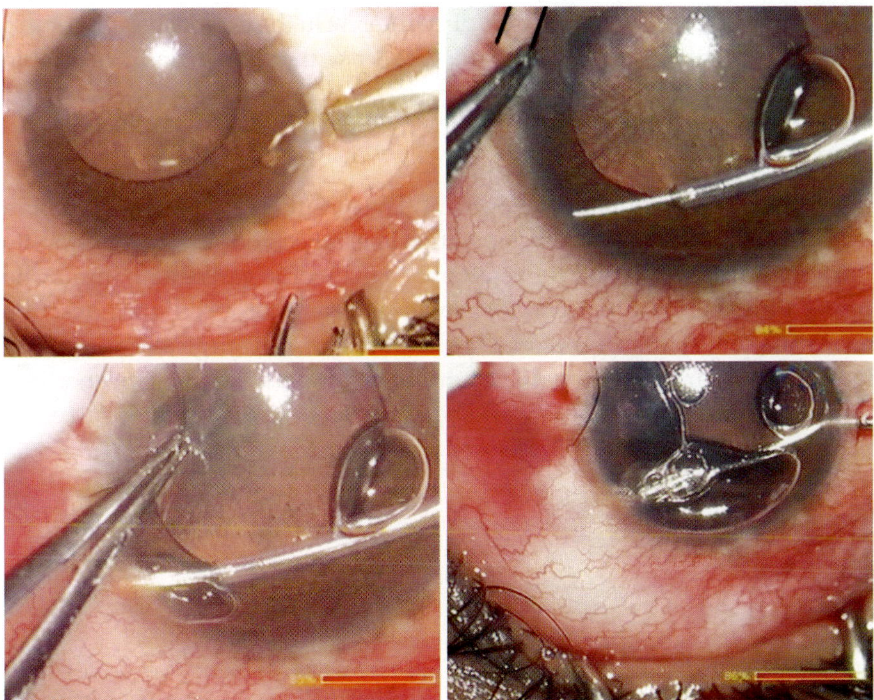

Fig.12: Ab interno filtration. A pocket incision is made, to allow the ablation tip to pass through. The tip touches the cornea endothelium then passes straight through the limbus in to subconjunctival space. Air is injected through the track and then to half fill the anterior chamber, followed by the deepening of the anterior chamber with sodium hyaluronate. No suture is needed in the end

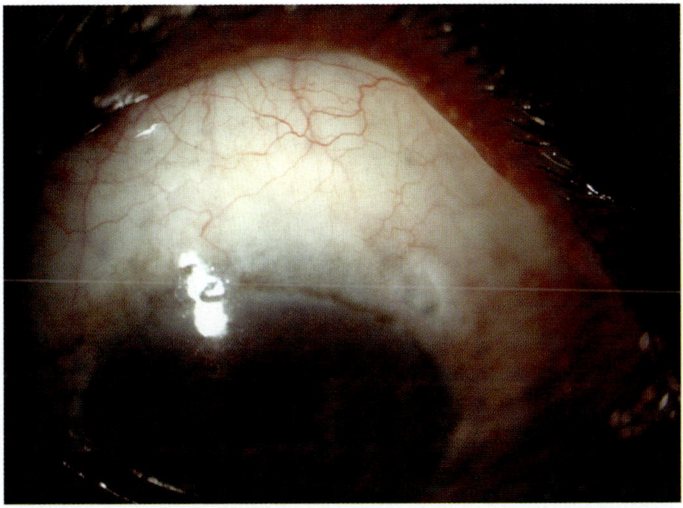

Fig. 13: Ab-interno filtration, four years postoperative. There is diffuse bleb formation

It is obvious that we should take deep interest in the normal lymphatics and we should conduct our anti-glaucoma surgery with minimal damage, keeping in mind the invisible lymphatic system.

To sum up

Fugo blade is an important development. The plasma energy from this tool can do any kind of classical glaucoma operation like trabeculectomy, non-perforating filtration, cyclodialysis and the fixation of a glaucoma valve, with unmatched finesse. Plus there are options for newer and simpler techniques described above. The failure after glaucoma has a lot to do with surgical trauma. Fugo blade reduces surgical trauma. The lymphatics and tissue saving properties of Fugo blade allows us to fail safe and be in a position to re-operate with ease at the same place or in an adjoining area.

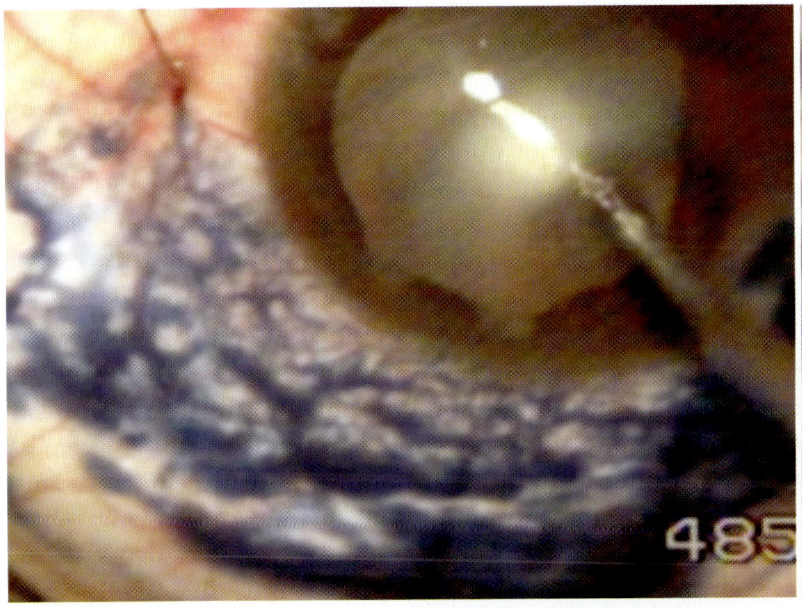

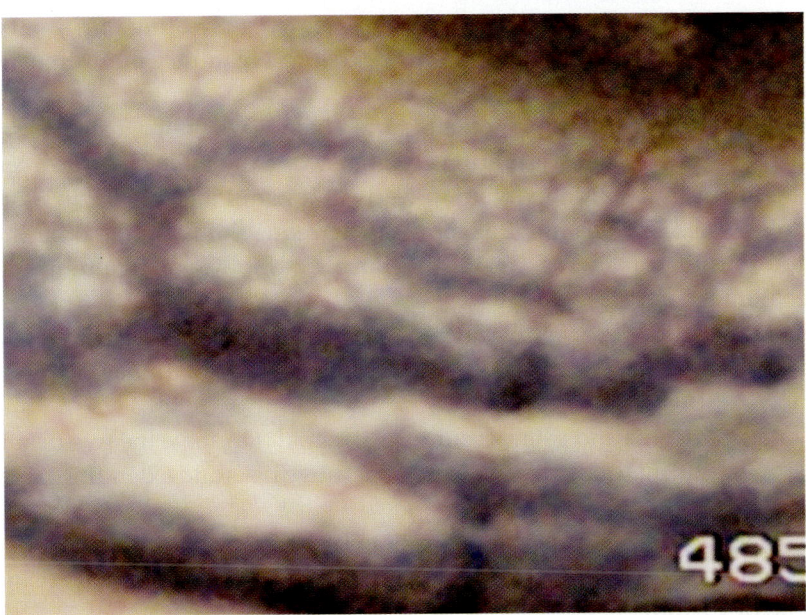

Fig. 14: Lymphatics of the conjunctiva outlined by injecting trypan blue dye in the pretenon potential subconjunctival space. The dye quickly enters the lymphatic system

37

Bimanual MicroPhaco and Deep Sclerocanalostomy (BMP and DSC): New Technique

Jerome Bovet (Switzerland)

INTRODUCTION/INDICATIONS

Cataracts and glaucoma have always been linked together.

The crystalline lens is responsible for most of secondary glaucoma, these come from a pseudo-exfoliation or a simple hypertrophy of the crystalline lens.

The diagnostic problem we find in combined surgery is to know what is the part played by each of these pathologies in ocular hypertension.

When should we feel the need to propose a combined operation when a simple cataract operation is enough.

A study by Jean-Marc Baumgartner has shown a lowering of 3 mm Hg of ocular tension in normal patients after a simple cataract operation using phacoemulsification.

In Europe, more and more patients suffer, because of their age, from pseudo exfoliation. The problem is important in cataract operations, because, in a certain number of cases, pseudo exfoliation leads to a zonulolysis that can develop into total lysis. The lens then falls into the vitreous fluid. On the other hand, pseudo exfoliation increases the pressure by deposit of hyaloids on the trabeculum level.

The crystalline lens, whilst increasing in size, can diminish the flow of aqueous humour, especially in the hypermetropic eye with narrow anterior chamber.

For all glaucoma and cataract surgery, the goal is to solve the two problems in one operation, without increasing postoperative risks and extending recovery time.

Nowadays, the new operating techniques for cataract allow intervention by paracentheses of less than 1.2 mm and an implantation of the lens using an incision of 1.7 mm.

This removes all problems of astigmatism induced by the operation.

This new technique allows less postoperatives checks and a faster visual recovery.

Non-perforating surgery techniques for glaucoma, not only have a small number of postoperative complications, but also have the advantage of producing a very rapid recovery.

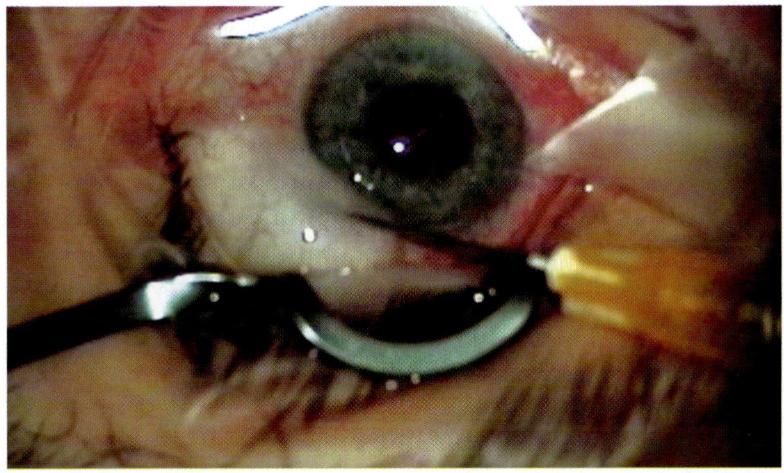

Fig. 1A: Scleral flap

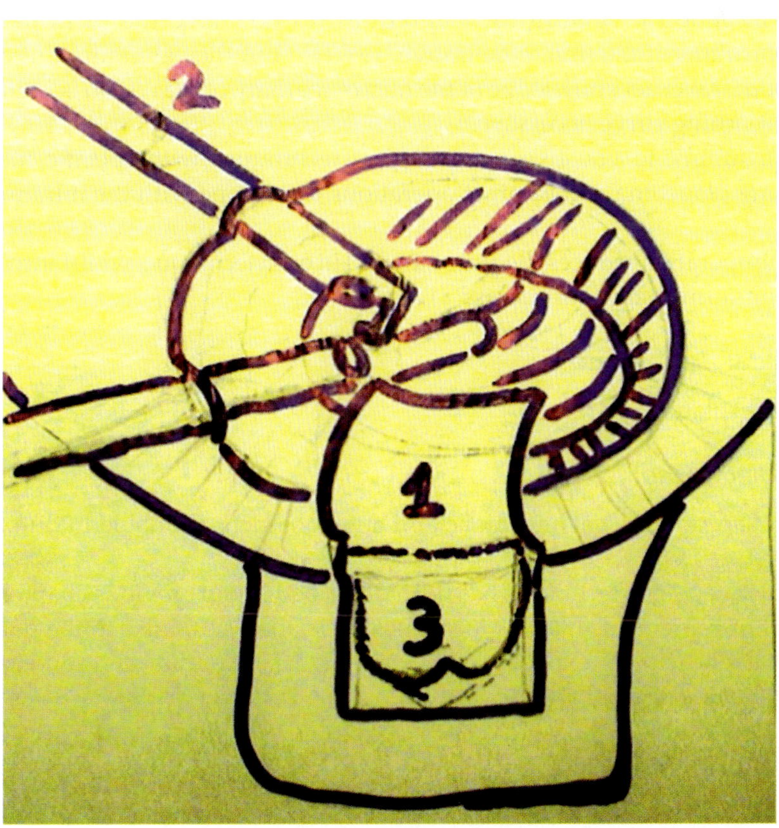

Fig. 1B: Scleral flap (animation)

We are going to describe our combined operation for cataracts/glaucoma using 2 new techniques

- one, Bimanual MicroPhaco technique for cataracts
- the other, deep sclerocanalostomy

In the combined operation, timing of the two operations is important.

Several authors prefer to perform each of these operations separately at different sites. After having tried multiple combinations, either on one or two sites, it seemed to us that the best solution was to start on one side by dissecting the first flap up to the scleral blade, then to do a bimanual microphaco on a temporal site, at the end, finishing the second flap and the canalostomy under viscoelastic solution in the anterior chamber.

This has several advantages: dissection of the first flap is done on an eye with healthy pressure, dissection is made easier, the cataract surgery is carried out without any risk of rupturing the Descemet and, in the end, the dissection of the second flap is carried out with weak intercamerular pressure, so diminishing risk of rupturing the Descemet.

Non-penetrative surgical techniques do not have the postoperative complications of the first, penetrative, surgery, but they are more difficult to carry out. An exact knowledge of the micro-anatomy of the region is important and a learning curve necessary.

We submit to you two new surgical techniques with specific timings, allowing glaucoma and cataract operations to be done with the minimum of risk.

The operation reduces the risks inherent in each technique, whilst increasing the long-term chances of success.

Surgical Technique

1st stage: glaucoma

1st Scleral Flap

Sclera flap under local anesthetic and sub-conjunctival bubble in outpatient surgery

This anesthetic technique has been described in the previous chapter.

Let us remember that this local anesthetic allows - thanks to the patient's ability to participate - exposure of the operative field for dissection and its best, and variable angles of work.

Choices for dissection

The path of dissection and flap's localization are chosen to spare the penetrating vessels and to search for the zone that is the most avascular.

The draining vessels are on the surface, as shown by Stegmann.

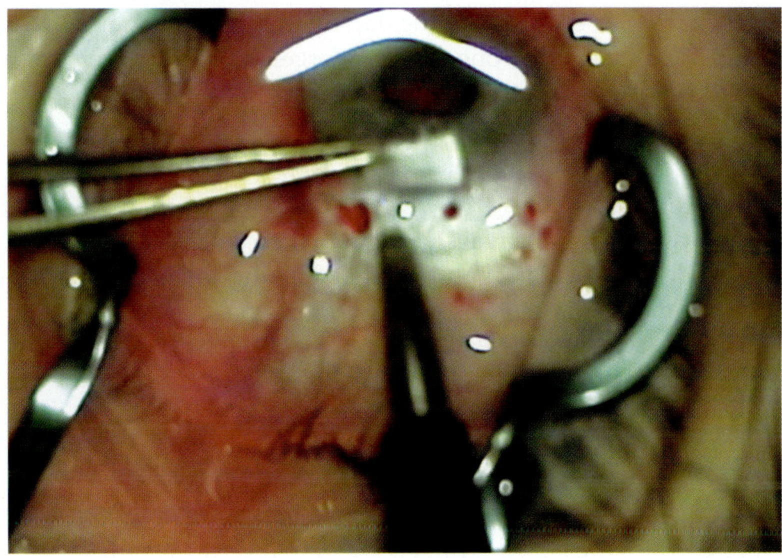

Fig. 2: Incision of scleral flap

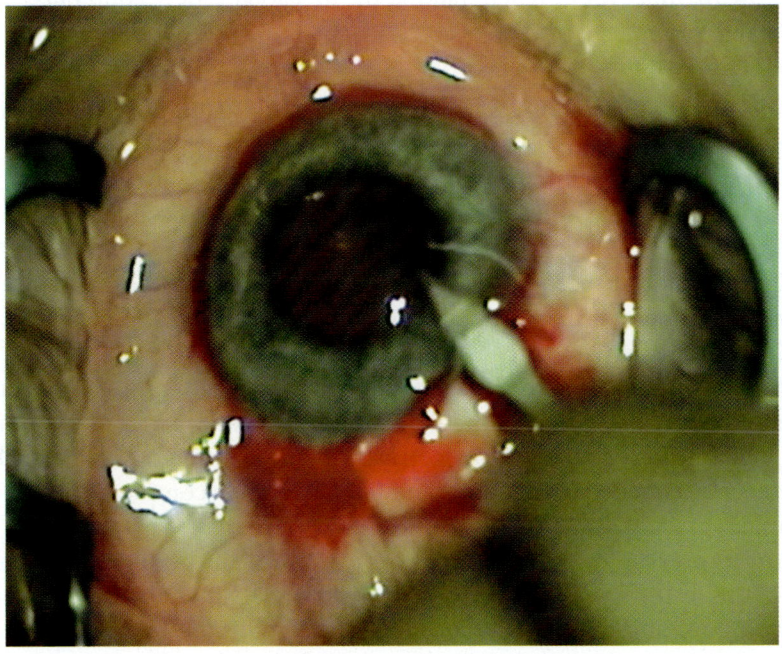

Fig. 3: Enlargement of paracenteses

The choice of the best place for the flap to spare the penetrating vessels to find the most avascular zone, one must not forget that the draining vessels are on the surface, as shown by Stegmann in his film.

Conjunctival shutter with limb

Stages are as follows:

Dissection of the conjunctival shutter with limb, not less than 10 mm, with Vescoat scissors. Dissection in an L shape allowing the conjunctival flap to relax in the opening.

Exposing the sclera by dissecting Tenon's capsule with care.

Use the lightest possible electro coagulation in order to spare the draining vessels as much as possible.

1st Scleral flap:

Incision of the scleral flap

- 6 × 4 mm, the width being of less importance than the length
- depth of 300 microns, cut with a 30° diamond (Meyco Switzerland) or with a diamond for KR (Meyco, Switzerland) up to the lames corneostromales

It is important to make a flap which is thick enough not to tear when one arrives in the corneal stroma.

It is important to dissect the lames corneennes, starting from the limb, the cut allowing more room when making the incision of the second flap.

2nd Stage Cataract

Bimanual MicroPhaco 19G 2 paracenteses are made at temporal level, with a 20 gauge diamond knife.

Then we make an intracameral injection of a solution of lidocaine diluted 0.2% without preservative. This allows the iris to be anesthetised in case of mobilization.

Enlargement of the 2 paracenteses to exactly 1.2 mm 19G and filling the anterior chamber with viscous.

Capsulorhexis with a special capsulorhexis cannula.

Hydrodissection and hydrodelineation of the nucleus and the epi-nucleus. Penetration in the anterior chamber, first with a Nagahara irrigation cannula of 19G, then introduction of our phacotip of 0.9 mm diameter, without sock. The difference between 19G (1, 2 mm) and 0.9 mm allows complete cooling of the cannula.

Any type of phaco-emulsification machine can be used for this new procedure, but the most appropriate are the machines that allow a strong aspiration mixing the peristaltic rotative force with the force of the Venturi pump.

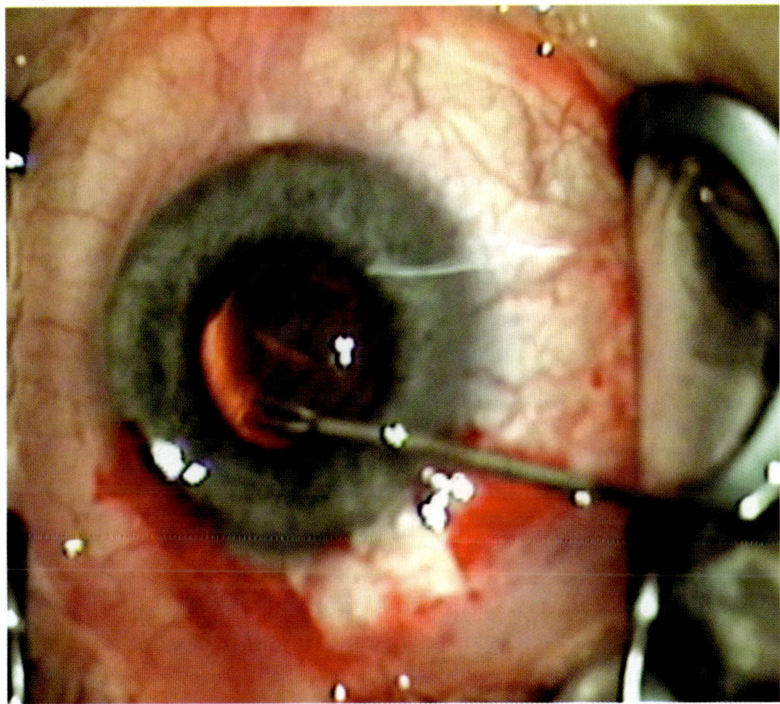

Fig. 4: Capsulorhexis with special capsulorhexis cannula

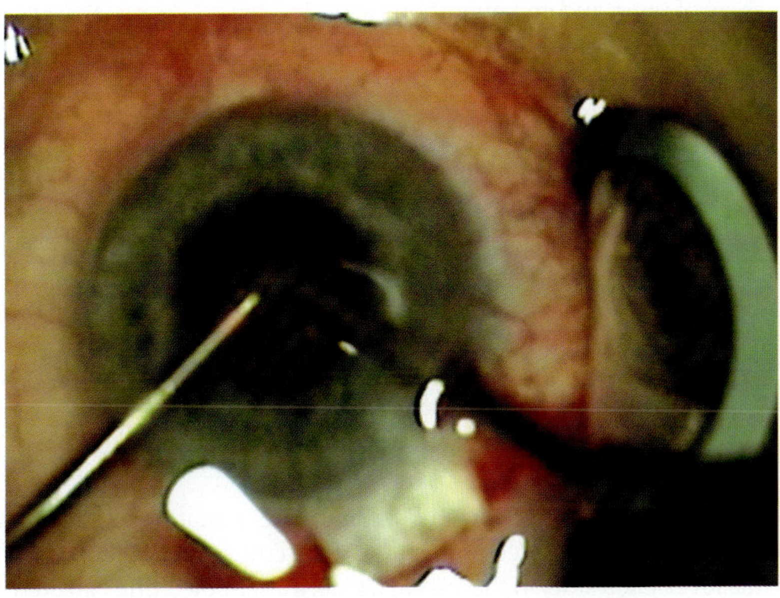

Fig. 5: Difference between 19G and 0.9 mm allows complete cooling of the cannula

The parameters are the following

- irrigation 65 cc/min
- aspiration strength minimal 150 mm Hg
- power 40%

Flip and chop phacoemulsification technique, after having aspirated the viscous and the superior cortex: We first make a groove using maximum aspiration, then we lift the nucleus slightly in order to pass the irrigation cannula behind it and break it into 1/8 slices that are each sucked up as we go along. We repeat this procedure until we have emulsified the nucleus in its entirety.

In order to avoid the collapse of the chamber, first, we remove the phacotip and only after that, do we remove the Nagahara irrigation chopper.

Then, we introduce the irrigation-aspiration cannula (de Duet 19G) to aspirate the cortex and occasionally the rest of the nucleus. Once this procedure is done, we fill up the anterior chamber with viscous.

Lens Implantation

We enlarge the paracenteses from 1.2 to 1.7 mm and an acrylic hydrophobe and hydrophile Acri Smart 36a implant is injected (Acritec Germany, inserted in a silicone special capsule). This enables us to avoid introducing the capsule into the anterior chamber and to inject solely the implant.

The implant is very easily positioned in the anterior chamber.

Once the implant is in situ, we leave in the viscous and proceed to the second stage of the glaucoma operation.

3rd Glaucoma

2nd Scleral flap

5 mm dissection, with a 30° diamond knife (Meyco, Switzerland), of the length of the second triangular flap of all the depth of the sclera leaving some scleral plates in order to just reveal the choroidien tissue. This allows getting exactly at the scleral spur, at the beginning of Descemet's membrane.

Dissection, holding on to the second flap, with a triangular swab in order to push back the stroma. In this way, we free Descemet's membrane. Those who practice deep lamellar keratoplasty ("keratoplastie lamellaire") operations will have no difficulty in finding the plane of dissection.

Separation of the Descemet from the stromal tissue is quite easy, so long as one is in the right plane.

The 1.5 mm incision in Descemet's membrane is made in order that the Schlemm's canal is not covered at the time of the cutting of the flap.

On this level, each side, in the scleral tissue, a slight bleeding can be seen at the cut in the drainage vein of the Schlemm's canal.

Removal of the second flap with the diamond.

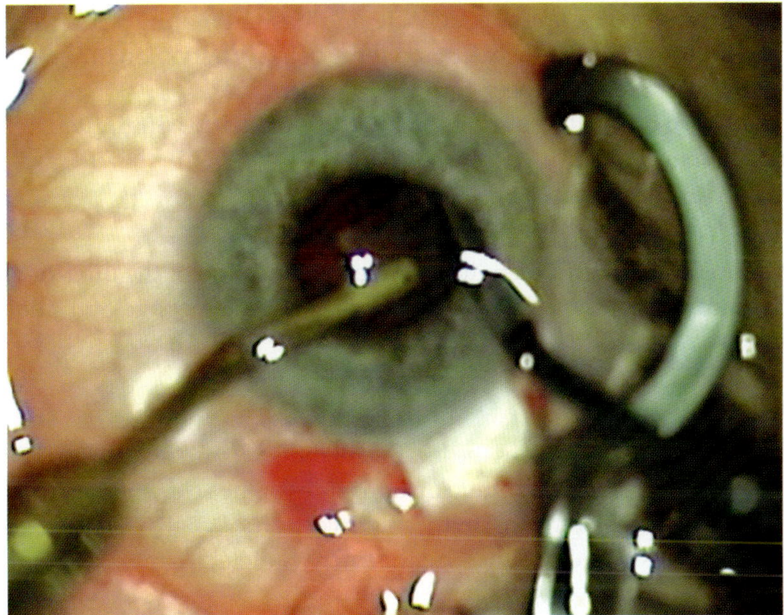

Fig. 6: Filling of anterior chamber with viscous

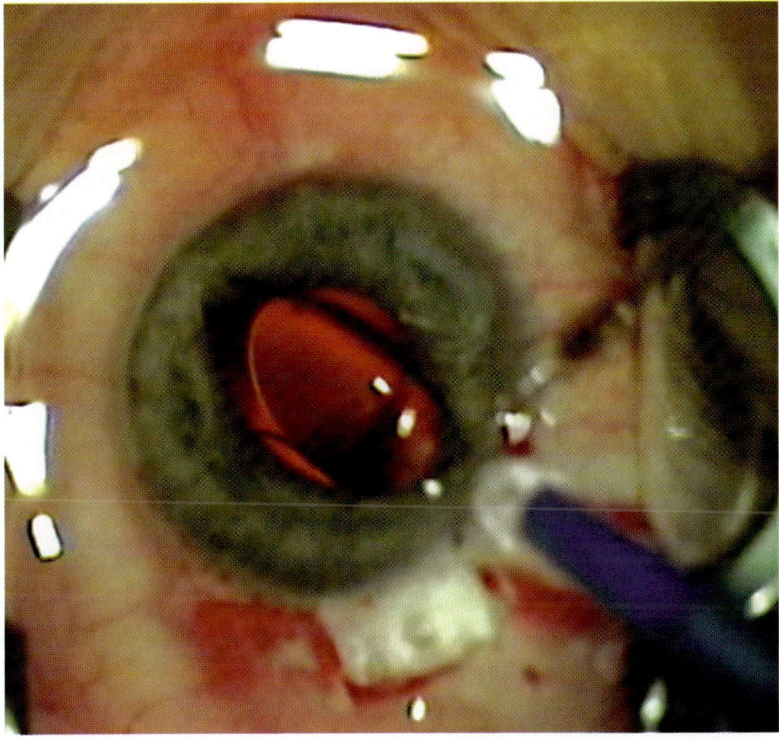

Fig. 7: Injection of implant

This part of the operation is delicate and has to be done with great care. Because, on a number of occasions, when using Vannas or other scissors, Descemet's membrane has been torn.

Cut up the scleral flap in half: one half is soaked for 5 minutes in 0.04% mytomicin, then rinsed.

Schlemm Canal Dissection

Using Bonn forceps with micro teeth, a 5 mm dissection of the interior wall of the Schlemm's canal is made, allowing us to see some seepage of the aqueous humour.

Canalostomy

The Schlemm's canal vein gives the location of the Schlemm's canal. Introduction of an extra fine Grieshaber cannula on both sides of the sclera of the Schlemm's canal until some resistance is felt. Slow injection of high viscosity viscous (Healon, G V AMO) whilst removing the micro catheter.

Implant/Mitomycin C

Put in place, in the bed of the second flap, the previously prepared implant, the implant having been, beforehand, soaked in Mitomycin and rinsed before being used.

Close the first flap with inverted stitches using nylon 10.0, at each corner of the flap pulling the stitches tight.

Close the conjunctive with 3 inverted stitches using 9.0 re-absorbable thread.

Remove the viscous from the anterior chamber, and also from behind the lens, in order to avoid any of the viscous remaining. Any left remaining could cause postoperative hypertension.

Postoperative treatment

This combined operation, is carried out as ambulatory surgery and with local anesthetic, there is no need to cover the eye with a dressing.

Patients are treated with cortisone and antibiotic drops.

Dosage is 1 drop 3x a day for 3 weeks.

Postoperative checkups.

The postoperative follow-up must be rigorous,

The patient is checked, one hour after the operation, before leaving the clinic, after 1 day, 1 week, and 1 month.

Usually, all eye hypotensor treatments are stopped, even if it's necessary for them to be re-introduced at a later date.

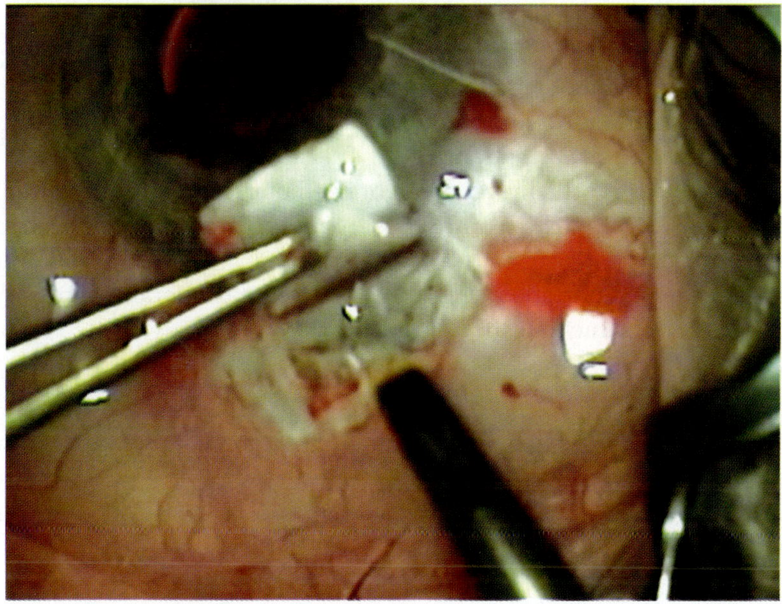

Fig. 8: Scleral spur at the begining of Descemet's membrane

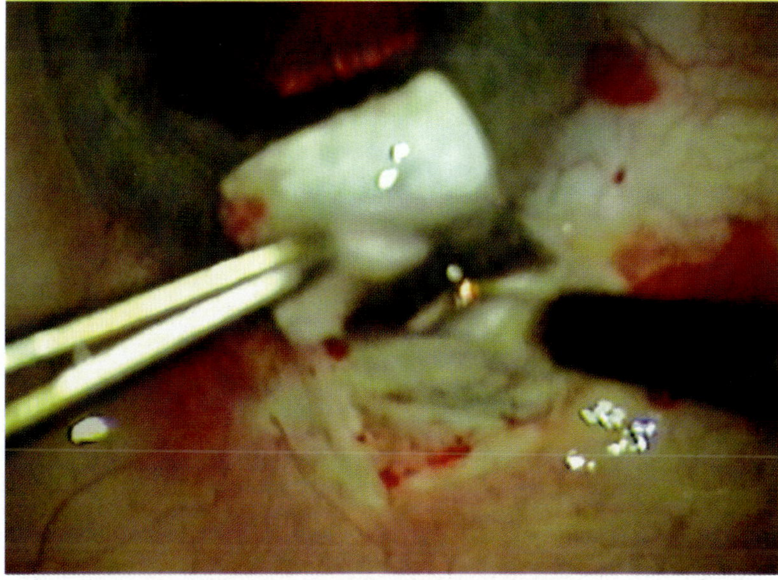

Fig. 9: Torn Descemet's membrane

The filtration bubble that is found when trabectomy is used, does not exist using this technique. As a result, the patient has to be checked controlling the ocular tension in both the eyes. If possible, the measure has to taken each time at the same hour, in order to avoid obtaining distorted results because of the curve of the nychthemeral ocular pressure.

Patients who are cortisone respondent need particularly special attention.

Continuous check-ups to control postoperative pressure are necessary in cases of glaucoma.

It is extremely important to check the pre- and postoperative pressures in the two eyes at the same times.

Complications during the Operation

Complications specifically connected with this combined operation consist in the rupture of the Descemet's membrane. This happens if the timing already described is not respected and if the second flap is done before operating on the cataract.

Postoperative Complications

The most frequent postoperative complication with this technique is an increase of pressure, more or less long-term, with the collapse or closing up/healing on the site of the operation. Our technique uses an autograft of the sclera, soaked in Mitomycin C which inhibits all fibrocyte proliferation. This produces the best results and the lowest costs in the long-term.

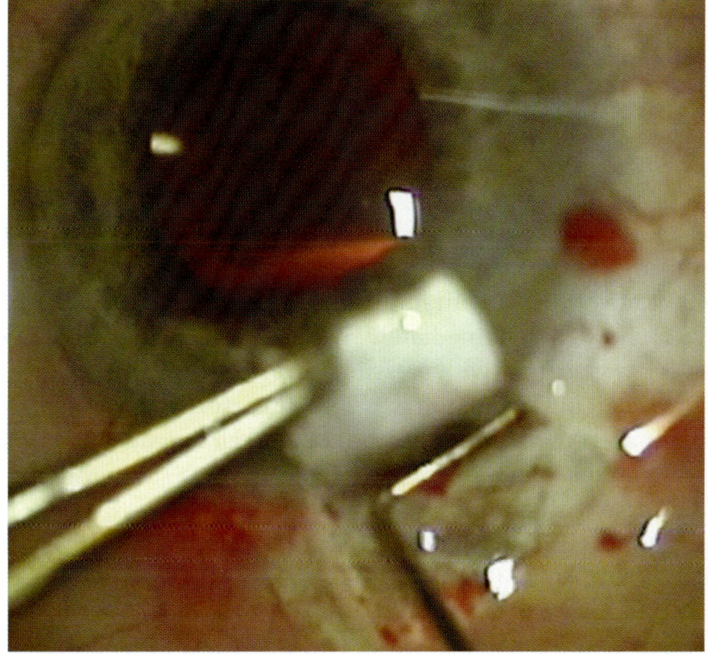

Fig. 10: Removal of micro catheter

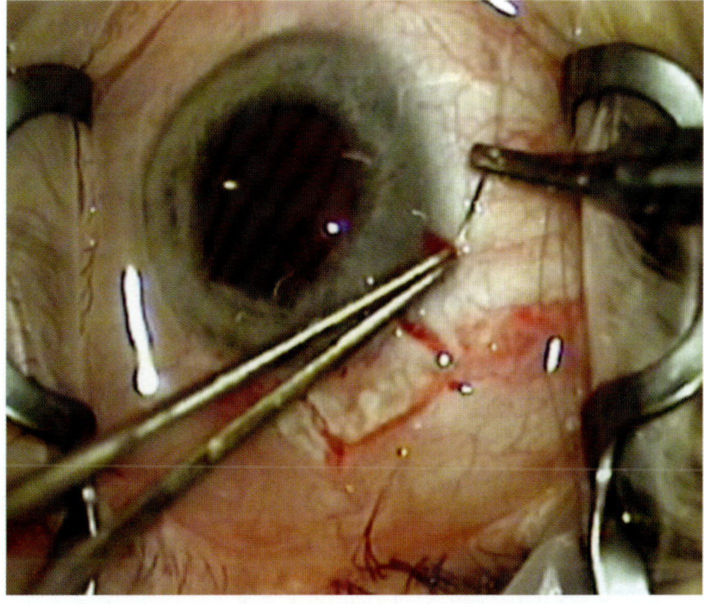

Fig. 11: Closing the conjunctiva with 3 inverted stitches

38

Modern Glaucoma Surgery

Jes Mortensen (Sweden)

In spite of more than one hundred years of treatment by pressure lowering medication in glaucoma there was no evidence that decreasing the IOP is beneficial, till now when the first results from the Early Manifest Glaucoma Trial (EMGT) shows that immediately treating people with early stages of primary open-angle glaucoma with pressure-lowering treatment can delay disease progression. Mean IOP reduction was 25%. Profesor Anders Heijl, the EMGT study director at the University Clinic at Malmö University Hospital, warned that the treatment used in the study was insufficient to stop progression of the glaumoca disease with rapidly progressing glaucoma.

The glaucoma disease is considered an opticusneuropathy, not only a disease of the chamber angle.

Glaucoma is observed in the older population , the prevalence in the Swedish population is 5% at the age of 75 years. In the black African population the disease occurs at a younger age and the IOP is much higher than observed in a white population.

Many different drugs have been developed to lower the IOP: Pilocarpin, betablockers, adrenaline drugs, carbonic anhydrase inbitors and recently, prostaglandin analogues. The older drugs facilitate the escape of aqueous humour through the trabecular meshwork; during the last twenty years drugs that diminish the aqueous production have been introduced and now recently drugs that facilitate the uveoscleral outflow have been used as weapon to fight high IOP in glaucoma.

In spite of the uncertainty of the pathogenesis the IOP retains a central position in the pathogenesis of the damage to the optic nerve: Directly by mechanical damage to the nerve fibers or through interaction with the bloodflow to the papilla. No specific level of the IOP that will cause damage to the nerve is known for each patient the sensitivity surely depends on the individual´s genes and a function of other risk factors.

Surgery for the management of glaucoma is much older than medication. Albecht von Graefe (1828 -1870) in Berlin operated on open-angle glaucoma back in the 19th century with iridectomy. Open-angle glaucoma was operated on to increase the outflow of the aqueous humour. Many different operations have been tried, lately the trabeculectomy has been regarded as the golden standard. The trabeculectomy is a well tested operation to lower the IOP, but has quite a few postoperative complications: Hyphema, shallow or flat AC, hypotony, choroidal detachment, hypotony maculopathy all due to excessive filtration, later cataract follows in 50% of the operated eyes.

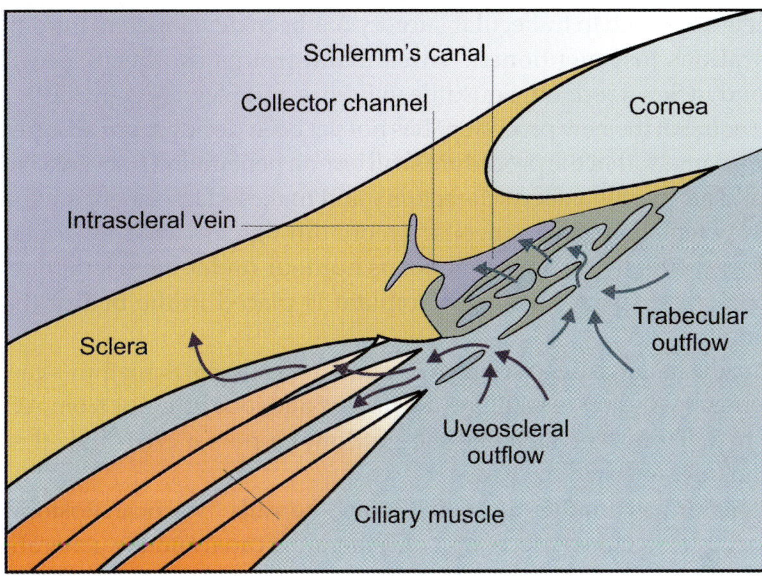

Fig. 1: Schematic illustration of the two outflows routes: the conventional one through the trabecular meshwork and the uveoscleral outflow routes (with permission from Pharmacia-Upjohn)

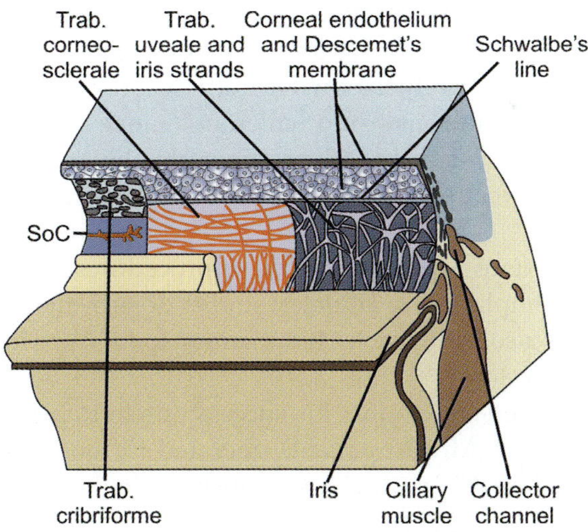

Fig 2: Three-dimensional structure of the trabecular meshwork in the human eye. The inner uveal meshwork extends towards the iris root and forms the so called ciliary meshwork separating the intermuscular spaces from the anterior chamber (with permission from the Pharmacia-Upjohn)

A new approach to trabecular surgery has been developed to minimize the complications just mentioned. Three main groups can been seen to day: Mermoud in Scwitzerland, Sourdille in France and Stegmann in South Africa.

The name of the new procedure has not yet been decided, but all agree upon one item, namely, that the procedure shall be non penetrating trabecular surgery. Mermoud advocates a deep sclerectomy and makes a Descement´s window to facilitate percolation of the aqueous humour through this window from the AC. To further facilitate the flow of aqueous humour under the scleral flap to the subconjunctival space, a collagen implant is placed in the bed of the deep sclerectomy.

Sourdille makes a deep sclerectomy and deroofing of Schlemm´s canal and a Descemet´s window to facilitate the flow of aqueous humour from AC to the scleral bed. To further facilitate the outflow he puts a cross-linked sodium hyaluronate implant in the bed.

Stegmann has another approach which he calls "viscocanalostomy". He uses a deep sclerectomy, deroofing of Schlemm´s canal and the generation of a Descement´s window. To facilitate the flow of aqueous humour, high -viscosity sodium hyaluronate (Healon GV) is injected into Schlemm´s canal to open the canal and after the superficial flap has been securely sutured the same is injected under the flap to prevent fibrinogen production that could prevent the free flow into the "lake" as the functioning space is named by Stegmann.

Sourdille and Stegmann agree that subconjunctival filtration is not required. In more than 80% of cases no filtration can be seen postoperatively. Stegmann thinks that the outflow occurs through collector channels and aqueous veins. Stegmann has intraoperatively shown that outflow through these routes occurs by injecting sodium hyaluronate into Schlemm´s canal.

Increase of the uveoscleral outflow might also be an explanation of the pressure lowering effect of the non penetrating procedures produce in the operated eye.

The most important aspect is that these procedures have very few and relatively limited complications. The latest studies done by the above mentioned investigators have also shown at least the same capability to lower the IOP as found after trabeculectomy.

Stegmann has even shown that his success rate in trabeculectomy of less than 20% in the black African patients operated for open-angle glaucoma, increases to more than 80% with viscocanalostomy in the same population.

METHODS

The first time I heard about viscocanalostomy was at the the ESCRS´s meeting in Gothenburg in the autumn of 1996. Professor Stegmann gave a lecture about his method and results.

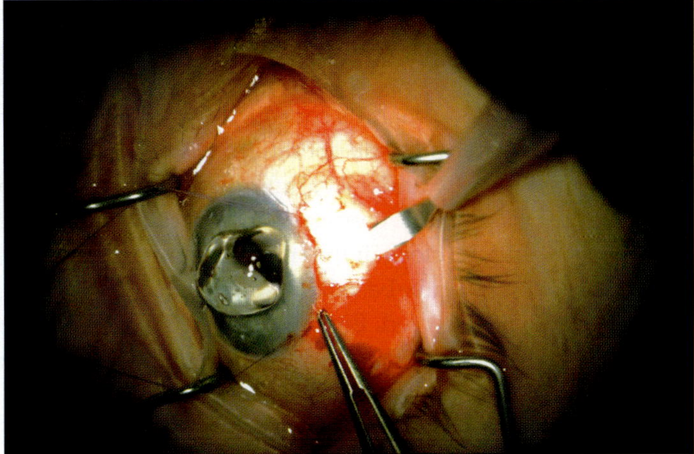

Fig 3: Sutures are placed at the cornea-scleral border

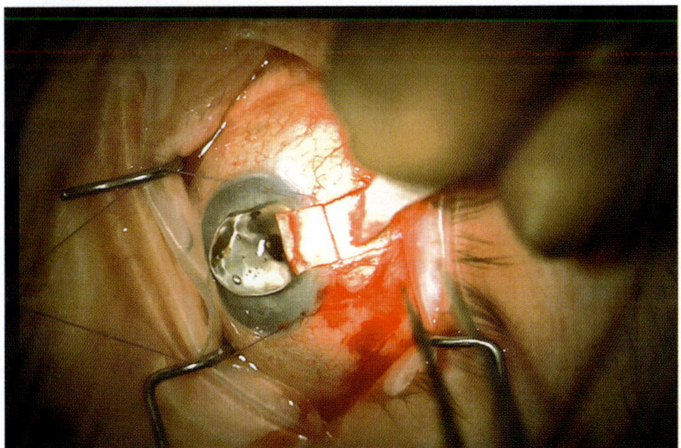

Fig 4: The flap is cut free and folded over the cornea

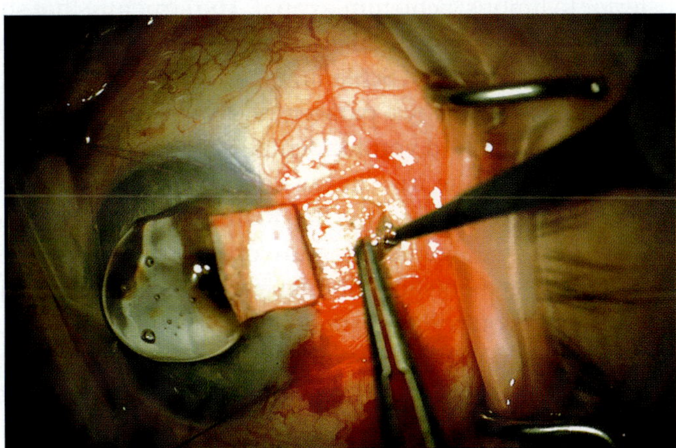

Fig 5: A second flap is dissected 0.5 mm inside the border of the superficial flap

I was thrilled and started in the spring of 1997 to perform viscocanalostomy—that is I tried hard to learn. Later that year I had the opportunity to have Stegmann as my teacher. That was really a hard learning curve still going on. First we did the operations according to Stegmann´s concept, but as we learned more from the other groups we have modified the operation.

We do the operations mostly under local anesthesia and use the subtendonal anestesia. Sutures are placed at the cornea-scleral border (if the operation is at 12 o´clock placed at 10 and 2 o'clock, if the operation is at 6 o´clock, sutures are placed at 4 and 8 o´clock). A fornix-based conjunctival flap extending from half past one to half past ten is dissected. Bipolar cautery is done very carefully. A parabolic flap is dissected 5 × 5 mm. I start with my guarded knife set at 200 - 250 microns cutting a curved incision parallel to the limbus at a distance of 5 mm. A crescent knife is then used to undermine the scleral flap in exactly the same way I do my phaco-flaps, but of course bigger. It is a time saving and procedure as I have made so many flaps in my life. The flap is cut free and folded over the cornea. Before surgery I always place a thick cover of Healon 5 to protect the cornea; this even helps me even to fixate the scleral flap.The flap is extended half a mm into clear cornea.

A second flap is dissected 0.5 mm inside the border of the superficial flap. This flap is dissected down to Descement´s membrane through Schlemm´s canal. That is the difficult part of the operation to describe if you are dissecting deep enough. If you go to deep you will see the coroid free in the bottom of the wound. That is no catastrophe, it can even serve as a marker, but that is only in the beginning of the dissecting. If you go to deep at the end you will perforate into the AC.

In the modestly pigmented eyes of the Swedish patients, you have to look very carefully. Your marker should be a thin layer of sclera covering the choroid shining through the almost translucent scleral layer, giving a gray-blue color.

As the inner-flap is dissected forward, the next stop will be approximately one mm posterior to limbus: Schlemm´s canal. The structure that should warn you is a cotton like fiber running parallel to limbus, when you pass through this layer a smooth interior surface of Schlemm´s canal reveals itself. Now stop!

Time for lowering the IOP by a paracentesis. Do lower the pressure so you get hypotony of the eye. Should you accidentally cut the Descement´s window, you will not end-up with the iris "in the knee". Dissect first with the same round knife you just used to dissect the flap to free the first part of the window, and you can then just put a gentle pressure on Schwalbe´s line with a spear sponge to separate Descements´ membrane from the corneoscleral junction. If you have done it right - you will now see aqueous humour percolating through the window. If you do not get percolation you must "peel" the roof off the Schlemm´s canal, an gently try to peel the tissue surpluce from the Descement´s window. I use the Tano´s brush which is used in the posterior segment to

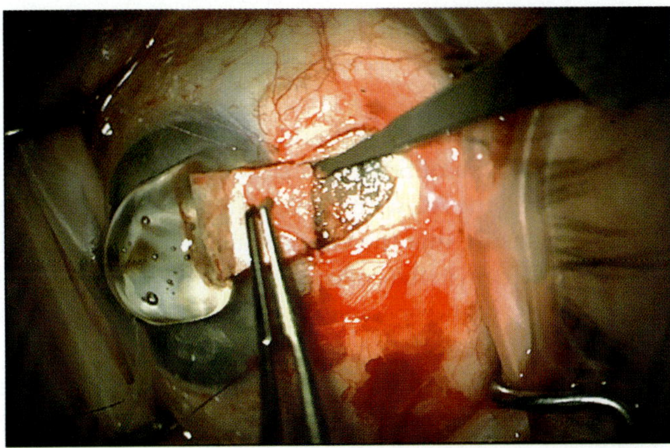

Fig 6: The structure that should warn you is a cotton like fiber running parallel to limbus

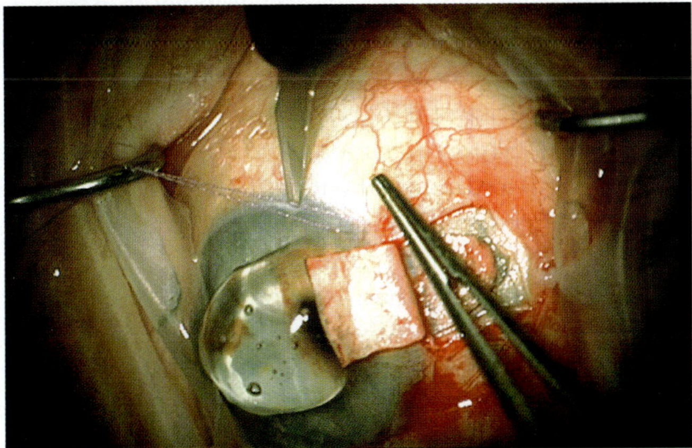

Fig 7: Time for lowering the IOP by a paracentesis

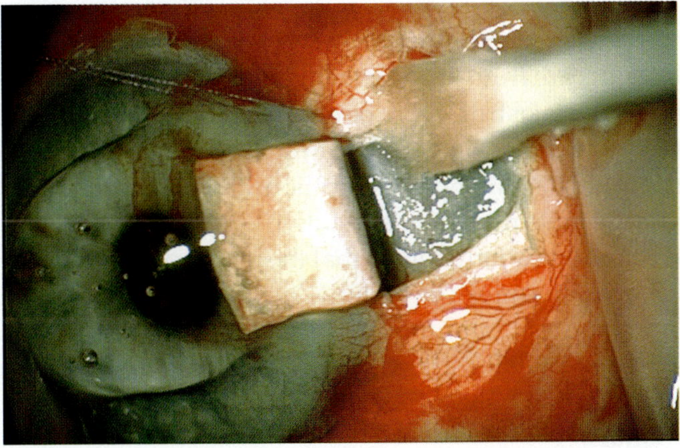

Fig 8: Put a gentle pressure on Schwalbe´s line with a spear sponge

peeling the ILM in operations for the macular hole. You can also use the diamont dust needle, which you also use to clean the posterior membrane in cataract surgery.

Viscocanalostomy is done both left and right with a 150 micron cannula introduced through the ostia of Schlemm´s canal. Be careful not to inject too forcefully as you might fill the AC with Healon 5 and that could give a very high pressure next day. To ensure that the viscocanalostomy is done right I always look to see if the blood-stream in the collecting venoles is broken by the absorbed Healon 5, that is clearly seen especially if you put a click of Healon 5 as a magnifying glass over the venoles.

The deeper flap is excised with Vanner´s scissors and now I place an implant. In the early days , I used Corneal´s Sk Gel 3.5, If the eye had no operation before. If the eye had earlier surgery I use the Staar´s collagen implant, as I then want to get a filtration. To day I use a 1.0 PDS monofil resorbable suture.

2001 I was in India and met Professor Meyer in South Africa who told me that Catgut was used by him in South Africa as they were not able to pay the high price for the Staar and Corneal implants . In Sweden we are not allowed to use Catgut because of the risk of BSE (bovine spongiform encephalopathy). In 2001 we began to use PDS (polydioxanon) suture material as an implant.

We cut a 4 mm length and suture it with a 10.0 suture under the scleral flap just like the Staar collagen implant. It is visible through a gonioscopy lens which makes it easier to locate the scleral window. The PDS material resorbs slowly, it lasts probably for more than 4-6 months. The price is $ 2!

The superficial scleral flap is tightly sutured in most cases to omit filtration; peroperatively corticosteroid and antibiotics are injected in the subtendonal space. Local steroid is given as eyedrops for 4 to 6 weeks 3 times a day. The follow-up: Day one , two weeks, one months. At the visit after one month I make a puncture of the Descemnets window in almost every case .

RESULTS

Stegmann´s results are from his operation on black Africans which according to Stegmann is the most difficult population to get success with filtering procedures for glaucoma. He presents an IOP reduction of 64% in 160 cases. The success rate is 82.7% without medication, and the mean follow-up was 35 months. These are quite remarkable results.

Personal communication showed that the results achieved when operating on the white population are even better.

Mermoud´s success rate in a study with 44 patients, probably white population, defined as IOP < 21,0 mmHg without medication, was 69% and in another group who had trabeculectomy the success rate was 57%. The follow-up was 24 months.

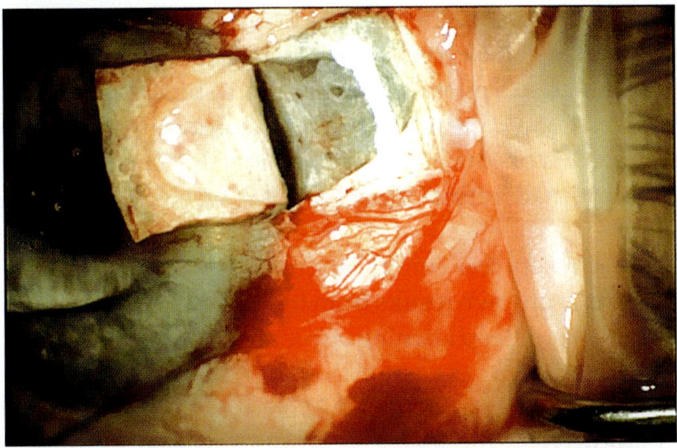

Fig 9: Aqueous humour percolating through the window

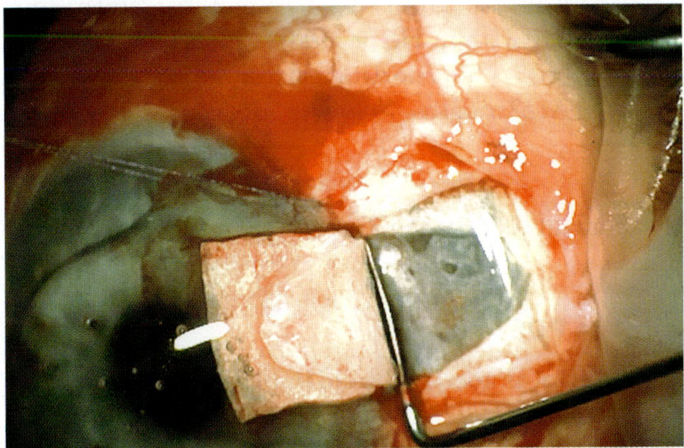

Fig 10: Viscocanalostomy is done both left and right

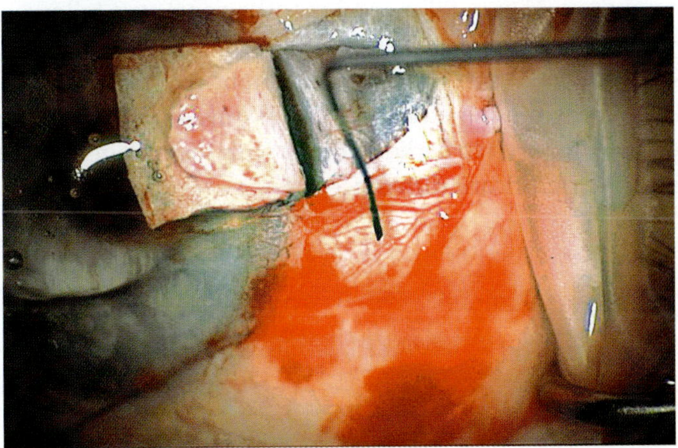

Fig 11: The blood-stream in the collecting venoles is broken

Complications: Hyphema 1 eye, flat AC zero eye, choroidal detachment 2 eyes, ocular hypertension 6 eyes, cataract formation 4 eyes.

Sourdille presents, in a pilot study of 72 eyes, a success rate of 72.2%, success defined as IOP less than 20 mm Hg without medication.

Complications: Hyphema in 7 eyes, choroidal detachment 1 eye, no flat AC was seen, one eye had retinal detachment 3 weeks postoperatively, was reattached.

As will be seen a very low complication rate.

Now I shall show my own results from the very begyinning: it is well known that the operation has a steep learning curve and that the complications are not unusual in the start up.

86 eyes operated , 67 eyes followed 3 months, 35 eyes followed 6 months and 10 eyes followed 12 months. The group consisted of different types of glaucoma. Exfoliation glaucoma was the most dominant, 63 % (see the figure). Duration of the glaucoma diagnosis mean 66 months, range 1 to 228 months. Success defined as IOP 21 mm Hg or less. At three months follow-up, 39 % without therapy and 60 % with one drug. At 6 months, 26 % without drugs and 54 % with one drug. At 12 months, 40 % without drugs and 60 % with one drug.

Complications

Choroidal detachment observed in 2 cases, high IOP first day in 22 cases and cataract in 1 case.

Results with the PDS suture

Is the new PDS implant as good as the old implants from Staar and Corneal? In a new study with 48 eyes (27 eyes with exfoliation syndrome,16 eyes with simplex syndrome, 1 eye with cong. Tarda and two eyes with sec. Glaucoma). All eyes were operated with PDS implant and YAG-laser punction of the Descement window. 24 eyes followed 3 months and 8 eyes followed 6 months. Mean IOP preop was 28 mm Hg. Mean IOP postop was 15 mm Hg. Mean IOP in the months group was 29 mm HG and after 6 months mean IOP was 15 mm HG. 21 eyes (88%) were without medication , 7 (88%) eyes were without medication after 6 months. Compared to earlier studies with the collagen implant did not show any statistic significant difference.

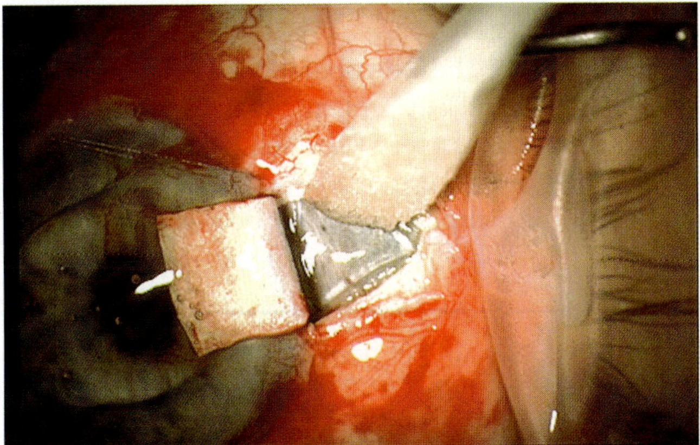

Fig 12: I used Corneal´s Sk Gel 3.5

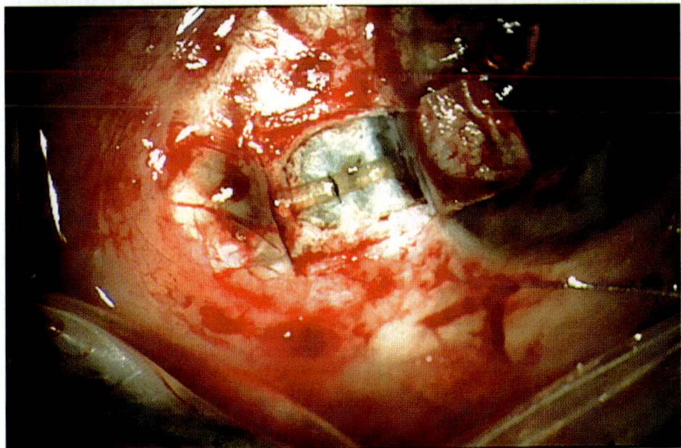

Fig 13: I use the Staar´s collagen implant

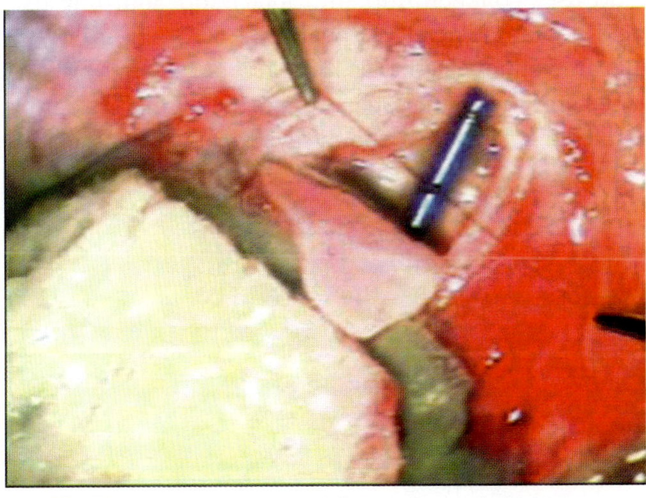

Fig 14: To day I use a 1.0 PDS monofil resorbable suture

Discussion

The learning curve is steep, but the operation is a real thrill to do.The first patients were all operated without implant; today we use an implant regularly and even YAG-laser punction of the Descement window.

Our success rate has improved and today almost all our patient are operated as out patients. Very little complications have been seen.

CONCLUSION

The riddle of glaucoma has not yet been solved. The glaucoma is caused by different factors not only the high IOP . The first results from the Early Manifest Glaucoma Trial (EMGT) shows that immediately treating people with early stages of primary open-angle glaucoma with pressure-lowering treatment can delay disease progression. Mean IOP reduction was 25%. Profesor Anders Heijl, the EMGT study director at the University Clinic at Malmö University Hospital, warned that the treatment used in the study was insufficient to stop progression of the glaucoma disease with rapidly progressing glaucoma.

The golden standard for many years has been the trabeculectomy, known for effectively lowering the pressure, but plagued not infrequently with quite severe complications, and this has led to a search for new operations. The nonperforating trabecular surgery, which has few and seldom severe complications, can be the answer. Time will show if the lowering of the IOP is as good as the trabeculectomy in the long run. Stegmann in South Africa has obtained results that are even better than ordinary trabeculectomy in the most difficult population to operate: black Africans. Mermoud in Scwitzerland and Sourdille in France have achieved similar results in a white population. Stegmann uses non implant but high-viscosity sodium hyaluronate (Healon GV), Mermoud uses collagen implant (Staar) and Sourdille use reticulated hyaluronic acid implant (Sk Gel, Corneal).

Our results are yet not as good as those of our teachers but are improving. We have reached one important issue: to quote Stegmann,"I sleep better because I am not afraid to look my patients in the eye the day after the operation".

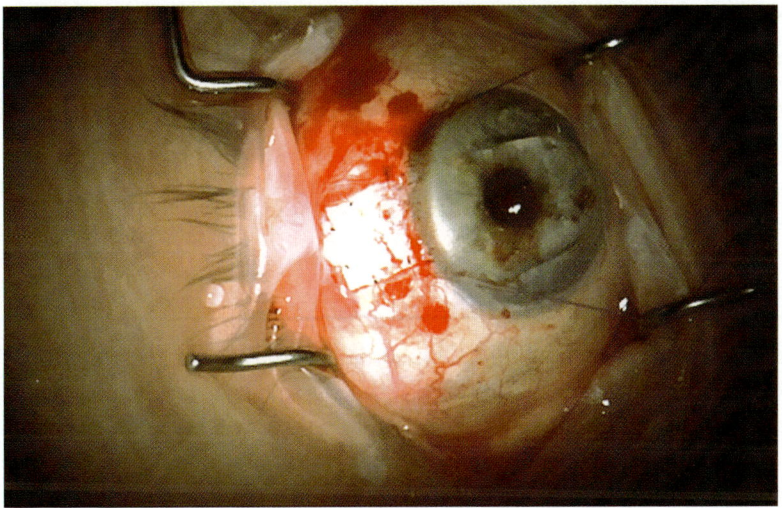

Fig 15: The superficial scleral flap is tightly sutured

39

Deep Sclerectomy with T-Flux Implant with "Outside In" Drainage

Ranjit H Maniar (India)

INTRODUCTION

Surgery for Primary Open Angle Glaucoma is usually a *last resort* option. Today we exercise this option less frequently, thanks to better medications that have not only a pressure lowering effect but also neuroprotective properties. When there is a need for surgery, it implies that medical management alone is not sufficient in controlling the disease process. One would expect that the surgical procedure, therefore, would deliver the goods each time, every time, for keeps. Unfortunately, surgical outcomes do not always match the need of the hour. Glaucoma surgery is known to fail over a period and trabeculectomy, once the gold standard, is now known to stop draining as time progresses. The chief culprit is fibrosis between the scleral bed and the flap that shuts down the drainage corridor.

NATURE'S DRAINAGE CHANNELS

Surgery for glaucoma is nothing but our attempt at duplicating nature's process artificially. However, it does not always work out quite the way we intend it to. Let us, therefore, take a fresh look at nature's drainage channels from the eye. Most of our focus these long years has been limited to structures within the anterior chamber, mainly the trabecular meshwork. We generally tend to ignore the fact that from the trabecular meshwork onward, fluid is gathered up by aqueous veins, which connect to the episcleral vasculature. *At no point is the aqueous allowed to flow naked and openly*. However, during all our surgical procedures we do exactly that – let the aqueous drain out uncovered by a sheath. Have we, even for a moment, considered the deleterious effects of such an event? Do we pause to deliberate on a cause-and-effect relationship between a bare unsheathed drainage and fibrosis induced failure?

ENSURE SURGICAL SUCCESS

The only way to ensure continuous drainage is to mimic nature as closely as possible, i.e. by providing covered or sheathed outflow from the eye. An early attempt in this direction was made with the introduction of the Ahmed Glaucoma Valve. It was, however, destined to fail, as it relied on the creation of an external drainage lake, which eventually filled up. Molteno designed an

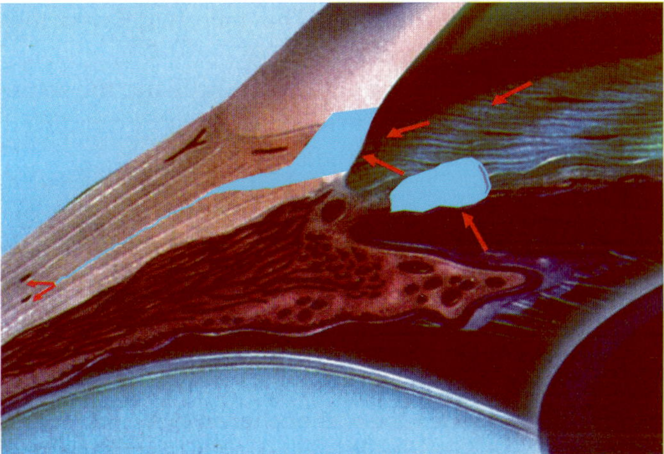

Fig. 1: Trabeculectomy

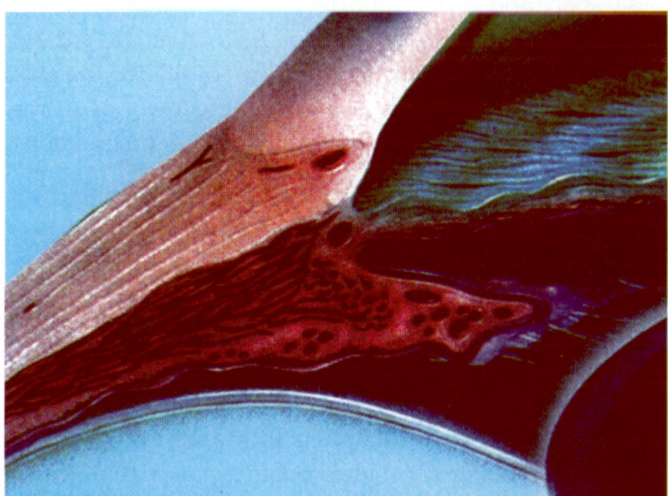

Fig. 2: Nature's enclosed drainage channels

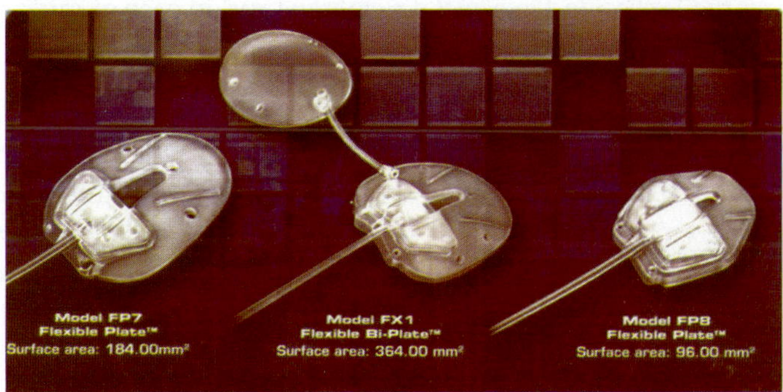

Fig. 3: Ahmed glaucoma valve

'extension' lake by having two plates. This merely delayed the inevitable pressure equalization that resulted in 'no-flow'.

While the concept of sheathed outflow was brilliant, the setting up of an artificial lake was flawed. I attempted to rectify this flaw by directing the aqueous outflow into the potential supra-choroidal space.

HISTORY OF THE PROCEDURE

In 2001, I used a non-valvular silicon shunt to carry fluid directly from the anterior chamber to the supra-choroidal space. This drainage device, in its initial avatar, consisted of a simple small-bore silicon tube that had sharp tapered ends. After creating a scleral flap, an opening was made into the supra-choroid 3 - 4 mm from the limbus. The tube was anchored to the scleral bed by a 10-0 nylon suture and one end was introduced into the supra-choroid. It was then flushed with an insulin syringe containing Ringer's, to open up the potential supra-choroidal space and 'charge' the device. This 'charging' served to remove any air pocket and permit a smooth capillary flow when this tube was made to puncture the anterior chamber next. Flap suture completed the procedure.

The procedure worked well in terms of IOP control overtime. The only disadvantage was that one had to open the anterior chamber. Then came along deep sclerectomy.

DEEP SCLERECTOMY WITH T-FLUX IMPLANT

As the procedure is well documented, I shall not attempt to reinvent the wheel. I shall reiterate, however, this procedure offers several advantages over trabeculectomy.

a. A proper and diligent technique ensures an *adequate* outflow.
b. There is an inherent *safety* in not opening the anterior chamber.
c. The T-Flux Implant, being a non-absorbable biocompatible acrylic polymer, helps to *maintain a permanent intrascleral space*. This is achieved by anchoring it to the scleral bed with a single suture.
d. It *stabilizes the Trabeculo-Descemet's membrane* and in case of micropunctures and prevents iris herniation.

THE FLIP SIDE

There is no denying the fact that deep sclerectomy is technically difficult. It has a steep learning curve. In the initial stages one often lands up converting to conventional trabeculectomy. It is no secret that this surgery places a great demand on surgical skill, which can be mitigated to some extant only by expensive diamond blades! The data on long-term results is often conflicting, at best equivocal.

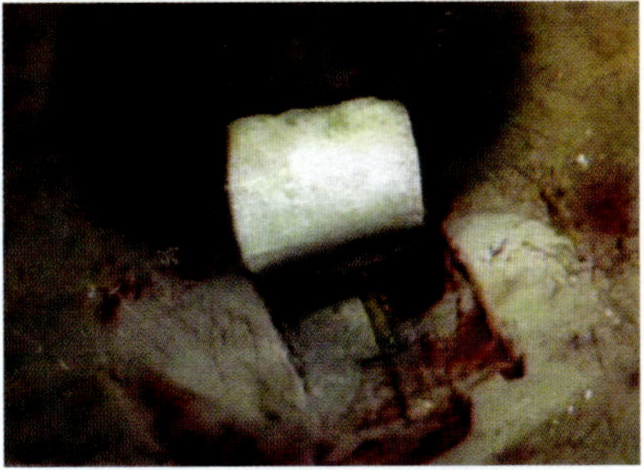

Fig. 4A: Non-valvular shunt

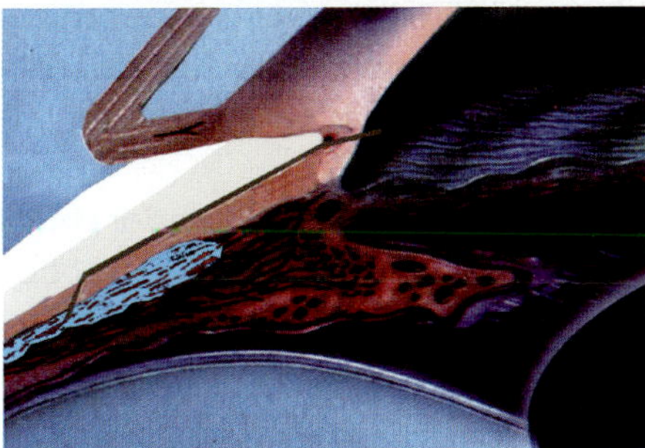

Fig. 4B: Non-valvular shunt

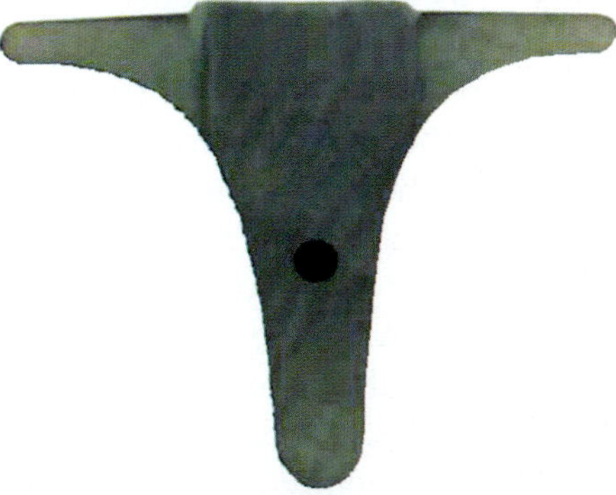

Fig. 5A: T-Flux

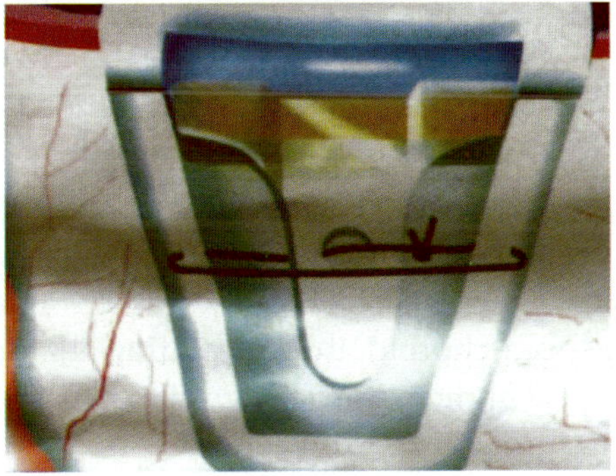

Fig. 5B: T-Flux in scleral bed

Given these constraints, why would one want to take up this procedure, that to with modifications?

DEEP SCLERECTOMY WITH T-FLUX IMPLANT WITH SUPRACHOROIDAL DRAINAGE

The plain and simple answer is that DS with T-Flux *with supra-choroidal drainage* is the surgery of the future. With the introduction of the T-Flux Implant one merely *enhances* the outcomes of a well done deep sclerectomy; however, with the added dimension of supra-choroidal drainage one virtually **ensures** perpetual outflow.

The key step in this procedure is to make an aperture in the sclera, 2 mm-3mm from the limbus, up to the supra-choroid and insert the foot of the T-Flux into this potential space. Being about 0.2 mm thick, it glides in easily.

In one procedure it combines.

a. **Safety** — One does not need to open the anterior chamber.
b. **Efficacy** — Performed painstakingly, the procedure offers adequate drainage.
c. **Sheltered Drainage** — One can largely circumvent the deleterious effects of naked outflow by placing the T-Flux upside down, thus providing a roof over outflow. There is also little chance of prolonged scleroaqueous contact to induce any degree of significant fibrosis.
d. **Continuous Drainage** — By inserting the foot of the T-Flux into the supra-choroid, one creates a channel along which fluid passively tracks down. *Nature does the rest*. This is perhaps the only surgery that can ensure perpetual drainage, by utilizing the inherent vascularity of the choroid and its ability to absorb and return fluid to the general circulation. There is thus, no fear of closure of the 'external lake' as with the AGV and Molteno designs.

During the period 2001-2002, I had an occasion to perform this procedure on five eyes in three patients. All patients also had significant cataract, necessitating combined surgery. All patients followed-up regularly as advised, on weekly, monthly, quarterly and annual basis for three and a half years. Patient 1 (2 eyes) passed away 42 months after surgery, while patients 2 and 3 continue their annual follow-up.

The mean preoperative IOP fell from a value of 28 to 13 mm at 1 month, stabilizing at 15 mm at end of 1 year, 17 mm at end of 2 years, and 18 mm at end of 3 years, 6 months. During his period field remained stable without any topical therapy.

My colleague, Dr. Deepak Bhatt, performed ultrasound Biomicroscopy (UBM) in late 2004, and documented patent passages from the intrascleral space up to the supra-choroid. He was also able to trace the outline of the T-Flux Implant all the way down to the supra-choroid, thus providing anatomical corroboration to the clinicophysiological findings and lend credence to my theoretical musings (I am deeply grateful to him for the same).

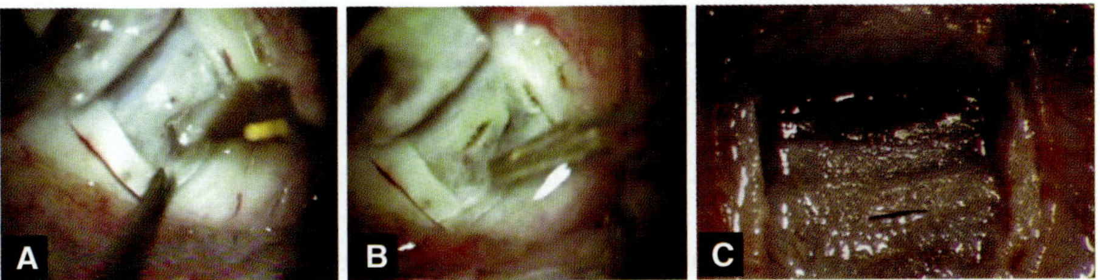

Figs 6A to C: (A, B) Suprachoroidal entry, (C) Deep sclerectomy

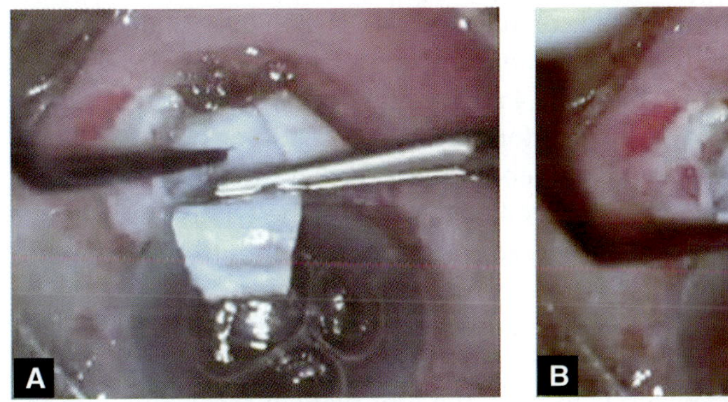

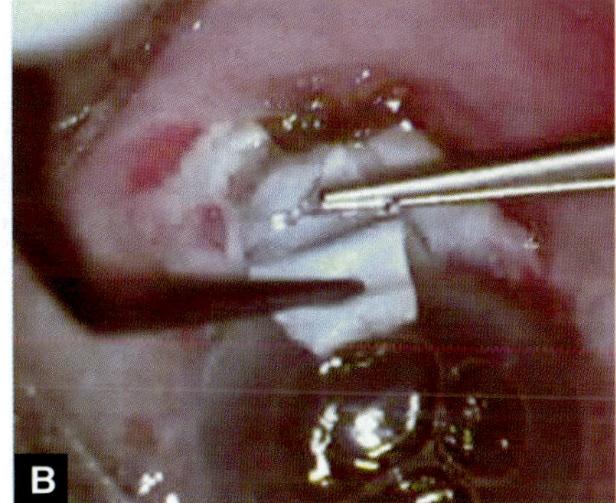

Figs 7A and B: Inserting foot of T-Flux in suprachoroidal space

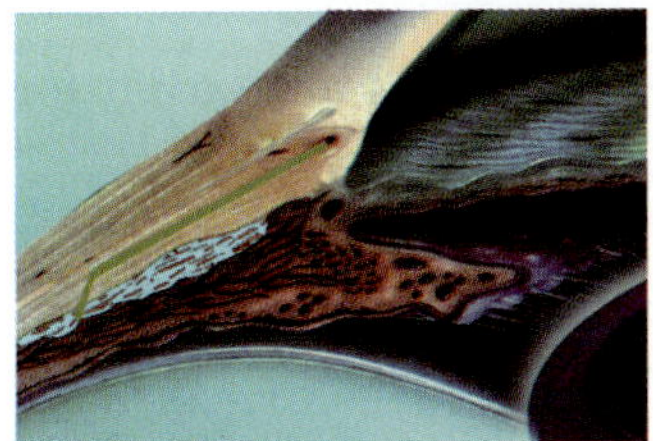

Fig. 8: T-Flux with suprachoroidal lake

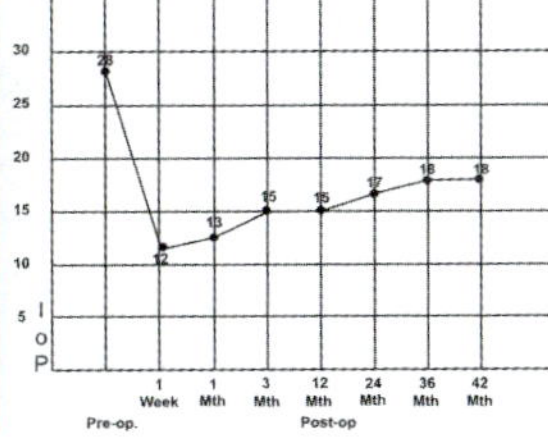

Fig. 9: Postop. IOP

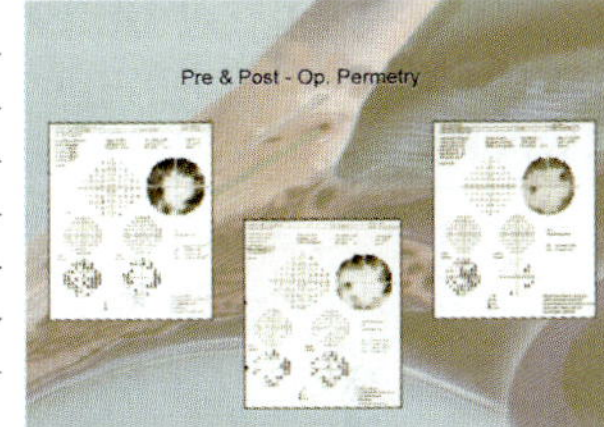

Fig. 10: Pre and Postop. perimetry

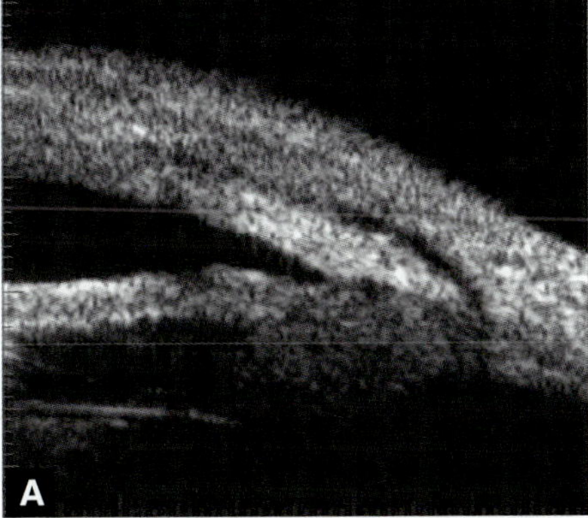

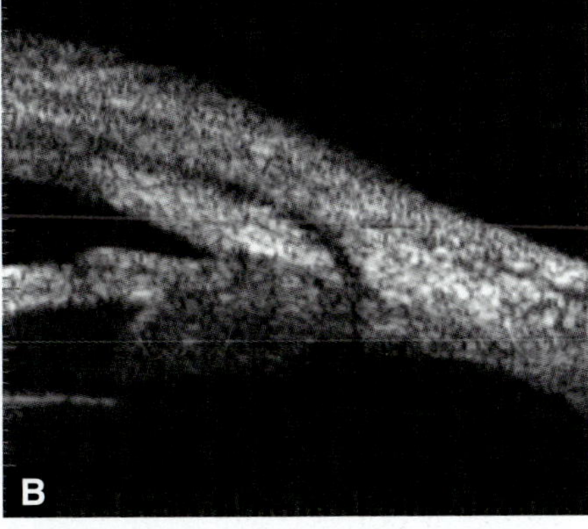

Figs 11A and B: UBM at 1 year

THE SURGICAL PROCEDURE

There are essentially four parts to the surgical procedure.

a. Deep sclerectomy;
b. Placing and anchoring of the T-Flux Implant;
c. Fashioning of the scleral aperture, and
d. Inserting the foot of the implant in to the supra-choroidal space.

1. I generally prefer a peri-bulbar block.
2. A superior rectus bridle suture follows.
3. A standard fornix-based conjunctival flap is then dissected.
4. The scleral flap has to be a minimum of 5 × 5 mm with 1/3rd depth.
5. Within this flap, another 4 × 4 mm scleral pocket is dissected.
6. Deep sclerectomy is then performed.
7. Next, side pockets are made above the level of the deep sclerectomy in order to accommodate and embed the arms of the T-Flux implant.
8. An opening is made into the sclera about 2 to 3 mm from the limbus. This is tunneled backwards, away from the limbus.
9. The T-Flux Implant is sutured upside down onto the scleral bed.
10. The arms embedded into the side pockets.
11. The next crucial step is to push the foot plate of the T-Flux into the supra-choroidal space with the help of a spatula.
12. All flaps are sutured.

Postoperative regime consists of steroid antibiotic drops 3-4 times a day for 2 weeks.

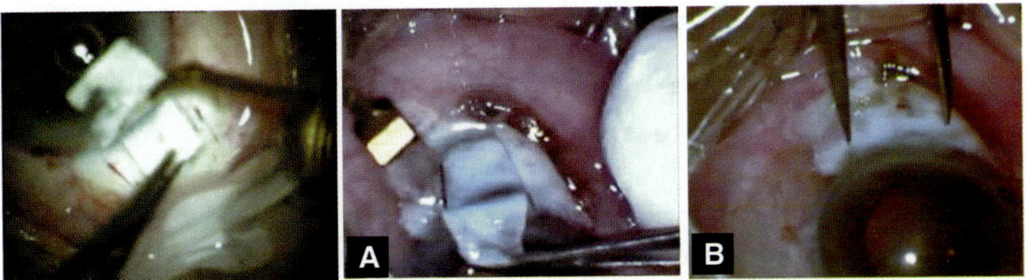

Fig. 12: Scleral pocket

Figs 13A and B: (A) Flap disection (B) Caliper

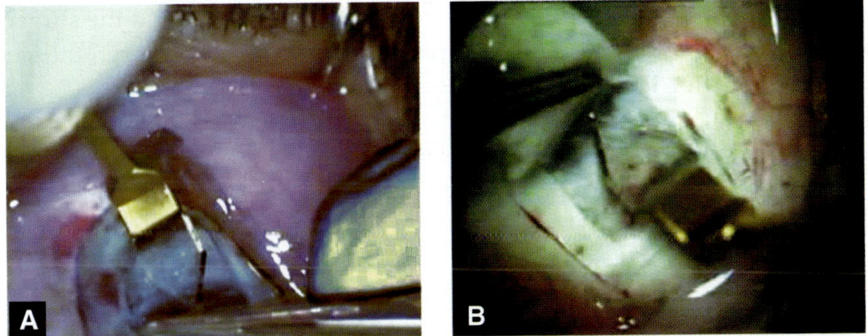

Figs 14A and B: Deep sclerectomy

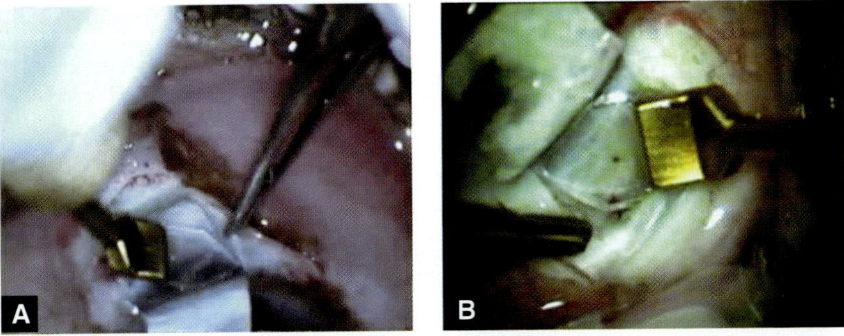

Figs 15A and B: Side pocket

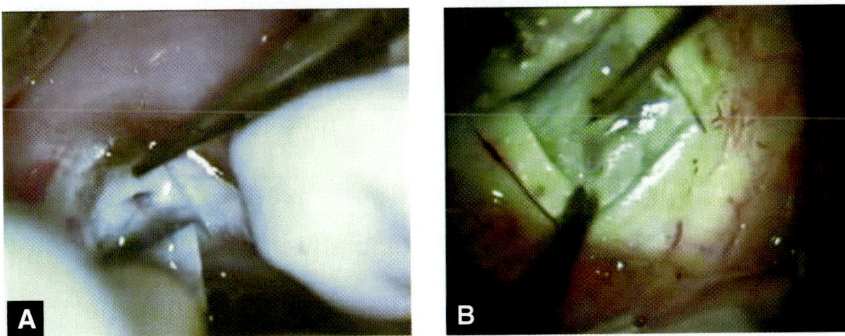

Figs 16A and B: Suprachoroidal aperture

Follow-up visit protocol is as under:

Next day, 1 week, 2 weeks, 1 month, 3 months (Repeat UBM), 6 months, 1 year, bi-annually thereafter.

CONCLUSION

The concept of supra-choroidal drainage is sound in theory. It also works in practice. In all the above cases, I have used an existing device (the T-Flux Implant) to provide a roof over the filtering aqueous. It is very well suited for this surgery. However, cost is a major limiting factor, both for the patient and the surgeon. I am currently working on an indigenous design which will serve the same purpose at an affordable cost.

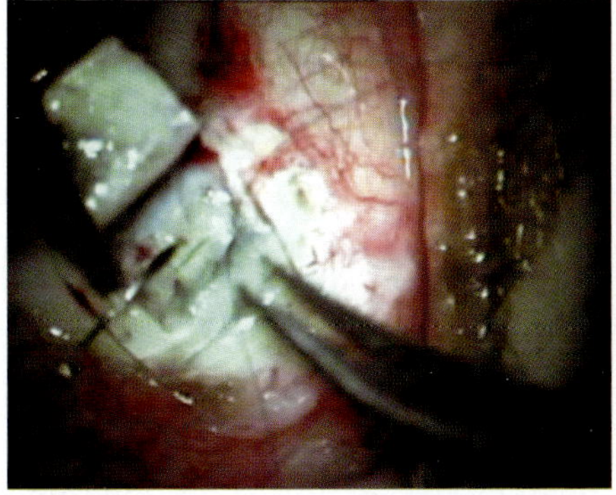

Fig. 17: Suturing T-Flux

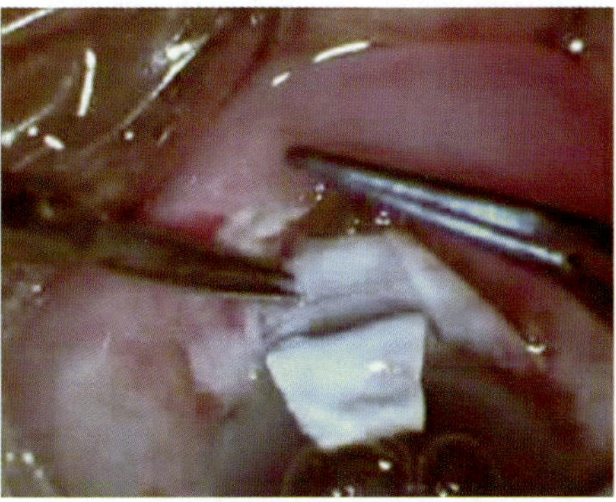

Fig. 18: Inserting foot of T-Flux into suprachoroidal space

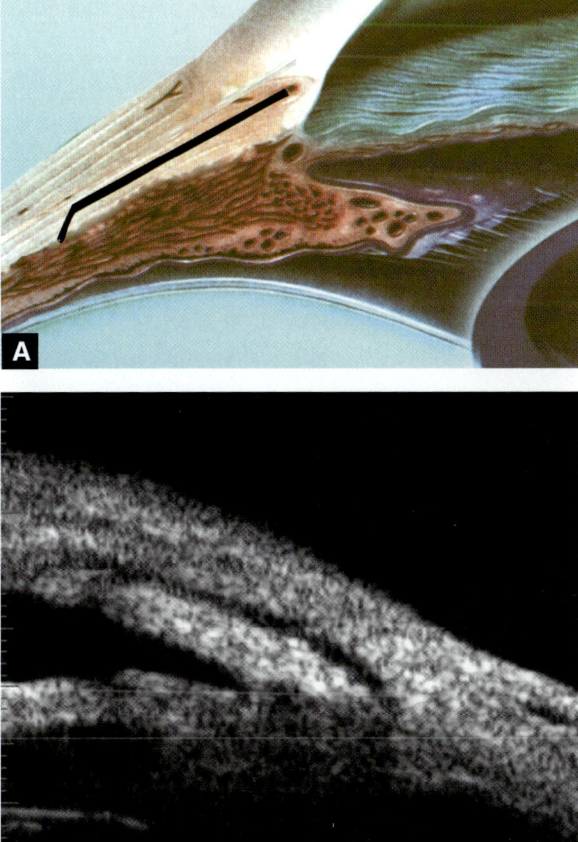

Figs 19A and B: T-Flux at 1 year

Index

A

B

C

D

E

G

H

I

L

M

N

O

P

S

T

V